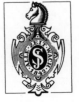

D. Krausé   J. L. Drapé
D. Maitrot   B. Woerly   J. Tongio

CT and MRI
of Disk Herniations

With a Foreword by Luc Picard

With 242 Figures in 606 Parts
and 3 Tables

Springer-Verlag
Berlin Heidelberg New York
London Paris Tokyo
Hong Kong Barcelona

Dr. Denis Krausé
Dr. Jean Luc Drapé
Professor Dr. Daniel Maitrot
Dr. Bernard Woerly
Professor Dr. Jean Tongio

C. H. U. Strasbourg-Hautepierre
Avenue Molière, 67098 Strasbourg
France

ISBN-13: 978-3-642-73593-6   e-ISBN-13: 978-3-642-73591-2
DOI: 10.1007/978-3-642-73591-2

Library of Congress Cataloging-in-Publication Data.
CT and MRI of disk herniations / D. Krause ... [et al.].   p.   cm.
Includes bibliographical references. Includes index.

1. Intervertebral disk-Hernia. 2. Intervertebral disk-Hernia-Tomography. 3. Intervertebral disk-Hernia-Magnetic resonance imaging. 4. Vertebrae, Lumbar-imaging. 5. Vertebrae, Cervical-Imaging. I. Krause, D. (Denis) [DNLM: 1. Cervical Vertebrae-anatomy & histology. 2. Intervertebral Disk Displacement-diagnosis. 3. Lumbar Vertebrae-anatomy & histology. 4. Magnetic Resource Imaging. 5. Thoracic Vertebrae-anatomy & histology. 6. Tomography, X-Ray Computed.
WE 740 C959] RD771.I6C8 1991 617.3'75-dc20 DNLM/DLC for Library of Congress 90-9932 CIP

Softcover reprint of the hardcover 1st edition 1991

2127/3145-543210

Acknowledgements

We would like to express our gratitude to the following:
Mr. Dany Vetter, for the beautiful photographic work;
Mrs. Monique Holterbach, Sonia Lienhardt, and Monique Funck,
for their excellent secretarial assistance;
Dr. Antonio Perez-Infante, for the translation;
and the firms Schering and Boots-Dacour,
for their encouragement and support.

Foreword

The ever-increasing interest in the spine and its pathology is not surprising. Acting as the main support of an erect posture unique in the animal kingdom, the human spine is, owing to its numerous articulations, at the same time a supple structure that can respond to the many stresses which are put on it. Constant movement is necessary to preserve its function, but regular and well-positioned rest is also essential. The high frequency of spinal disorders resulting from misuse is easily explained by day-to-day reality.

Among the disorders that result from misuse of the spine, herniated disk, leading to radicular compression, is one of the most frequent. New techniques, less invasive and yielding more precise information, have been progressively developed for the diagnosis of this disease and at the same time new methods of treatment have appeared, giving us a much broader range of choices and decisions to make.

In the face of this evolving, complex situation, a multidisciplinary team from Strasbourg decided to clarify the topic. A single man's experience, whatever his qualities, would certainly have been insufficient and the necessarily limited views of a single speciality would also have been a handicap. This remarkable work is thus the result of collaboration between clinical and interventional radiologists and a neurosurgeon.

Denis Krausé, Jean-Luc Drapé, and Bernard Woerly, all in the radiology department headed by Professor Jean Tongio, have been working for a long time to assess precisely the symptoms of disk herniation, especially on CT scans and MR images. This innovative team was the first to use an oblique view centered on the nerve roots in MRI, first at the lumbar level and later at the cervical level, which led to instructive correlations with the already known findings on myelograms.

Obviously, this special interest has also led to developments in percutaneous methods of treatment, mainly chemonucleolysis. In fact, Denis Krausé and his colleagues were among the first to use chemonucleolysis at the cervical level. The technique that was developed led to a very high success rates, higher than are generally obtained at the lumbosacral level. The contribution of Daniel Maitrot on surgery is a reflection of his wide knowledge and expertise.

The enthusiasm and competence of this multidisciplinary team has led to a real *tour de force*. The reader has before him the whole of current knowledge necessary to a full understanding of the problems, especially concerning the therapeutic approach. As everyone knows, we do not treat a lesion but a human being, and for this the understanding of the links between the visible radio-anatomical lesions and the clinical findings provided by this book is mandatory. The book will thus permit both nonspecialist and specialist alike to find all the clinical, anatomical, radiological, and therapeutic data necessary for the best possible decision making.

CT and MRI of Disk Herniations is a timely book. The text is clear and the abundant illustrations facilitate reading and understanding. I would like to thank and congratulate my friends from Strasbourg, and wish this book all the success it deserves: it should become *the* modern state-of-the-art reference work on a difficult topic where the success of intervention has such important individual as well as social consequences.

Nancy, September 1990   Luc Picard

                                               Professor of Neuroradiology,
                                               Faculty of Medicine of Nancy,
                                               Head of Department of Diagnostic
                                               and Interventional Neuroradiology,
                                               University Hospital of Nancy

Contents

Magnetic Resonance Imaging

Contributors

F. BUCHHEIT
Professeur, Chef du Service de Neurochirurgie
Centre Hospitalier et Universitaire, Strasbourg-Hautepierre
France

J. L. DRAPÉ
Chef de Clinique, Service de Radiologie III
Centre Hospitalier et Universitaire, Strasbourg-Hautepierre
France

D. KRAUSÉ
Praticien des Hôpitaux, Service de Radiologie III
Centre Hospitalier et Universitaire, Strasbourg-Hautepierre
France

D. MAITROT
Professeur, Service de Neurochirurgie
Centre Hospitalier et Universitaire, Strasbourg-Hautepierre
France

J. TONGIO
Professeur, Chef du Service de Radiologie III
Centre Hospitalier et Universitaire, Strasbourg-Hautepierre
France

B. WOERLY
Radiologue
Clinique de l'Orangerie, Strasbourg
France

Computed Tomography

Cervical Disk Herniations

Introduction

The most common expression of cervical disk herniation is cervicobrachial neuralgia (CBN).

Until a few years ago, the classic diagnostic workup of a CBN consisted solely of cervical myelography. This very sensitive but invasive neuroradiological examination permits the demonstration of nerve root lesions using oblique projections (amputation of a radicular sheath, possibly associated with dural sleeve compression by diskal or disko-osteophytic material).

Routine CBN workups now include computed tomography (CT) as a supplementary examination, to the detriment of cervical myelography; the sensitivity of CT is equal to if not greater than that of subarachnoid opacification.

At the cervical level, the absence of epidural fat and the small size of the spinal canal make the performance and especially the interpretation of the investigations more difficult. This is clearly illustrated by the fact that, before the advent of CT, soft cervical disk herniations were considered less frequent than osteophytic lesions.

The value of CT lies in its ability to perform scans of 1-mm-thick sections both in the plane of the disk and, especially, at the level of the intervertebral foramina, thus differentiating between soft disk herniations and uncodiskarthroses.

Clinical Study [47, 137, 145, 171, 240]

Cervicobrachial neuralgia combines a painful cervical syndrome with pain of radicular origin. Its onset is sudden, and the pain is severe from the start. A sensory or muscular deficit may also be present. CBN is more likely to be found in individuals under 50 years of age; the most frequent etiology is soft disk herniation.

One should differentiate this neuralgia, seen in young individuals and monoradicular in origin, from cervical arthrosis, with its chronically evolving, truncated, polyradicular pain, which often occurs in association with a significant cervical syndrome. Patients with cervical arthrosis are on average older and routine X-rays show numerous signs of arthrosis.

Clinical Signs of Cervicobrachial Neuralgia

Two major syndromes are associated in CBN:

1. *A cervical syndrome of diskal origin* gives rise to cervical pain. The pain is usually located in the interscapular region, but a clinical picture of upper dorsal pain or nuchal pain is not uncommon. Whatever the presentation, the pain is continuous and dull and is exacerbated by neck movements. Localized muscle spasm may lead to torticollis. The diagnostic orientational value of these pains of diskal origin is only slight.
2. *The radicular syndrome* results from the mechanical compression of a nerve root. The CBN involves a neural segment corresponding to the compressed root. Paroxysms occur against a background of continuous pain. Associated paresthesias are sometimes observed. The added presence of motor deficit signs due to motor root compression results in a sensorimotor syndrome; the purely sensorimotor type of syndrome is the most common (Fig. 1).

Cervical disk rupture may evolve in three phases which correspond to three degrees of lesion: cer-

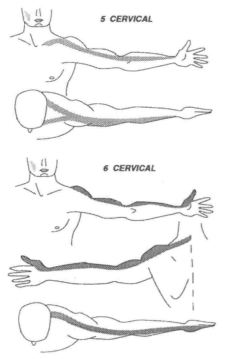
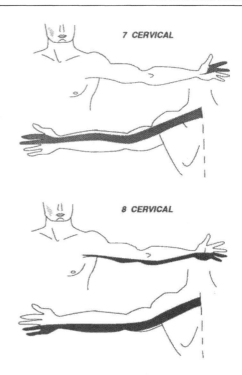

Fig. 1. Signs of involvement of cervical nerve roots C5–C8. Root signs

C5 *Pain distribution:* external portion of arm proximal to elbow
   Muscular impairment: deltoid
   Sensory impairment: external aspect of shoulder and arm

C6 *Pain distribution:* anterior portion of arm and external part of forearm, down to first and second fingers
   Muscular impairment: biceps; anterior brachialis; long supinator
   Sensory impairment: Hypoesthesia and/or paresthesia of fingers
   Reflex involvement: bicipital and stylo-radial reflex

C7 *Pain distribution:* posterior aspect of arm and forearm, down to second, third, and fourth fingers
   Muscular impairment: triceps, long and short radial extensor muscles of wrist, extensor muscles of fingers
   Sensory impairment: hypoesthesia and/or paresthesia of fingers
   Reflex involvement: triceps

C8 *Pain distribution:* internal aspect of arm, down to fifth finger
   Muscular impairment: flexor muscles of fingers, interosseous, small muscles of hand
   Sensory impairment: hypoesthesia and/or paresthesia of fifth finger
   Reflex involvement: ulnar reflex

vical pain, CBN, and brachialgia, which is sometimes isolated with attenuation of the cervical pain.

Clinical Examination

Neurological examination of patients suffering from CBN permits accurate determination of the site of nerve root compression. Some components of the clinical picture suggest a radicular origin.

The sensory deficit is especially pronounced for heat and pain; it is more pronounced distally, and is sometimes accompanied by vasomotor and trophic disturbances.

The reflex deficit usually precedes the motor deficit.

The motor deficit is clear-cut in acute forms but less defined in chronic forms. With respect to motor segmental activity, one tests the strength of the biceps and triceps muscles, which depend on the C6 and C7 nerve roots.

Electromyographic examination reveals objective signs of nerve root involvement and determines the topography; however, this is more likely to be possible during the chronic phase of the evolution of a CBN, i.e., from 3 weeks after onset.

Signs of spinal cord irritation are routinely sought: hyperreflexia or motor disturbances of the lower limbs, Babinski's sign, Brown-Séquard syndrome.

In general, the fewer nerve roots compressed, the more accurate the topographic diagnosis. Nevertheless, topographies may be partial or incomplete, in which case correlations between the clinical signs and the affected level are imperfect. Certain anatomical variations, such as anastomoses between the posterior rootlets of two contiguous levels, may perhaps explain these problems [56].

Clinical Types

Various general types of CBN may be differentiated:

Types which regress spontaneously after several weeks of medical treatment: these are frequent and are not investigated further.

Types requiring surgical treatment: these are the hyperalgesic, insomniac, disabling types, found in young adults, which lead to deterioration in general health and dependence on potent drugs such as corticosteroids or even morphine or its derivatives.

Types with motor deficit: these are found relatively frequently on routine investigation.

Types associated with a spinal cord irritation syndrome: these rarer forms are caused by large posteromedian disk herniations; emergency investigation is called for and the CBN is of secondary importance.

Differential Diagnosis

The medical history, clinical examination, and diagnostic workup should exclude brachial or cervicobrachial pain of nonradicular origin – elbow lesions, epicondylalgia; wrist lesions; nerve trunk lesions of the median nerve in the carpal tunnel or of the ulnar nerve at the front of the elbow surface (Guillon's zone).

Brachial plexus pain as part of a scalenus syndrome is manifested by neurological and vascular signs, which should always be sought. A chest X-ray is valuable in ruling out compression of the plexus (tumor of the lung apex; Pancoast's syndrome). The possibility of cervical rib should not be neglected.

Etiology of Cervicobrachial Neuralgia

In Young People (under 50 years)

Cervicobrachial neuralgia in young people most commonly arises from soft cervical disk herniations. This has been shown by the routine performance of CT. Numerous other etiological factors have been reported, but they remain rare if not completely anecdotal, and we have only come across a few isolated case in which CBN in younger individuals was caused by anything other than soft cervical disk herniation. When the CBN is only secondary, the clinical context and the course of the radicular pain lead one to expect a different etiology.

It is evident that in these very specific cases, the diagnostic workup does not begin with CT of a particular cervical level.

Cervical Arthritis

Generalized. Among the obvious etiologies of CBN are the manifestations of generalized cervical arthritis: diskal protrusions and multilevel, bilateral lesions of the posterior vertebral bodies or foramina. These generally result in chronic symptoms with various successive forms of cervical pain and bilateral, tiered cervical complaints which may or may not be accompanied by signs of spinal cord involvement. In the advanced form there is myelopathy due to the cervical arthritis, and the CBN is of secondary importance compared to the medullary syndrome.

The signs are sometimes comparable to those of CBN evolving in a hyperalgesic fashion. Routine plain films are invaluable, since they demonstrate the spread of the multilevel, bilateral uncovertebral arthritis.

Our experience has been that the patients with CBN from generalized cervical arthritis are older; in these cases we use cervical myelography, which permits a more detailed investigation of all the nerve roots emerging from C4 to C8 thanks to oblique projections.

Localized. In rare cases involving young individuals, CT has demonstrated a narrowing of the uncovertebral joint limited to the intervertebral foramen and resulting in a typical CBN. These patients may benefit from foraminotomy. This operation is infrequent in comparison to disk surgery.

Soft Disk Herniation
[33, 66, 67, 83, 115, 177, 221, 233]

Definition

Soft disk herniation involves the extrusion of the nucleus pulposus through a fissured anulus fibrosus.

The definition of hard disk herniation is less precise, resulting from degenerative spinal changes such as calcified hernias in association with significant uncovertebral arthritis. Uncomplicated diskal bulging involves only the anulus fibrosus. Bulging disks do not perforate the posterior longitudinal ligament, since this ligament and the anulus form an anatomical unit.

CT-surgery correlations in 75 patients whose herniations were operated on solely on the basis of CT findings established the following points:

— Soft disk herniations almost always perforate the posterior longitudinal ligament and leave there a nuclear fragment, the free fragment.
— The herniation almost always migrates upward and laterally toward the intervertebral (neural) foramen, compressing the nerve root; purely ascending or descending migrations like those found at the lumbar level are exceptional.

The term "free fragment" denotes the presence of nuclear material extruded from the anulus fibrosus and found either in the substance of the posterior longitudinal ligament or posterior to the perforated ligament. This has been established directly during surgery using the operating microscope. In effect, the surgeon approaches the disk anteriorly. After an initial diskectomy followed by placement of a Cloward retractor, the surgical microscope is used to visualize the nuclear fragment within the perforated posterior longitudinal ligament. It must be pointed out that in most cases this free fragment is not entirely separated from the disk; it remains in contact with the anulus fibrosus and the perforation channel.

Mechanisms

Various pathogenetic factors have been implicated in soft disk herniation.

Mechanical factors such as trauma or repeated microtrauma may result in fissuring of the anulus, giving rise to bulging of the nucleus; soft disk herniations are abrupt and severe in onset and the resultant CBN is hyperalgesic. Sudden eruption of the disk material and tensing of the anulus following trauma or exertion may explain the painful paroxysms occurring against a background of more chronic symptoms. In all such cases, fissure formation and repeated microtrauma favor disk degeneration.

Early *disk degeneration* is considered by some to be the major promoting factor in hernia formation, the real cause of apparently spontaneous herniation. The process is identical to that seen in aging, but with an earlier onset and more rapid evolution; it may commence when the patient is no more than 20 years old, more often toward the age of 40. The nucleus becomes dehydrated and hard, less homogeneous, and less distinguishable from the deeper layers of the anulus. It no longer plays a role in pressure distribution, resulting in additional mechanical stresses. Having become fibrous and inelastic, the nucleus tends to fragment. Our experience, however, has been that herniations usually involve an apparently undegenerated disk, with no history of significant trauma - though some postulate a category of apparently "primary" hernias involving a disk which may have been rendered more fragile by trauma that originally went unnoticed.

Posterolateral herniations appear to be more frequent than medial ones. Two facts may account for this:

— The distinctive shape of disks at the cervical level, due to the presence of uncinate processes: in effect, the disk turns back upon itself at the uncinate processes, creating vulnerable lateral zones at the folds.
— The structure of the posterior longitudinal ligament, which consists of two layers: the deep layer is reinforced only in its medial portion by the superficial layer, leaving a weaker lateral zone through which the disk may exit.

Lower cervical herniation involves the C5–C6 (30%) disk or space and the C6–C7 (50%) disk, and can be explained by the fact that this is a transition zone between the mobile cervical spine and the rigid thoracic spine, as already pointed out by others [164, 289].

Spontaneous Evolution

Regression of the hernia: Fissuring of the anulus fibrosus results in dehydration of the disk, which decreases in height, as well as in localized inflammatory reactions that eventually resorb the nuclear fragment and permit healing of the fissure. Because of this, the compressed nerve root is partially freed. This is precisely what has been found in patients with typical soft disk herniations who were not operated upon because of regression of the clinical signs. In these patients, follow-up CT scans showed complete disappearance of the hernia. This process takes at least 6 months.

Disk degeneration is inevitable in herniated disks and progresses until complete. The disk substance is replaced by fibrous tissue and, especially, by intradiskal gas.

Calcification: A chronically evolving hernia may also become calcified, resulting in the formation of localized osteophytes and giving rise to the classic disko-osteophytic nodules (hard disk) well known to rheumatologists. This stage supposedly precedes that of cervical arthrosis; in fact, postural disturbances create supplementary strains at the posterior apophyseal and uncovertebral joints, thus favoring osteophyte formation. This could in effect provide a link between the conditions we have differentiated, namely soft disk herniations in young subjects and generalized foraminal arthrosis in older individuals.

Anatomy of the Lower Cervical Spine
[125, 222, 233, 248, 266, 277, 287]

Spinal Canal

The spinal canal is triangular in shape. It is bounded anteriorly by the vertebral bodies and the uncinate processes, which are the extensions of the lateral portion of the superior vertebral surfaces at each cervical level, and laterally by the pedicles, which have an oblique posterolateral orientation, and by the articular pillars. The laminae and ligamenta flava lie posterior to the spinal canal; the transverse processes form a groove, and contain the transverse foramen, through which the vertebral nerve and vertebral artery pass. Between the oval-shaped spinal cord and the anterolateral wall of the spinal canal there is an angle occupied by veins and a small amount of fat.

Spinal Cord and Meninges

The spinal cord is oval or circular in shape, with a cervical enlargement extending from C4 to T1. It is enclosed by the meninges – from within outward the pia mater, the arachnoid, and the dura mater.

The subarachnoid space is easily identified on CT scans provided the cervical spinal canal is of normal size. The spinal cord is attached to the dura mater by the denticulate ligaments; these structures cannot be entirely differentiated on CT scans.

Intervertebral Disk

The intervertebral disk is a biconvex fibrocartilaginous structure molded onto the concave portion of the upper and lower surfaces of the vertebral end-plates. It serves as a shock absorber and a distributor of mechanical stresses. A normal adult disk consists of three parts:

— The cartilaginous surface, in contact with the opposing surfaces of the vertebral end-plates and thinnest covering the nucleus pulposus.
— The peripheral anulus fibrosus, composed of obliquely oriented collagen fibers, which has two roles, that of a strong link between neighboring vertebrae and that of a shock absorber, and thus ensures vertebral stability while permitting spinal mobility.
— The nucleus pulposus or gelatinous nucleus, which is found in the central portion of the anulus and is well hydrated; thanks to its deformability and low compressibility, it serves as a distributor of mechanical stresses.

Disks at the cervical level have a distinctive shape because of the presence of uncinate processes. In effect, the disk turns back upon itself at the two uncinate processes, creating lateral folds which are considered by some to be constitutionally weak zones.

Epidural Space

The epidural space is the space between walls of the spinal canal and the thecal sac, it contains blood vessels (especially veins), ligaments, and fat.

The posterior longitudinal ligament links the posterior surfaces of the vertebral bodies and extends from the occipital bone to the sacrum. It is wide and ribbonlike, adhering to the posterior surface of the intervertebral disks as far as the entrance of the intervertebral foramen and to the adjacent margins of the intervertebral bodies; it is composed of two layers [124]:

— A deep, anterior layer which sends short fibers toward the anulus, thus joining two contiguous vertebrae.
— A superficial layer composed of long fibers running the length of several vertebrae and adhering to the deep layer medially as well as laterally.

At the disk level, the posterior longitudinal ligament appears to be more solid in the midline, the lateral zone being weaker; as we shall see, the latter is the site of most soft disk herniations.

The importance of the epidural veins has been underlined by the studies performed by Theron [285, 287], who opacified them in order to investigate cervical spine lesions. At the level of each vertebral body, blood drains into the disploic basivertebral veins, which join the transverse retrovertebral plexuses found anterior to the posterior longitudinal ligament. These plexuses link the two anterior longitudinal veins (Fig. 2).

The longitudinal axes also drain laterally into the vertebral plexuses surrounding the vertebral artery, via the foraminal veins. These large veins, the main content of the upper and anterior portion of the intervertebral foramen, form a sleeve around the spinal nerve. The number and caliber

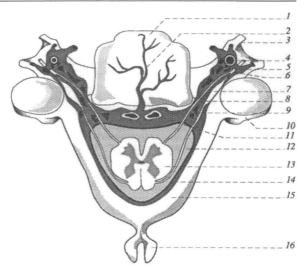

Fig. 2. Transverse section through a cervical intervertebral foramen. The anterior and posterior nerve roots pass through the foramen, completely surrounded by the numerous intervertebral veins. The dorsal root ganglion is anterior to the articular facet. The entire epidural space is lined with veins, also posterior to the thecal sac. *1*, Vertebral body; *2*, basivertebral vein; *3*, transverse process; *4*, vertebral artery; *5*, foraminal veins; *6*, neural root; *7*, neural ganglion; *8*, motor root; *9*, sensitive root; *10*, articular pillar; *11*, medial epidural veins; *12*, CSF (subarachnoid space); *13*, spinal cord; *14*, posterior epidural vein; *15*, lamina; *16*, spinous process

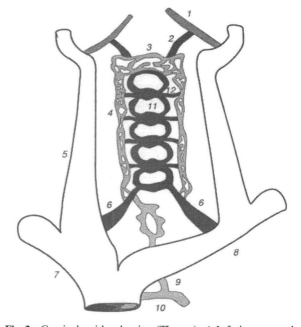

Fig. 3. Cervical epidural veins (Theron). *1*, Inferior petrosal sinus; *2*, anterior condylar emissary veins; *3*, suboccipital venous plexus; *4*, vertebral plexus, surrounding the vertebral artery; *5*, internal jugular veins; *6*, vertebral veins; *7* and *8*, right and left brachiocephalic veins; *9*, right intercostal vein; *10*, azygos vein; *11*, basivertebral veins; *12*, intervertebral veins

of these veins may vary; they are not valular, thus permitting the flow of blood in either direction. Anatomic sections clearly show both the anterior epidural veins and the foraminal veins, as well as their relationships with neural and disk structures. These venous structures are of importance in that they mark the boundaries of the epidural space at the level of the lateral portion of the disk and the uncinate processes (Fig. 3).

Cervical Spinal Nerves

The cervical spinal nerves (Fig. 4) are mixed nerves each composed of an anterior motor root and a posterior sensory root, both of which comprise several rootlets. Three segments of the root are described:

— The intradural segment, formed by the rootlets: The latter originate well above the disk, whereas the root emerges via the foramen at the same level as the disk.
— The extradural segment within the spinal canal: Each root has a dura mater sheath which is continuous with the epineurium of the spinal nerve. Both the anterior and posterior roots emerge from the thecal sac above the level of the disk, surrounded by their respective sheaths. They traverse the fat of the epidural space, enclosed by the venous plexuses,

to reach the intervertebral foramen. The lower cervical roots follow a more ascending path toward the intervertebral foramina, which are widened by extension of the head (which lowers the spinal cord) [239].
— The foraminal segment: The intervertebral canal, which has a vertical axis and is oval-shaped, has an average length of 20-25 mm; it runs anteriorly and downward at an angle of 45° with respect to the axial reference plane. Anteriorly, it is crossed by the transverse foramen, which contains the vertebral artery and nerve enveloped in the vertebral venous plexus. The internal orifice of the intervertebral canal is called the intervertebral foramen. This foramen is bounded anteriorly by the lateral portion of the intervertebral disk, and posteriorly by the uncovertebral joint. The lateral limits consist of the interspinous processes and the anterior portions of the articular pillars. In the intervertebral foramen the anterior and posterior roots come into contact with both the intervertebral disk and the uncinate process. Combined, the roots occupy approximately 40%-50% of the cross section of the foramen, the remaining volume being mostly occupied by the foraminal veins. The posterior sensory root is three times larger than the anterior motor root [222]. The roots fuse distal to the spinal ganglion to form the spinal nerve.

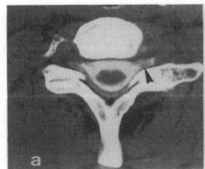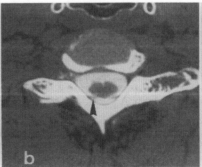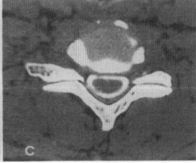

Fig. 4 a–c. Normal anatomy of the cervical spinal canal as seen on CT after the administration of contrast medium (iopamidol). The contrast enhancement permits more accurate visualization of the spinal cord and subarachnoid space within the cervical spinal canal. **a** Foraminal section. Radicular sheaths are visible at the neural foramen entrance *(arrowhead).* The opacification of the radicular sheaths is very variable from one investigation to the next. **b** Diskal section. The vertebral cartilaginous plate is partially seen. The posterior sensory nerve roots are clearly identifiable within the subarachnoid spaces *(arrowhead).* **c** Diskal section. Because of the relative narrowness of the cervical spinal canal, the subarachnoid spaces are smaller

Topography of Cervical Roots

One should be familiar with the topography of the cervical roots [169] in order to be able to investigate the dermatomic areas affected by root compressions. The cervical plexus consists of eight roots, while there are only seven vertebral bodies. The first root exits above the body of C1. In contrast to the lumbar spine, each root exits via the intervertebral foramen above the vertebra having the same number as the root. Thus, the C7 nerve root exits via the C6-C7 foramen and the C8 root via the C7-T1 foramen. Only roots C5 to T1 are capable of giving rise to CBN; the higher roots provoke neck pain.

CT Scanning Techniques

Although lumbar herniations are currently the subject of extensive CT studies, attention is less frequently paid to the cervical spine. Nevertheless, on both anatomic and clinical grounds, CT scanners are perfectly suitable for investigating CBN and for detecting soft disk herniations in particular. A well-conducted clinical examination both identifies those patients who are highly likely to have a herniation and focuses attention on the affected cervical level, thanks to the dermatomic correlations between the pain, the deficits that may be present, and the compressed root. Thus, only two or three levels, usually C5-C6 and C6-C7, are explored; this helps limit the duration of the examination. The inadequacies in the sensitivity of cervical CT scans noted by early authors were due to the absence of structures serving to mark the epidural space in the way that the fat does at the lumbar level. The foraminal epidural veins serve as markers when opacified by the intravenous injection of a contrast medium; their displacement and the venous stasis caused by a herniated disk and its free fragments provide the basis of a new radiographic semiology which we have refined over the past 4 years.

The technique should be adapted to the delicate anatomical structures examined when searching for disk herniations, which are sometimes manifested only by small free fragments migrating in the foramen.

Parameters

The best image resolution is obtained with a large matrix and the smallest investigation field possible. We therefore use a 131-mm field with a 512×512 matrix. In order to improve density resolution and especially to diminish partial volume effects, in common with many other authors we obtain scans of thin (1-mm) noncontiguous sections every 2 mm.

Sections

The detection of root compression of diskal origin relies on thin sections through the disk (in order to identify a herniation), as well as through the intervertebral foramen, which is small and located partly above the plane of the disk (Fig. 5). The performance of scans above the disk is justified on three grounds:

— The root should be explored along the entire length of its oblique course from the thecal sac above the level of the disk to the intervertebral foramen.
— We know from experience that small free fragments can make their way to the center of the intervertebral foramen.
— We routinely look for foraminal venous stasis, a very reliable sign of cervical herniation.

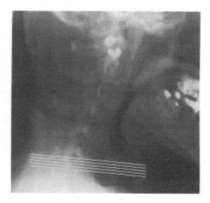

Fig. 5. Lateral scout view. Sections pass above the disk, thus investigating the overlying foramen. It is necessary to pull on the patient's arms in order to free the C6-C7 and C7-T1 levels from the plane of the shoulders. In practice, four or five 1-mm-thick sections 2 mm apart are sufficient for investigating a particular level (C5-C6 or C6-C7)

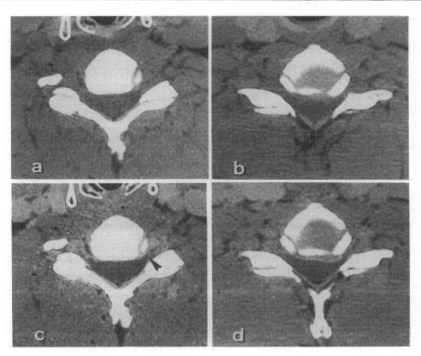

Fig. 6 a–d. Reasons for the use of intravenous contrast medium: normal anatomy. **a** The nerve roots are otherwise poorly visualized within the foramina. **b** The posterior margin of the disk appears blurred and poorly defined. **c** Contrast enhancement permits good identification of the origins of both left and right C6 roots *(arrowhead).* **d** Contrast enhancement of the posterior longitudinal ligament and the longitudinal veins clearly shows a left diskal asymmetry

A level at which disk herniation is suspected will thus be scanned from the intervertebral foramen, 4–5 mm above the diskal plane, through the disk down to the superior surface of the underlying vertebral body.

In contrast to the situation at the lumbar level, there is no point in performing supplementary cephalad or caudad sections, given the absence of ascending or descending migratory herniations.

Intravenous Injection of Contrast Medium

Intravenous injection of contrast medium is absolutely essential [11, 61, 162, 217, 234, 251] (Fig. 6). The anterolateral epidural veins and the foraminal veins occupy almost the entire epidural space. The enhancement of these veins provides an ideal marker for the posterior margin of the disk and the intervertebral foramen, far superior to the fat that serves the same purpose at the lumbar level.

Examination

A single intravenous injection of 100 ml iodinated contrast medium is performed immediately just before the investigation. At present, we use the nonionic medium iopamidol (Iopamiron 300, Schering).

The patient is positioned supine on the table and must remain immobile. In order to avoid artifacts stemming from projection of the shoulders over the intervertebral spaces, we pull down on the patient's wrists, thus separating the scapular plane from that of the lower cervical spine. This permits one to free the shoulders by an average of 1–2 cm at the level of C7–T1.

To identify the site, we perform a scout view, which provides a digital image of the cervical spine. The incidences are centered parallel to the plane of the disk.

One should remember that the scans begin in the intervertebral foramen above the disk and then pass through the disk itself. In everyday practice, two levels are investigated, generally C5–C6 and C6–C7, usually with four or five sections scanned for each level examined.

Radioanatomy [123, 125, 160, 222, 310]

Foraminal Plane

The foraminal plane (Figs. 7, 8) is located several millimeters above the diskal plane. Without intravenous injection of contrast medium, it is very difficult to differentiate the structures in the nerve root–vein complex. After injection, the foraminal veins take up the contrast medium and appear as hyperdensities enveloping the roots. The roots themselves appear hypodense and are only visible intermittently from one section to the next, because they take oblique courses forward and downward. Under good conditions, one may clearly identify the dorsal root ganglion, in contact with the articular process.

The distribution of the hyperdense veins and the hypodense nerve roots in the intervertebral foramina is not always the same from one patient to the next. This underscores the value of thin sections passing through the intervertebral foramina on both sides, permitting comparison. In

case of doubt, one should perform scans of contiguous 1-mm sections between the standard sections.

The intervertebral foramen is limited anteriorly by the transverse canal and the vertebral artery, laterally by the posterior margin of the body of the overlying vertebra, and posteriorly by the articular pillars. The more anterior articular facet is that of the subjacent vertebra.

Diskal Plane

Given the bowl-like appearance resulting on the one hand from the presence of the uncinate processes and on the other from the slight difference in thickness between the lateral and medial parts of the disk itself, an intervertebral disk is not often visualized in entirety in one section. Under normal conditions, the nucleus pulposus is indistinguishable from the anulus fibrosus.

Following the intravenous injection of contrast medium, the disk is seen to be limited later-

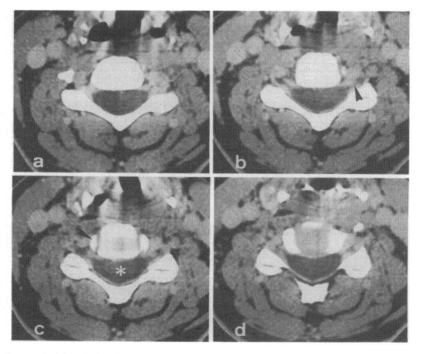

Fig. 7 a–d. Study of a cervical level after intravenous injection of 100 ml Iopamiron 300: normal anatomy. **a, b** Sections through the neural foramen. The foraminal veins are opacified, and the hypodense nerve root can be distinguished from the surrounding venous structures *(arrowhead).* **c** Section through uncinate processes and upper part of disk. The uncinate processes are lateral to the disk *(arrowhead).* The spinal cord is recognizable (✳). **d** Diskal section. The posterior margin of the disk is well delineated (enhancement of the posterior longitudinal ligament and the longitudinal veins)

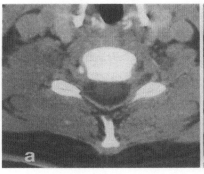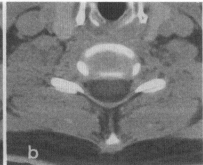

Fig. 8 a, b. Foraminal plane: normal anatomy. In young patients (ideal conditions), the foramina, the spinal cord within the subarachnoid space, and the posterior margin of the disk are clearly visualized

ally by the uncinate processes and posteriorly by a hyperdense rim; it is separated from the spinal cord by the hypodense anterior subarachnoid space. The epidural fat is sometimes visible at the entrance to the foramen, but is usually very sparse.

The contrast medium opacifies the epidural veins. Both the dura mater and its vessels and the posterior longitudinal ligament are enhanced. This permits clear identification of the posterior margin of the disk and differentiation of the subarachnoid spaces from the extradural structures, which are almost small at the cervical level and in the diskal plane.

The foraminal uptake of contrast medium is symmetrical, and under normal circumstances never extends beyond the anterolateral angle of the cervical spinal canal.

Pedicular Plane

The pedicular plane passes through the superior surface of the underlying vertebra. On this section, one can study the size, form, and structure of the spinal canal, which is limited anteriorly by the vertebral body and the uncinate processes, laterally by the pedicles and the articular pillars, and posteriorly by the laminae and the ligamenta flava.

The spinal cord is usually visualized as a homogeneous oval structure which appears denser than the cerebrospinal fluid. Under good conditions, the outline of the cord is easily distinguished. Detailed study obviously calls for the intrathecal injection of contrast medium, but this is only exceptionally done in investigations of CBN. Nevertheless, the pedicular plane is one to bear in mind. Indeed, it permits demonstration of stenosis of the cervical spinal canal when present.

Radiographic Investigation of Soft Cervical Disk Herniations

Conventional Investigations

Plain Films

Plain films in anteroposterior, lateral, and left and right oblique projections should be routinely obtained. These radiographs may show a possible posterior diskal defect, an arthrosis, or especially, our experience, loss of the cervical curvature. Functional radiographic methods are of little value. The same is true for signs of disk degeneration on routine plain films, as we now know that a disk may be degenerate and not herniated, and, conversely, that a herniation may involve a healthy disk: Routine plain films are especially useful in evaluating the extent of arthrosis between vertebral bodies, spinous processes, or of foraminal uncarthrosis. The latter even when severe, is not necessarily the cause of coexisting CBN.

These are common lesions, and numerous patients with uncarthrosis are completely asymptomatic. Nevertheless, routine plain films serve to show the bone structure (which is usually normal), and to rule out infectious, inflammatory, or (bone) tumor etiology.

Myelography with Nonionic Water-soluble Contrast Media

Myelography using nonionic water-soluble contrast media [4, 12, 24, 87, 92, 255, 269] is laterocervical, with injection of the contrast medium at C1–C2 under fluoroscopic control. Anteroposterior and oblique projections show root compressions well, in addition to the amputation of the arachnoid sheath accompanying the root and of the lateral perimedullar space. However, myelography is an invasive examination and has often been questioned both by patients and by their physicians, despite the excellent images it is capable of providing. It has not enjoyed widespread use in the investigation of CBN.

Apart from its invasive character, the major drawback of myelography is its low sensitivity when it comes to small foraminal herniations. In effect, the radicular sheath is short at the cervical level involved, so thorough examination of the foramen is not possible.

If uncarthrosis is present, it will be difficult by means of myelography to determine whether the cause is the protrusion of bone or a possible additional soft disk herniation. On the other hand, myelography is valuable in that it furnishes an overall view of the spine, explores all the nerve root emergences on both sides and shows the diameter of the spinal cord, all in one examination.

Cervical Diskography

Cervical diskography [55, 192] was introduced to France by Massare in 1974. At present it is enjoying a resurgence of interest, especially in combination with CT scans during cervical chemonucleolysis; this therapeutic aspect will be discussed in a later section of this chapter.

CT Signs of Cervical Herniations

The CT signs of cervical disk herniation, recently elaborated, are readily recognized; any remaining doubt can be cleared up by scans of contiguous 1-mm sections after the intravenous injection of contrast medium [11, 61, 82, 160, 162, 200, 204, 251, 310].

CT scanners are capable of identifying a disk herniation and its immediate impact upon the root, located a few millimeters higher at the entrance to and within the intervertebral foramen. This is made possible by the stasis of the foraminal veins.

Stasis of the Foraminal Veins: The Basic and Pathognomonic Sign

Because the herniation occurs laterally, below the veins, at the entrance to the intervertebral foramina, the veins are compressed and displaced upward. The result is foraminal venous stasis that is readily visualized as a poorly delineated hyperdensity (100–120 HU) on CT scans after the intravenous injection of contrast medium. The stasis is visible on several sections, and is clearly different from the contralateral side. A comparison of both intervertebral foramina is very important; they are not always located in the same axial plane. The venous stasis obliterates the intervertebral foramen and is also visible in the anterolateral angle of the spinal canal. When the stasis is considerable, it extends upward to the diskal plane, and should be looked for there.

In our experience this venous stasis, resulting from displacement and compression of the epidural veins by nuclear material is the most characteristic sign. One finds it in all instances of nerve root compression by disk material involving a posterolateral soft disk herniation, but it is never observed with foraminal uncarthrosis, even in extremely severe cases. The explanation for this is that with herniation the nucleus is forcibly extruded, resulting in a congestion of these venous structures that is impossible with uncarthrosis, which develops over a period of several years.

The herniation is found a few millimeters below the nerve root and is always sharply defined, posterolateral, and involves the intervertebral foramen.

While these semiological considerations apply to the vast majority of herniations occurring at the cervical level, we have encountered very occasional cases in which only the stasis is evident on CT, the posterior margin of the subjacent disk appearing normal. The stasis is well delineated, punctiform, and confined to the interverte-

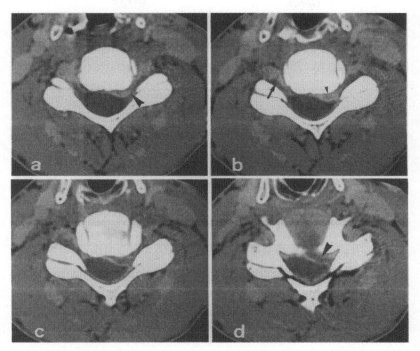

Fig. 9 a–d. Common posterolateral herniation. Left C6 cervicobrachial neuralgia: CT study at C5–C6. **a, b** Foraminal sections. Existence of a left foraminal hyperdensity extending into the anterolateral angle of the spinal canal. This is an expression of stasis of the foraminal veins *(arrowhead)*. On the right, the intervertebral foramen only shows the nerve root and its ganglion (→). *Note* the existence of small hypodense structures within the venous stasis; these are slightly along the disk and indicate nuclear migration towards the foramen *(arrowhead)*. **c, d** These sections are lower and pass through the disk. They demonstrate a midline herniation shifting to the left. The nucleus is recognizable within the herniation as a hypodense area *(arrowhead)*. *Operative findings:* median perforation of the posterior longitudinal ligament and a free fragment on the left

bral foramen. A herniation has occurred, but the herniated disk material is detached from the disk and has migrated into the intervertebral foramen, where it is obscured by the dilated veins (see below).

Cervical Herniation

Cervical herniations are readily visualized on sections passing through the disk. Posterolateral herniations are bounded by a thin hyperdense rim, permitting clear identification of the posterior structures, consisting of the cerebrospinal fluid and the spinal cord. This rim represents the posterior longitudinal ligament, the dura mater and its blood vessels, and, especially, the anterior epidural veins, which have been enhanced by the injection of contrast medium. The posterior longitudinal ligament cannot be differentiated from the other structures. The posterior margin of the herniation usually appears uniform. Several types of cervical herniation are found.

Posterolateral Herniation

Posterolateral herniation (Figs. 9–13) is the type most frequently found. It presents no diagnostic problems, as the signs are plentiful; the associated overlying venous stasis is readily recognized.

The herniation is clearly visible in sections passing through the diskal plane as a large posterolateral structure oriented upward toward the intervertebral foramen and filling in its entrance. The herniation may even slightly displace the corresponding anterolateral spinal tract (usually without any clinical signs).

In most cases a relative hypodensity (40–50 HU) can be seen within these large herniations. This hypodensity, representing the nucleus pulposus, may be oval-shaped, round, or sometimes linear, it is distinguished thanks to the

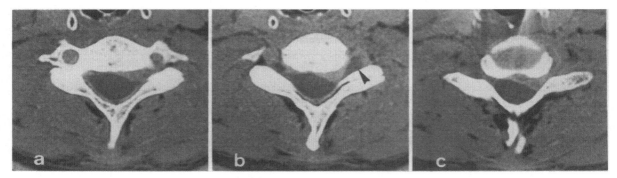

Fig. 10 a–c. Common posterolateral herniation. Left C7 cervicobrachial neuralgia: CT study at C6-C7. **a** Section through C6 pedicles and foramina above shows asymmetry, with left hyperdensity; this represents ascending venous stasis. **b** Foraminal hyperdensity (venous stasis) is clearly seen. Easily distinguished ganglion (perhaps edematous) in distal part of foramen *(arrowhead)*. *Note* the obliteration of left anterolateral subarachnoid space. **c** Disk herniation is visible in this section; its hypodensity corresponds to the herniated nucleus. *Operative findings:* median perforation of the posterior longitudinal ligament with lateral migration of the free fragment

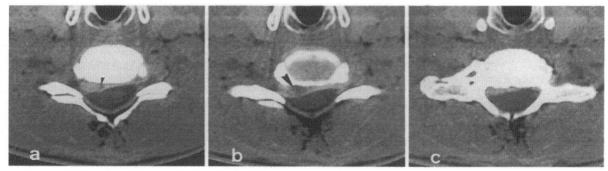

Fig. 11 a–c. Common posterolateral herniation. Right C7 cervicobrachial neuralgia: CT study at C6-C7. **a** Venous stasis at entrance to right foramen, combined with a punctiform hypodensity *(arrowhead)*. **b** Diskal section: the easily identified herniation has a central, rounded hypodensity *(arrowhead)*. **c** Persistence of the venous stasis below the disk, representing pathologically obstructed longitudinal and anterior epidural veins. *Operative findings:* perforated ligament and lateral free fragment

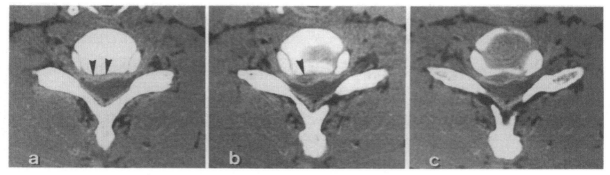

Fig. 12 a–c. Common posterolateral herniation. Right C7 cervicobrachial neuralgia: CT study at C6-C7. **a** Venous stasis at entrance to right C7 foramen. The clearly visible stasis corresponds to the foraminal veins, as well as to the more median transverse plexus *(arrowhead)*. **b, c** Small, paramedian disk herniation with a central hypodensity *(arrowhead)*. *Operative findings:* perforated ligament and two free fragments, one median and the other more lateral

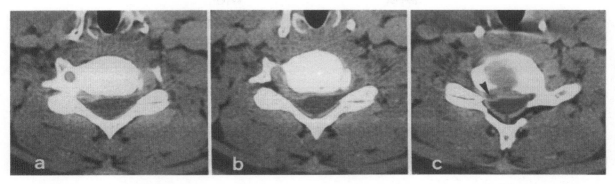

Fig. 13 a–c. Common posterolateral herniation. Right C7 cervicobrachial neuralgia: CT study at C6-C7. **a, b** Right foraminal hyperdensity extending above the foramen and visible at the level of the pedicles of the vertebra above. **c** Small median right herniation with small, well-defined hypodensity corresponding to nuclear fragments; the herniation seems to be within the ligament *(arrowhead)*. *Operative findings:* free fragment and perforated ligament

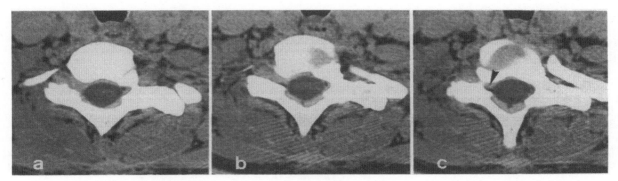

Fig. 14 a–c. Small lateral herniation. Right C8 cervicobrachial neuralgia: CT study at C7-T1. **a** Venous stasis seen as a foraminal hyperdensity extending a considerable distance upward. **b, c** Very small homogeneous disk herniation without hypodensities, quite lateral and just behind the horizontal C7-T1 uncinate process *(arrowhead)*. *Note* that at this level, the collapsed disk has a normal posteromedian border. *Comment:* Small, lateral herniations are often homogeneous, even when there is a free fragment which perforates the posterior longitudinal ligament

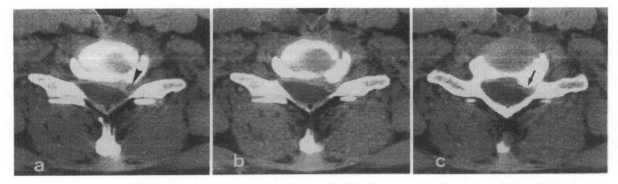

Fig. 15 a–c. Small lateral herniation. Left C7 cervicobrachial neuralgia: CT study at C6-C7. **a, b** Rounded hypodensity belonging to the disk, at the foraminal entrance *(arrowhead)*. **c** Small left retrovertebral osteophyte below the hernia (→). *Comment:* This very small herniation was readily found at surgery

thin (1 mm) sections and, especially, the intravenous injection of contrast medium. When the herniation is significant, the hypodense nucleus travels upward, toward the intervertebral foramen, and is therefore visible within the foraminal venous stasis. When the amount of nuclear material herniated is considerable, the hypodensity is

seen on the CT scans of all the foraminal and diskal sections.

Small Lateral Herniation

The small lateral type of herniation (Fig. 14) is always found at the entrance to an intervertebral foramen. The CT appearance varies, but gener-

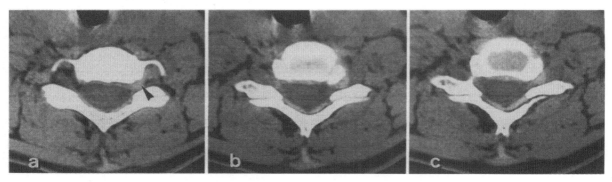

Fig. 16 a–c. Migratory free fragment. Left C7 cervicobrachial neuralgia: CT study at C6–C7. **a** Punctiform foraminal venous stasis far removed from the intervertebral foramen and far lateral with respect to the uncus *(arrowhead)*. **b, c** The posterior border of the disk is strictly normal. *Surgical findings:* The perforated ligament is revealed by the surgical mi-

croscope. The free fragment is in the intervertebral foramen, far removed from the lateral border of the disk; it is an example of a migratory free fragment. *Comment:* Being obscured by the foraminal vein stasis, the free fragment is not directly visible

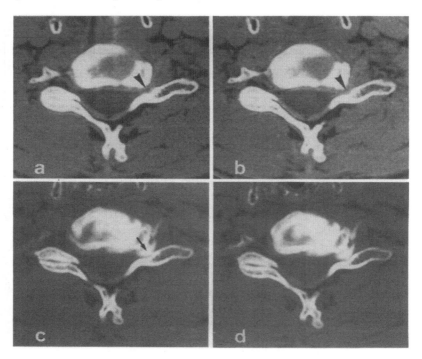

Fig. 17 a–d. Migratory free fragment. Left C7 cervicobrachial neuralgia: confirmation by postdiskography CT. **a, b** Localized, left, foraminal venous stasis indicating the existence of a free fragment *(arrowhead)*. **c, d** Postdiskography CT scans following chemonucleolysis at C6–C7. The contrast medium

opacifies the free fragment, distant from the disk in the left C6–C7 foramen (→). *Comment:* The chemonucleolytic agent reaches the migratory free fragment even in the midportion of the foramen

ally the herniation is hyperdense and homogeneous and is entirely contiguous with the posterolateral margin of the disk. This type of herniation is characterized by its attachment to the disk. Venous stasis is evident. In general, no nuclear hypodensities can be visualized, as the portion of nucleus extruded is too small to be differentiated within the herniation. In a few cases, however, a diskal hypodensity can be discerned (Fig. 15).

Migratory Free Fragment
The migratory free fragment (Fig. 16) must be differentiated from a very small lateral herniation that is still attached to the disk. Such fragments are completely invisible on laterocervical myelography, and are the most difficult type of herniation to identify on CT. The posterior margin of the disk is absolutely normal; one sees only an isolated punctiform foraminal hyperdensity appearing on two or three sections. This indicates the presence of a small nuclear fragment which has detached itself from the disk and migrated into the intervertebral foramen. The fragment is therefore not directly visible: since it is small and obscured by the congested veins, there is no hypodensity. Only the intravenous injection of contrast medium enables identification of the fragment, along with the asymmetric appearance of the two intervertebral foramina examined. The free fragment is always opacified on postdiskography CT (Fig. 17).

Abnormality of the posterior disk margin on CT is thus not always present in root compression of disk origin. In rare cases, a foraminal hypodensity may be observed when the free fragment is large (Figs. 18, 19).

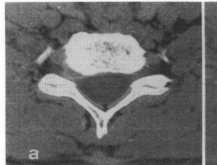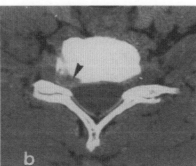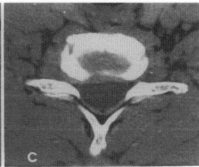

Fig. 18 a–c. Migratory free fragment. Right C7 cervicobrachial neuralgia: CT study at C6–C7. **a** Right foraminal venous stasis. **b** Hypodensity differentiable within the stasis, in the midportion of the foramen *(arrowhead).* **c** The posterior margin of the disk is straight. *Comment:* Given the large size of the hypodensity it is a migratory free fragment

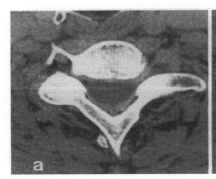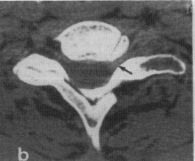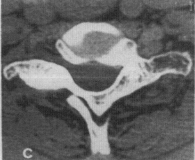

Fig. 19 a–c. Migratory free fragment. Left C7 cervicobrachial neuralgia: CT study at C6–C7. **a, b** Foraminal stenosis due to uncinate process hypertrophy. Punctiform hyperdensity at the foraminal entrance (→). **c** *Note* the posterior border of the absolutely normal appearing disk. *Surgical findings:* Perforated ligament and free fragment at the foraminal entrance. Given the very small size of the fragment, which is obscured by the stasis, no hypodensities are visible. *Comment:* The 1-mm-thick sections permit detection of a small fragment responsible for CBN in an elderly patient with a narrowed intervertebral foramen

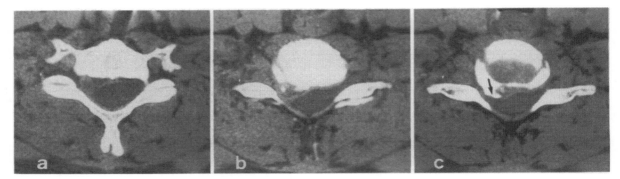

Fig. 20 a–c. Herniation with uncarthrosis. Right C7 cervicobrachial neuralgia: CT study at C6–C7. **a** Right foraminal venous stasis with a foraminal hypodensity. **b** Narrowing of the neural foramen due to foraminal uncarthrosis. Soft disk herniation comprising a hypodense fragment combined with punctiform calcifications. **c** Both the herniation and a retrovertebral osteophyte remain visible (→). *Surgical findings:* perforation of the posterior longitudinal ligament and free fragment combined with small, ossified nodules. *Comment:* This is a soft hernia in a predisposed individual; foraminal uncarthrosis and calcifications (probably ligamentous) in contact with the hernia. CT scans permit one to differentiate between soft and calcified structures

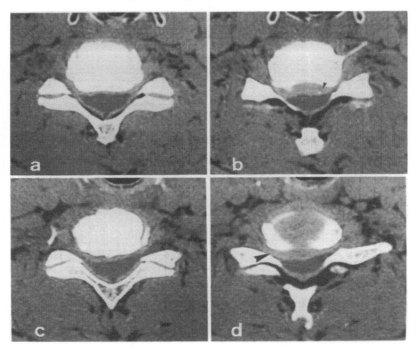

Fig. 21 a–d. Two-level herniation. Right C7 cervicobrachial neuralgia: two-level CT study. *At C5–C6:* **a** Bilateral foraminal uncarthrosis; no evident venous stasis. **b** Significant posteromedian disk herniation following degeneration. Small, left, posterolateral ligamentous calcification *(arrowhead).* Being collapsed, the disk is less visible. *At C6–C7:* **c** Right foraminal stasis above a posterolateral herniation. **d** Disk herniation is visible below the diskal plane, along with dilated veins *(arrowhead). Comment:* Given the large median herniation at C5–C6, surgery was performed at both levels. In fact, only the right C6–C7 herniation was responsible for the CBN

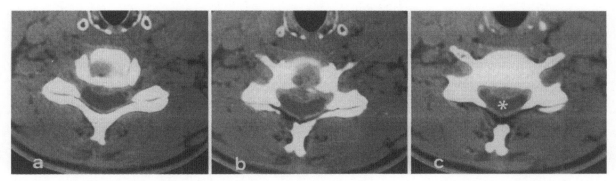

Fig. 22 a–c. Median herniation. Bilateral dysesthesias involving the first two fingers of both hands: CT study at C5–C6. **a** There is no foraminal venous stasis, neither left nor right. **b, c** A median herniation with a free fragment (diskal hypodensity). The median herniation presses the spinal cord (✷) against the posterior arch, probably resulting in strained nerve roots; this could well explain the dysesthesias observed. *Surgical findings:* Median free fragment. Remember that this was not a case of typical CBN

Other Types of Herniation

Calcified Herniation

The term "calcified herniation" is applied to several abnormalities. A soft disk herniation may become partly calcified (hard disk). Of course, there is venous stasis. In most cases one finds ipsilateral or contralateral isolated foraminal uncarthrosis at the level of the herniation. Finally, retrovertebral osteophytes or ligamentous calcifications may also be observed (Fig. 20). Combinations of these elements may also occur without calcified herniation being present.

Thin sections easily differentiate disk material from hard osteophytic components, and may distinguish it from a preexisting foraminal stenosis. In these very specific cases, CT is vastly superior to laterocervical myelography, which merely shows nonspecific radicular amputation. The ability to identify calcified herniations is of great value for a neurosurgeon who has a diskectomy to perform.

Double Herniation

Simultaneous herniation at two levels is rare in the cervical spine; in our population it accounted for two of 75 cases operated on over a period of 3 years (see Fig. 21). Identification of a double herniation may be quite arduous; while monoradicular CBN generally stems from herniation at one level only, it is rather difficult to entirely absolve the overlying or underlying level at which a second herniation may be present.

A radiologist can confirm the level responsible for the CBN on the basis of the venous stasis; in practice, neurosurgeons prefer to operate on both levels, given the possible risk of subsequent recurrence (Fig. 21).

Median Herniation

Median herniation (Fig. 22) usually gives rise to cord symptoms, consisting of paresthesias associated with dysesthesias and affecting both upper extremities. However, the clinical picture is most often one of tetraparesis with a cord irritation syndrome spreading to all four extremities. CT scans may reveal a large median herniation with a hypodensity. There is no foraminal venous stasis since there is no direct compression of the root by the disk.

In practice, MRI is the first examination performed in the presence of medullary irritation, since it shows the spinal cord compression and identifies the level responsible. The entire cervical spinal cord is investigated using sagittal sections.

Smaller median herniations may be found during the investigation of typical CBN. Such a herniation alone cannot explain the radicular pain; it is important to search for an overlying foraminal venous stasis indicating migration of disk material originating from the median herniation (Fig. 23).

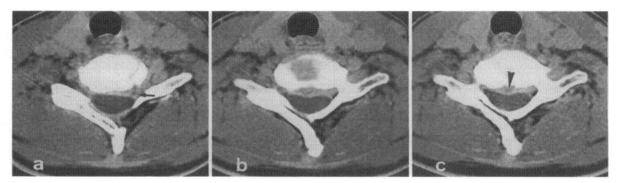

Fig. 23 a–c. Median herniation with migratory free fragment. Left C7 cervicobrachial neuralgia: CT study at C6-C7. **a** A left foraminal venous stasis with a quite punctiform hypodensity, which fills in the intervertebral foramen (→). **b, c** Median disk herniation, also with a hypodensity *(arrowhead) Surgical findings:* All these elements were readily found, as always in combination with a perforated ligament. *Comment:* Median herniations such as this are not responsible by themselves for unilateral CBN: however, in this case the neuralgia can be explained by the small migratory free fragment detached from the herniation and now in the foramen

Herniation Without a Free Fragment

Herniations without a free fragment (Fig. 24) appear to be relatively rare. They involve nuclear material which is entirely subligamentous. Their existence may be suspected on CT, but the overlap and hernial bulging are minimal, and above all no hypodensities are visible. Nevertheless, the diagnosis of a subligamentous herniation without a free fragment can be made only on the basis of CT-surgical correlations.

Interpretation of CT Scans

The CT scans of cervical herniations are best understood using the radiographic-anatomical correlations established in a group of 75 patients with cervical hernias who underwent surgery on the basis of CT findings alone. In the vast majority of these cases, the posterior longitudinal ligament was perforated and there was a free fragment in a transligamentous position. This applies to all the types of cervical herniations which we have just described.

By "free fragment" we refer to a fragment of the nucleus pulposus which has escaped from the disk, and is located somewhere within the various layers of the posterior longitudinal ligament.

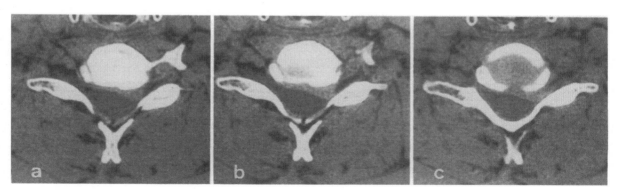

Fig. 24 a–c. Herniation without a free fragment. Right C7 cervicobrachial neuralgia: CT study at C6-C7. **a, b** Punctiform venous stasis found only at the entrance to the foramen. **c** Lateral disk herniation without hypodensities; the border is very uniform. *Surgical findings:* absence of perforated ligament or free fragment. *Comment:* Our experience has been that such cases are extremely rare. In the vast majority, there is an accompanying perforation of the posterior longitudinal ligament

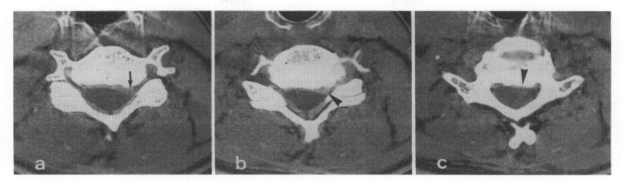

Fig. 25 a–c. Herniation with arthritis. Left C7 cervicobrachial neuralgia: CT study at C6–C7 (collapsed C6–C7 disk seen on plain films). **a** Extensive bilateral foraminal uncarthrosis. CT is capable of distinguishing the venous stasis at the neural foramen entrance from the arthrosis (→). **b** Far lateral and dense small disk herniation *(arrowhead)*. **c** Calcifications within the posterior longitudinal ligament *(arrowhead)*. *At surgery:* This small hernia was easily found. *Comment:* Foraminal uncarthrosis alone cannot result in venous stasis. There is inevitable also a small, soft herniation which suddenly produces the CBN

The free fragment may be visualized directly as a hypodensity in the middle of a large herniation; it may also be suspected from a very lateralized location of the herniation. An isolated foraminal venous stasis with an apparently normal disk may be the only sign of a nuclear fragment which has migrated some distance. The hypodensity represents the free fragment still in contact with the annulus fibrosus of the disk, and embedded in the fibers of the posterior longitudinal ligament.

A hypodensity in the middle of a common herniation is tantamount to free material associated with a ligamentous tear.

Conclusions based on the CT appearance of a herniation should, of course, be tempered by the clinical findings. This having been said, there is no direct correlation between the two: very large herniations with free fragments may have a spontaneously favorable outcome, and those with small free fragments at a distance may evolve unfavorably. The indication for surgery depends mainly on the clinical findings.

Herniation and Arthrosis

[10, 56, 92, 149, 165, 208, 224, 267, 274]

Younger People

Soft disk herniations may be associated with foraminal arthrosis, especially when the herniation is calcified – though in our opinion this association is relatively rare. CT scans show the calcification of the hernia, the presence of retrovertebral osteophytes, and possibly a concomitant arthritic foraminal stenosis. The presence of an apparently isolated uncarthrosis should prompt one to search the level in question for a small soft disk herniation which may have simply tipped the balance in a subject predisposed to arthritis (Fig. 25).

In more general terms, clear signs of arthrosis on routine plain films should prompt a search for a soft disk herniation if the clinical findings are suggestive; not only at the level affected by arthritis, but also at the levels above and below (Fig. 26).

In our experience, it is truly exceptional for typical monoradicular neuralgia in a young subject to be caused by isolated foraminal uncarthrosis limited to the intervertebral foramen through which the root passes (Fig. 27). These rare patients may, of course, benefit from operation (foraminotomy).

In cases of severe arthrosis with a typical neuralgia, the free fragment can be demonstrated by postdiskography CT (Fig. 28).

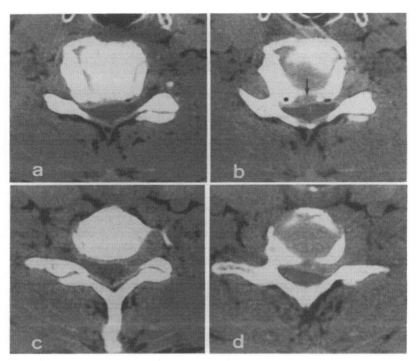

Fig. 26 a-d. Herniation and arthritis. Left C7 cervicobrachial neuralgia: two-level CT study (considerable C5-C6 disk degeneration seen on plain films). *At C5-C6:* **a, b** Very considerable stenosis of the right C5-C6 foramen resulting from uncarthrosis combined with degenerative bulging of the disk (→). This does not account for the left C7 neuralgia. *At* *C6-C7:* **c, d** These sections confirm the existence of a left posterolateral herniation one level below the discopathy. *Comment:* Plain films show a considerable degenerative C5-C6 discopathy which could not explain the neuralgia. The herniation is located at a lower level which appears normal on plain films

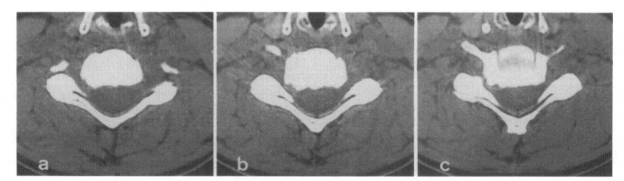

Fig. 27 a-c. Isolated foraminal uncarthrosis. Right C6 cervicobrachial neuralgia: CT study at C5-C6. **a** In this young woman, there is no clear-cut foraminal venous stasis. **b, c** The posterior margin of the disk is normal; there is only one calcification of the posterior longitudinal ligament. No subjacent venous stasis. *Surgical findings:* No disk herniations. A simple foraminotomy was performed. *Comment:* In our experience, uncarthrosis without an accompanying disk hernia or free fragment never leads to venous stasis

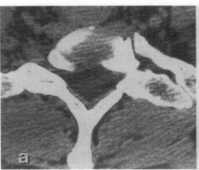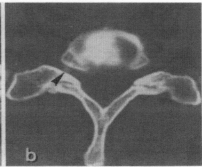

Fig. 28 a, b. Uncarthrosis and free fragment. Right C8 cervicobrachial neuralgia resistant to medical treatment: confirmation of diagnosis by postdiskography CT. **a** CT shows only a severe right foraminal uncarthrosis at C7–T1, without any venous hyperdensities. **b** Postdiskography CT at C7–T1: contrast medium injected at medial part of intervertebral space. A punctiform image is seen within the foramen *(arrow-* *head). Surgical findings:* The minute fragment was perfectly identified. *Comment:* In cases of severe foraminal stenosis, it is difficult to render small venous stasis visible because of partial volume effects. Even under such circumstances, however, postdiskography CT can demonstrate a minute migratory free fragment

Older People

The problem of CBN in an older subject with known multilevel bilateral arthritis is quite different. Oblique projections show narrowed intervertebral foramina in the lower cervical spine. Furthermore, pronounced anterior and posterior arthrosis of the vertebral bodies is usually found.

CBN is less common in this population. When present, it affects the upper extremity more severely and radiates less toward the hand. The neuralgia evolves gradually over a long period, and does not feature the hyperalgesia and insomnia characteristic of neuralgia in young subjects.

In these patients with arthrosis involving several levels, laterocervical myelography has the great advantage of demonstrating multilevel root amputations, whether uni- or bilateral.

Cervical Arthrotic Myelopathy

Cervical arthrotic myelopathy (Table 1, Fig. 29) presents a picture of advanced cervical arthrosis. In these circumstances the CBN is of lesser importance than the spinal cord involvement, the signs of which are very characteristic:

— intermittent neurogenic claudication
— weakness of the lower extremities
— paraparesis, tetraparesis
— hyperreflexia of all four extremities
— bilateral Babinski's sign

In the diagnostic workup of cervical arthrotic myelopathy, the spinal cord is the major consideration; MRI should be the first examination performed. T2-weighted sagittal sections can show both a narrowed spinal canal and a diskal or osteophytic component compressing or displacing the spinal cord against the posterior arch. MRI still has certain limitations, especially with respect to axial sections; indeed, it is quite difficult to show osteophytes or signs of diskopathy accurately in the transverse plane. Laterocervical myelography combined with metrizamide CT is more capable of demonstrating the existence of osteophytes associated with disk degeneration (Figs. 30, 31). Their exact location can be identified much more precisely thanks to the 1-mm-thick sections. A lateralized posteromedian osteophyte is readily detected, and the size of the spi-

Table 1. Diagnostic approach in the case of cervicobrachial neuralgia

Clinical findings	Cervical spine	Examination	Objective
Typical CBN	No hypertrophic changes	CT	Search for soft disk herniation
Typical CBN	Limited uncinate process hypertrophy, narrowing of only one foramen	CT	Confirm stenosis: search for accompanying soft disk herniation
Typical CBN	Hypertrophic changes at only one level	CT	Search for soft disk herniation above or below level exhibiting hypertrophy
More or less typical CBN	Advanced, generalized hypertrophic changes at more than one level	Myelography; possibly postmyelography CT of most pathogenic level	Evaluate all disko-osteophytic protrusions. Evaluate nerve root sheath amputations.
Cord syndrome with background CBN	Advanced hypertrophic changes in most cases	1. MRI: sagittal sections at affected level(s) 2. Postmyelography CT (preoperatively)	Search for cord compression, amputation of subarachnoid spaces Keep in mind: • Disko-osteophytic lesions of degenerated disk associated with ligamentous calcification • Value of accurately knowing size of cervical spinal canal and condition of spinal cord (atrophy at one or two levels) • Possibility of isolated herniation (rare) • Value for neurosurgeon of 1-mm axial sections

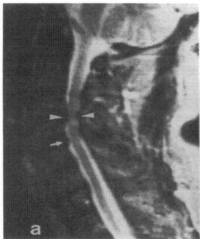 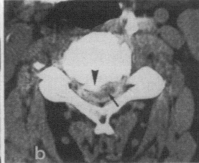 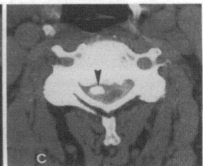

Fig. 29 a–c. Cervical myelopathy: 71-year-old patient with spastic quadriparesis. **a** MRI: sagittal T2-weighted section (TR 1800, TE 40, four echoes). This median section confirms spinal canal stenosis at C3–C4 with medullary compression secondary to disk degeneration *(white arrowhead).* There also exists a less severe diskal osteophytic bulging at C4–C5 (→). **b, c** CT myelography at C3–C4 as part of the presurgical workup. The right paramedian osteophyte is clearly visible *(black arrowhead),* and its relation to the spinal cord is apparent; the osteophyte is pedicled and has a descending retrovertebral projection. The spinal cord is deformed by the bony projection displacing it (→). *Comment:* Axial CT myelography is always superior to axial MRI in identifying the diskal osteophytic degenerative lesion

nal canal is also better evaluated, which is particularly useful for the neurosurgeon. Finally, atrophy of the cervical spinal cord involving one or two levels is easily recognized. We believe that in the future there will be fewer indications for metrizamide CT, especially with the advent of better cervical surface coils. It is important to note that in case of cervical arthrotic myelopathy, metrizamide CT should only be performed if neurosurgery has been decided upon [31, 91].

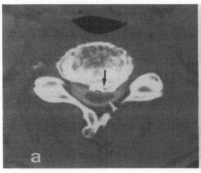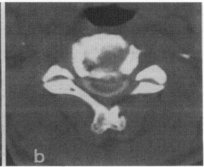

Fig. 30 a, b. Cervical myelopathy: gait disturbances and intermittent medullary claudication, paresthesia of both thumbs and both index fingers. Workup: Lateral cervical myelography, metrizamide CT scans at C4-C5, C5-C6, and C6-C7. *CT study at C5-C6:* **a** Foraminal plane: Narrow cervical canal combined with a median osteophyte (→). Absence of the anterior subarachnoid space; compressed spinal cord *(white arrowhead).* **b** Diskal plane: No herniations present. *Comment:* Metrizamide CT assesses the size of the spinal canal very accurately an indicates the location of osteophytes within the canal. The consequence is obvious: atrophy of the cervical spinal cord

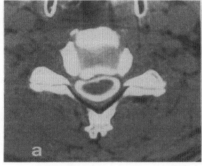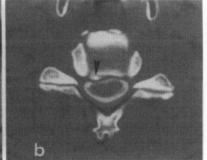

Fig. 31 a, b. Cervical myelopathy. Atypical right C6 cervicobrachial neuralgia, hyperreflexia of the right lower extremity. Workup motivated by incipient medullary symptoms: lateral cervical myelography and metrizamide CT focused on the most seriously affected levels. **a, b** C5-C6 diskal plane: deformed right anterior corticospinal tract opposite a retrovertebral osteophyte *(arrowhead),* no disk herniations present. *Comment:* Clinically, the CBN is less evident. Spastic paralysis is evident upon neurological examination. Workup confirms the existence of incipient medullary disease, reorienting the neurosurgical approach

Evolution of Unoperated Soft Disk Herniations
[163, 310]

A certain proportion of patients with typical cervical soft disk herniations (Fig. 32) are not operated on simply because there is regression or even disappearance of the painful symptoms, especially the C6 or C7 motor deficit after medical treatment. Physicians have long been aware of this phenomenon. We have performed follow-up CT at 6 months and 1 year in a number of patients whose CBN regressed with medical treatment. In all cases, the first sign of improvement was the disappearance of the foraminal venous stasis. After 6 months of natural evolution, the soft disk herniation itself may be considerably decreased in volume; it may even have totally disappeared after a year. The disappearance of herniated material has also been observed at the lumbar level using CT scans.

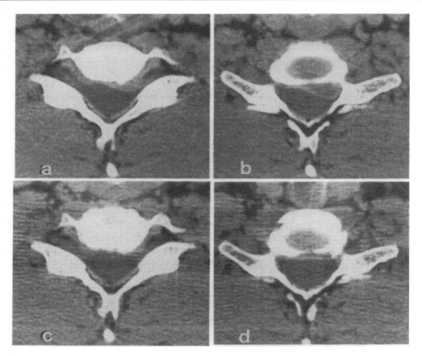

Fig. 32 a–d. Spontaneous evolution of disk herniation. Left C7 cervicobrachial neuralgia: CT study at Ç6–C7. **a, b** Large, left posterolateral herniation with a hypodensity. Venous stasis is easily recognizable above the disk. Given the clinical regression under medical treatment, the patient was not submitted to operation. After 10 months without treatment the patient was clinically well and CT showed **a** disappearance of foraminal venous stasis and **d** disappearance of the herniation. *Comment:* A large herniation with a free fragment can completely disappear over a period of several months. Follow-up CT scans can show the quality of the healing and give anatomical confirmation that complete healing at the cervical level is indeed possible

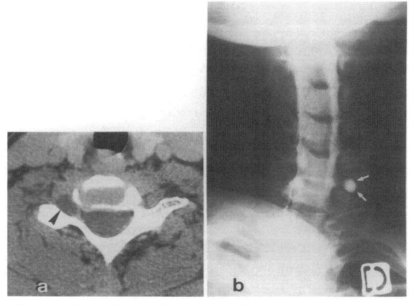

Fig. 33 a, b. Differential diagnosis in right C7 cervicobrachial neuralgia. **a** CT in the foraminal plane shows a large hypodensity occupying the entire foraminal canal. It is not a free fragment, the densities being liquid in nature *(arrowhead).* The disk appears normal. **b** Plain myelograms confirm a radicular cyst (→). *Comment:* Radicular cysts are common following microtrauma and may be responsible for CBN. They are clearly identifiable on CT

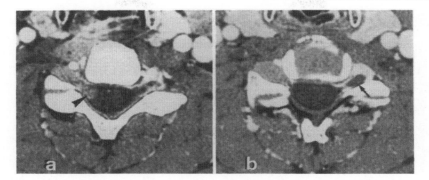

Fig. 34 a, b. Differential diagnosis in right C7 cervicobrachial neuralgia: CT study at C6–C7. **a** Dense tumoral mass in the right C6–C7 foramen enhanced by intravenous injection of contrast medium; it corresponds to a classic hourglass neurinoma. The contents of the spinal canal are readily identifi-able (arrowhead). **b** The disk is normal. *Note* the normal left C7 root, in contrast to its counterpart (→). *Comment:* Our experience has been that neurinomas are rarely implicated in CT investigations of CBN

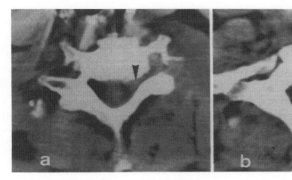

Fig. 35 a, b. Differential diagnosis in left C8 cervicobrachial neuralgia: CT study at C7-T1. **a** Filling in of the neural foramen and part of the anterolateral epidural space *(arrow-head).* **b** Tumor of the pulmonary apex resulting in a classic Pancoast's syndrome (✱)

Differential Diagnosis

The question of differential diagnosis on CT scans seldom arises: when faced with a hypodense structure within the intervertebral foramen, one should not mistake a radicular cyst (Fig. 33), which has a liquid density, a very rounded shape, and is located distal to the intervertebral foramen, with either a migratory free fragment or a large ganglion. If there is any doubt, myelography may be performed.

After the injection of contrast medium, a neurinoma appears as a hyperdense structure (Fig. 34). It usually has a component outside the intervertebral foramen, and one which juts into the spinal canal. When the neurinoma is small, there is no bone erosion; it is necessary to distinguish a small neurinoma from an isolated venous

stasis provoked by a migratory free fragment, the latter having a very characteristic appearance which has already been described above. Myelography is not helpful, since in both cases it shows nerve root amputation.

When confronted with CBN which cannot be attributed to a disk lesion, one should think of examining the structures outside the intervertebral foramen, particularly the soft tissues anterior to it. There may be nerve root compression by a neighboring process such as a tumor of the pulmonary apex with spread to the cervical plexus (Fig. 35); a spinal nerve may also be subjected to intraforaminal compression by a tumoral metastasis within the epidural space, whether isolated or associated with malignant or benign bone lesions (Fig. 36).

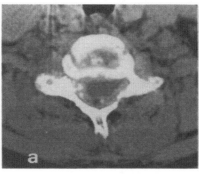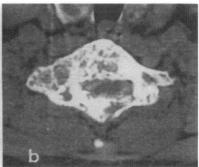

Fig. 36 a, b. Differential diagnosis in right C7 cervicobrachial neuralgia: CT study at C6–C7 (appearance on plain films typical of vertebral angioma). **a** Foramen and disk: filling in of the neural foramen by soft tissue. **b** This high-resolution scan confirms the invasion of the spinal canal by the vertebral angioma, indicating its aggressive nature

Magnetic Resonance Imaging

Magnetic resonance imaging appears very attractive for the examination of the cervical spine. Sagittal sections portray the spinal cord, the anterior and posterior subarachnoid spaces, and the posterior margins of both the disks and the vertebral bodies. Needless to say, a relatively large soft disk herniation can be readily diagnosed on sagittal MRI sections.

Nevertheless, we believe that given the present inadequacies of surface coils, axial sections at the cervical level are insufficient for very clear differentiation between soft diskal material and any associated osteophytes. Furthermore, the image quality on axial sections is still inadequate compared with that of CT after intravenous injection of contrast medium.

The oblique sections which are now available appear attractive for investigating the nerve root within the intervertebral foramen; however, the thickness of the sections (5 mm) probably renders illusory the hope of diagnosing a small free fragment next to the root in the first part of the foramen.

At present, we retain CT as the first radiological exploration in cases of typical CBN.

Cervical Chemonucleolysis

Introduction

Although the indications for lumbar chemonu-cleolysis in young subjects are being extended to take in cases where medical treatment of sciatica due to a disk herniation has failed, this procedure is proposed less often at the cervical level. Admittedly, CBN is less frequent than sciatica, but it is often very incapacitating, causing hyper-algesia and insomnia.

A high proportion of cases of CBN are caused by herniations [310], and analysis of 100 cervical soft disk herniations examined by CT and subjected to surgery over a 4-year period has demonstrated that the herniation usually consists of a free fragment of nucleus pulposus found in a tear of the posterior longitudinal ligament [160, 162].

The recently introduced technique of cervical chemonucleolysis requires close and ready collaboration between neurosurgeon and neuroradiologist and is presently performed only by a limited number of teams. Some use chymopapain [170], whereas others prefer aprotinin (Iniprol) [173] or the intradiskal injection of corticosteroids [303].

Microsurgical diskectomy via an anterior approach, the procedure most widely employed at present, is a relatively minor intervention which permits the exploration of the posterior longitudinal ligament and the ablation of the one or more free fragments found within it [8, 54, 117, 138, 179, 256]. The results are good; in most patients, nerve root pain decreases upon recovery from anesthesia. Postoperative nuchal pain usually disappears in 2–3 weeks. If a bone graft is not performed, postoperative cervical immobilization with a brace is not necessary; nevertheless, a brace may be used to reduce the residual cervical pain of the first few weeks. The hospital stay is short, less than 1 week. Complete resumption of normal activities is usually possible during the 2nd month following the operation; the

exact point varies slightly from patient to patient [268].

To be considered as an alternative to a simple operation with infrequent complications, then, cervical chemonucleolysis had to prove its therapeutic efficacy without significant risks for the patient. The following questions had to be answered:

- Does the method entail certain risks of a technical nature because of the anterior percutaneous approach, passing between on the one side the jugular and carotid vessels and on the other the aerodigestive passages? Might the thyroid gland be pierced during puncture of the lower cervical disks?
- How does the nucleolytic agent injected into the intervertebral disk diffuse? Can the enzyme reach the free fragment, which is a distinctive anatomical feature of soft disk herniations at the cervical level? This fragment is almost always in a transligamentous position.
- Does the possibility of enzyme diffusion into the epidural space present a danger, given the abundant venous plexuses which occupy this space, facing the posterior disk margin, and also the intervertebral foramina?
- Is treatment by chemonucleolysis possible under the same conditions as surgical treatment?

Being aware of these potential difficulties, we have always performed diskography before chemonucleolysis. This examination detects any leakage of contrast medium into the spinal canal or intervertebral foramen and, especially, opacification of the subarachnoid space, which would contraindicate injection of the nucleolytic substance, in our case chymopapain. However, diskography is incapable of accurately evaluating the dispersal of contrast medium outside and around the posterior disk margin, particularly if there is a foraminal free fragment, which we consider important to assess by means of direct opacification.

It was this that led to the idea of combining CT and diskography. For technical reasons, it was impossible to perform this examination before chemonucleolysis. Thus we established the following sequence: diskography, chemonucleolysis, and then CT 30 min after chemonucleolysis in order to verify the diffusion of the injected contrast medium, and therefore the enzyme, to the center of the disk.

Patient Selection

The first factor to be taken into consideration is the clinical picture. Chemonucleolysis is likely to be helpful only in the case of severe CBN resisting medical treatment for at least 2–3 weeks.

An associated partial motor deficit, which is a frequent finding, does not constitute a contraindication to chemonucleolysis [170].

Evidently, it is necessary to be able to attribute the nerve root compression to a soft disk herniation. The investigation of the CBN should obviously involve CT, which permits a complete study of the disk and the intervertebral foramen, as well as clear differentiation between soft disk herniation and possibly associated uncinate process hypertrophy.

Chemonucleolysis is feasible regardless of the anatomical type of herniation found on CT scans: large posterolateral herniation; lateralized, small herniation; distant migratory fragment within the intervertebral foramen.

The principal contraindications to chemonucleolysis are the following:

— pregnancy;
— known allergy to chymopapain or allergic reaction to previous chemonucleolysis;
— known allergic or atopic background [201];
— paralyzing CBN or cord compression of diskal origin in which the radicular pain is of secondary importance;
— chronic cervical pain not linked to a disk herniation;
— demonstration of localized uncinate process hypertrophy at the segment and side corresponding to the clinical symptoms;
— congenital spinal stenosis or a narrow cervical spinal canal;
— excessively severe disk collapse [173].

Techniques: Diskography

Positioning of Patient

Chemonucleolysis is performed in a vascular radiologic unit. The disk to be punctured is localized using televised fluoroscopy; this requires a mobile arc for the rapidly obtaining of frontal and lateral views. The patient must lie strictly supine with the head straight. It is often necessary to pull on the upper limbs in order to lower the shoulders and expose the last two cervical intervertebral spaces, C6–C7 and C7–T1. Asepsis is just as strict as in an operating room. Our patients are treated under narcolocal analgesia induced by Hypnovel, which combines phenoperidine and midazolam. The sedation facilitates patient cooperation, in maintaining the absolute immobility which is essential for disk localization and injection.

Disk Puncture

For frontal localization, it is necessary to tilt the incident beam parallel to the plane of the disk in order to expose it better and to insert the needle correctly in its center. Under ideal conditions, the tip of the needle appears in the middle of the intervertebral space in both projections, frontal and lateral. The disk is punctured using a thin 22-gauge needle whose tip has been bent by 1.5–2 cm in order to reach the nucleus pulposus at the center of the disk.

After palpation and manual displacement of the jugular and carotid vessels, with the sternocleidomastoid muscle laterally and the digestive and respiratory tracts medially, an anterior, laterotracheal approach is used, with the needle directed slightly medially. The intervertebral disk is reached very rapidly, since only a few centimeters separate the spinal column from the surface of the skin. Slight resistance may be felt when the needle penetrates the disk.

Diskography

Diskography entails the intradiskal injection of 0.4–0.6 ml water-soluble contrast medium (iopamidol; Iopamiron 300). The resistance encountered upon injection is usually moderate.

The examination may suddenly evoke the patient's radicular pain, confirming the responsibility of the corresponding disk for the CBN [12, 119, 134, 154, 155].

Frontal, lateral, and (possibly) oblique views frequently show an epidural leakage of contrast medium toward the intervertebral foramina which, however, does not contraindicate enzyme injection. The spinal cord and nerve roots are effectively protected by the dura mater.

Foraminal extravasation of the contrast medium, when it occurs, may be ipsilateral, bilateral, or contralateral (Fig. 37).

On frontal views, the opacified nucleus pulposus frequently exhibits a layered and bilobed appearance. This seems to correspond to the opacification of the lateral fissures of a degenerative nature which are very frequent in cervical disks and constitute the uncovertebral or Luschka's joints [220].

The appearance on lateral views varies. Contrast medium is sometimes visible in the most anterior portion of the spinal canal, possibly corresponding to the opacified herniation. This is difficult to confirm.

Chemonucleolysis

The chymopapain (Chymodiactin) should be injected slowly over 10 min, using a small graduated syringe and increasing by tenths of a ml. All our patients were given a dose of 2000 units Chymodiactin, regardless of the size of the herniation on CT scans. Gradual injection serves to avoid enzyme reflux along the path of the needle as well as excessive extradural or foraminal spread. Actually we reduce the dose: 1500 units in association with decreasing of Muchal pain.

Postdiskography CT

Postdiskography CT is routinely performed approximately 30 min following chemonucleolysis at the level of the segment which was opacified and treated. This examination demonstrates the dispersion of the contrast medium within the disk, and also, in the case of free fragment herniation, in the anterior epidural space, thanks to a tear in the posterior longitudinal ligament containing the fragment. Neurosurgeons have pointed out that of this ligamentous lesion at the cervical level.

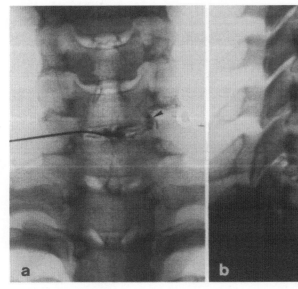

Fig. 37 a, b. Discography. **a** Plain film, frontal projection. Intradiskal contrast enhancement: the frequent lamellar appearance of the nucleus pulposus results from the opacification of the lateral diskal fissures (very frequent, degenerative lesions). Extravasation of contrast medium towards the left foramen (same side as the herniation) *(arrowhead)*. **b** Plain film, sagittal projection. Even, rounded intradiskal enhancement in the midportion of the intervertebral space

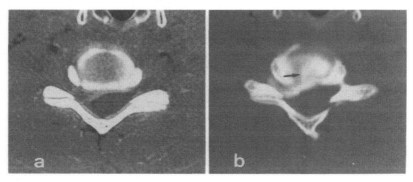

Fig. 38 a, b. A 34-year-old man with right C7 cervicobrachial neuralgia with an 8-week-old motor deficit: no response to medical treatment. **a** CT: right posterolateral C6–C7 herniation with a hypodensity. **b** Postdiskography CT after nucle-olysis: median leakage; perforation of the anulus fibrosus (—▶) and passage of the contrast medium around the free fragment as well as farther into the foramen (tear of the posterior longitudinal ligament)

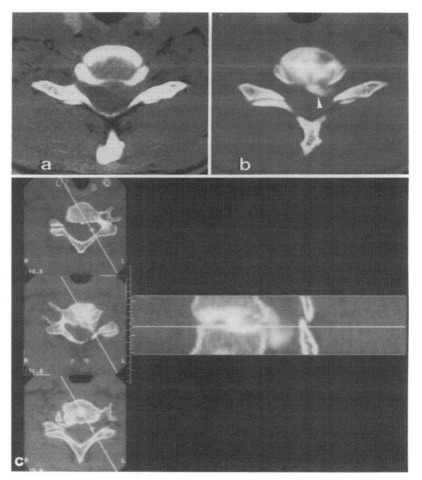

Fig. 39 a–c. A 26-year-old woman with recurrent torticollis. Right C7 cervicobrachial neuralgia had been causing insomnia for 6 weeks, necessitating the use of opiates. C7 motor deficit associated with hypoesthesia. **a** CT: classic left posterolateral herniation. **b** Postdiskography CT after chemonucle-olysis: median channel through the anulus fibrosus and com-plete opacification of the free fragment *(white arrowhead)*. *Comment:* Clinical remission in 12 h. **c** Sagittal oblique reconstructed section, perpendicular to the foramen. The herniation height is directly identified at the foramen entrance. The contrast opacification shows the sagittal shape of the fragment within the canal

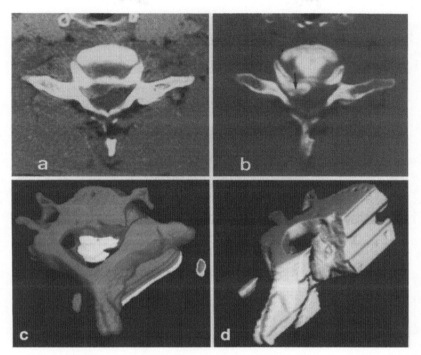

Fig. 40 a–d. A 38-year-old man with right C7 cervicobrachial neuralgia which had been resisting medical treatment for 5 months (epidural injections). **a** CT: posterolateral herniation with a transligamentous free fragment. **b** Postdiskography CT after chemonucleolysis: median channel through the anulus fibrosus; free fragment still visible in the anterior epidural space (—►). **c,d** 3 D Reconstruction: The volume of the herniation is better evaluated. These views are very attractive, but of poor diagnostic value

Cephalad to the disk, laterally located contrast medium may be observed within the foramen. This is indicative of a rupture of the posterior longitudinal ligament permitting the extradural passage of contrast medium and its spread at a distance from the disk.

On the diskal plane, one may observe a well-defined linear image of posteriorly directed leakage of the contrast medium to the herniated fragment. This is usually found in common posterolateral herniations. Median or paramedian sagittal leakage of contrast medium shows the free fragment's migration channel through the ruptured anulus fibrosus. The fragment itself is opacified only subsequently, in a lateral location (Fig. 38).

When there is a large herniation, the contrast medium outlines the herniated fragment on the CT scans. In this particular situation, the central hypodensity observed on the initial CT scans is still visible after diskography, and corresponds very accurately to the free nuclear fragment.

Sometimes this hypodensity fades away, due to the direct opacification of the hydrophilic free fragment, which seems to become saturated with contrast medium. The herniated fragment then becomes entirely opaque (Fig. 39).

Very large fragments appear to be more easily outlined by the contrast medium than directly opacified, in contrast to small herniations. Nevertheless, they come widely into contact with the Chymodiactin (Fig. 40).

Very lateral herniations are completely opacified, as if saturated by the contrast medium, as are migratory fragments farther away in the intervertebral foramen (Fig. 41).

Postdiskography CT scans almost always show the median or paramedian site of the anulus fibrosus rupture in cases in which a posterolateral herniation has secondarily lodged in the anterolateral angle of the spinal canal, in contact with the nerve root. The associated rupture of the posterior longitudinal ligament is probably located opposite the path of the fragment through the

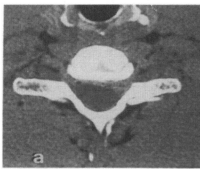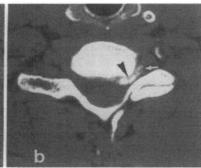

Fig. 41 a, b. A 44-year-old man with hyperalgesic left C7 cervicobrachial neuralgia which had been resisting medical treatment for 3 weeks. Clear EMG signs of denervation, evident reduction of the muscle strength of the hand. **a** CT: small, left C6–C7 herniation without hypodensity. **b** Postdiskography CT after chemonucleolysis: total and immediate opacification of the small free fragment, which was situated very far laterally *(arrowhead);* leakage of the contrast medium into the foramen and the length of the left C7 radicular sheath (→)

anulus fibrosus. This tendency of the free fragment to migrate laterally into the fibers of the posterior longitudinal ligament has already been observed by neurosurgeons, who use an operating microscope to locate the median breach of the ligamentous plane and the more remote and more lateral herniated fragment.

Results after Chemonucleolysis

Clinical Findings

In the course of clinical observation immediately after chemonucleolysis, one must be particularly alert to any signs of side effects. We have never observed any allergic reactions. The hospital stay is short, averaging 3–4 days, and the patient may resume work 4 to 6 weeks after the chemonucleolysis.

Pain. The regression of radicular pain after the intradiskal injection of chymopapain is both constant and rapid. The pain recedes within a few hours after the chemonucleolysis, at any rate within 24 h. sometimes residual nuchal pain or interscapular pain is observed during the first 15 days after the therapeutic procedure.

Paresthesia. These gradually regress within 2–8 weeks after the procedure. In certain patients they disappear rapidly, within 24 h after the intradiskal injection of the enzyme.

Motor deficit. Segmental muscle strength is usually found to be normal on clinical examination at 6 weeks, and normalization may occur earlier.

CT Appearance

All patients undergo follow-up CT between 2 and 4 months after chemonucleolysis. There is an almost constant reduction in the height of the treated disk. Residual posteromedian bulging of the disk and vacuum disk phenomenon are each observed in one fifth of cases. This examination especially shows the rapid regression of the venous stasis and the subjacent disk herniation, whether the fragment is posterolateral or lateral (Figs. 42, 43). This is quite the opposite of what is observed at the lumbar level, where follow-up CT 6 months after chemonucleolysis often still shows a herniation despite the fact that the patient is clinically considered to be cured.

In Conclusion

Although less frequent than lumbosacral sciatica, CBN in young subjects is often much more painful. Such acute nerve root involvement at a specific level is in most cases of diskal origin. After the acknowledged success of lumbar chemonucleolysis, the prospect of being able to treat these patients effectively by means of the intradiskal injection of, for instance, chymopapain was sufficiently attractive to neurosurgeons and neuroradiologists for this technique to be extended to the cervical level.

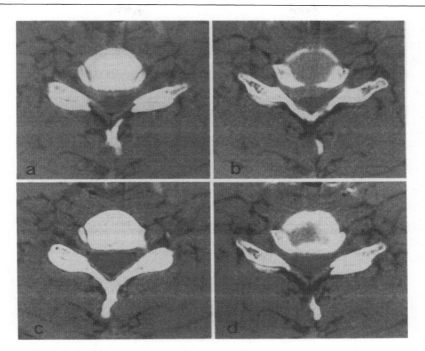

Fig. 42 a–d. Right C6 cervicobrachial neuralgia in a 34-year-old woman; existence of hyperalgia and a partial motor deficit. **a, b** CT: right posterolateral C5–C6 herniation, moderate compression of the spinal cord opposite the herniation. **c,** **d** Follow-up CT 10 weeks after chemonucleolysis: clinical remission, good regression of the discal herniation and of the foraminal venous stasis

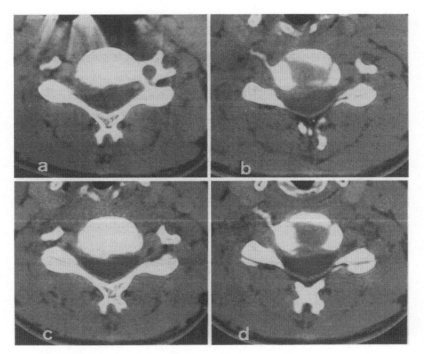

Fig. 43 a–d. A 34-year-old man with shoulder pain and hypoesthesia (C5–C6 cervicobrachial neuralgia?). **a, b** CT: right posterolateral C6–C7 herniation. Discordance between CT appearance and clinical findings. **c, d** Follow-up CT 8 weeks after C6–C7 chemonucleolysis: complete regression of the herniation and the overlying venous stasis

The effect of cervical chemonucleolysis on the radicular pain may be considered to be very satisfactory; the pain disappeared within 72 h after the therapeutic procedure in the vast majority of 130 patients treated. During the years 1987 to 1990, we observed not any significant treatment failures or recurrences of CBN in the same or an adjacent territory (9 clinical failures including 5 interventions). Patients whose CT examinations showed uncinate process hypertrophy associated with the soft disk herniation and narrowing the intervertebral foramen also responded very well to chemonucleolysis. This confirms the commonplace nature of foraminal uncinate process hypertrophy, which is associated with symptoms only when an associated soft disk herniation is present.

Conclusion

The accepted indication for cervical chemonucleolysis is the typical picture of hyperalgesic CBN. The CT investigation always shows a soft disk herniation. A single administration of 2000 to 1500 units Chymodiactin has a therapeutic effect which is both constant and rapid, sometimes even immediate. This is in contrast with chemonucleolysis at the lumbar level, where, despite strict selection of patients, there persists a failure rate of 15%–20% [17, 46, 101, 291]. The cervical disk is smaller than the lumbar disk. Morphologically cervical herniations are stereotyped: they always involve a small nuclear fragment, in a lateral position within the cervical spinal canal but usually remaining in contact with the disk. Completely extruded fragments at some distance in the intervertebral foramen are seldom found.

Rapid regression of the disk herniation following cervical chemonucleolysis is consistently observed on CT 2–4 months after the procedure, in contrast to what is observed at the lumbar level [101, 250].

Finally, CT after cervical diskography confirms all the CT findings after a simple intravenous injection of contrast medium:

— The predominance of common posterolateral disk herniations, whose central hypodensity corresponds to the free fragment. The latter may be distinct, or may be completely saturated with the contrast medium (i. e., hydrophilic).
— The lower incidence of very lateral soft disk herniations, which are always opacified.
— A small, isolated migratory fragment in the intervertebral foramen, at some distance from the disk.

Postdiskography CT especially permits direct visualization of the track of the herniated nuclear fragment through the ruptured anulus fibrosus. This channel has a median or paramedian location when the posterolateral herniation is relatively large. In small lateral herniations, contrast medium leakage occurs at the posterolateral portion of the disk, close to the uncinate process, where the contrast medium is then usually found. Finally, among the indirect signs of ligamentous rupture, which may be clearly demonstrated, is the presence of contrast medium in the anterior epidural space or the foramen.

We have emphasized the high success rates of cervical disk surgery and the value of microdiskectomy via an anterior approach. In order to become more widespread, cervical chemonucleolysis needs to achieve results close to those of surgery. This new technique already yields a success rate which may be considered comparable, while sparing patients the rigors of a surgical procedure under general anesthesia. The hospital stay is shortened to 2 or 3 days in almost all cases. The nuchal pain observed in the wake of chemonucleolysis constitutes a minor inconvenience which can be resolved by temporarily wearing a Chantz neck brace. On average, patients can resume work after a 1-month rest period. Cervical chemonucleolysis thus appears likely to replace or redefine the role of disk surgery at the cervical level in cases of typical CBN. There is long-term conservation of the intervertebral space.

Finally, cervical chemonucleolysis significantly accelerates the natural evolution of free fragments, which usually dissolve spontaneously only after 8–10 months.

Thoracic Disk Herniations

Introduction

Thoracic disk herniations are rare conditions occurring in middle age and equally affecting both sexes. They usually involve only one spinal segment.

They are known for a slow progressive clinical onset and a poor operative prognosis, which accounts for the relative infrequency of surgical indications [173, 174]. Nevertheless, these concepts should be examined in the light of recent advances in imaging (i. e., CT and MRI) and of new operating techniques.

Clinical Findings

Classically, posterior thoracic disk herniations have a progressive evolution. The initial clinical signs are polymorphous and depend upon the site of the lesions; they may include isolated or more-or-less associated signs of spinal, nerve root or cord involvement. This results in varied clinical pictures, which may sometimes be misleading. Radiological examinations are the only means to confirm the diagnosis.

Central thoracic disk herniations result in spinal cord involvement, with the latter being compressed between the herniation anteriorly and the laminae and dentate ligament posteriorly.

Lateral thoracic disk herniations, in theory, spare the spinal cord and compress the nerve roots directly, giving rise to radicular pain which remains isolated for a long time.

Centrolateral thoracic disk herniations result in combined cord and nerve root involvement.

In fact, the signs also depend upon the extent of the herniation and the anteroposterior diameter of the bony spinal canal. Thus, thoracic disk herniations may manifest themselves by:

- *Spinal signs,* such as focalized or diffuse back pain, either permanent or punctuated by activity.
- *Radicular signs* involving unilateral pain. The sites affected depends on the herniation site:
  - T1: internal margin of the forearm to the little finger; there may be an associated Claude Bernard-Horner syndrome.
  - T2: pain involving the axilla and the internal aspect of the arm.
  - T3-T8: segmental thoracic pain.
  - T9-T11: pain with a lumboabdomino-inguinal radiation.
  - The pain may radiate towards the areas of the lumbar roots or even the first sacral roots, when the compression involves the superior portion of the conus medullaris.
- Infrequently, *spinal cord pain* may suddenly become apparent in the wake of an extreme effort, and result in a decompensation in the form of flaccid-spasmodic paraparesis. It is sometimes possible to deduce a disk herniation from a compression of Adamkiewicz's artery. Lazorthes has shown that this artery usually originates on the left side of the body (i. e., 85%) and between T9 and T12 (75%) [169-171]. Spinal cord arteriography may confirm compression of the anterior spinal artery. *Vascular compression* is a dreaded complication of thoracic disk herniations; it is unpredictable and may result in major and definite neurological signs with a clinical picture of spinal cord section. Even if there is subsequent improvement, ischemic recurrence is always possible. If there is a lack of concordance between the volume of the her-

niation and the neurological disorders, one should consider a dual compression (i. e., mechanical and vascular). Surgery may be indicated [39, 173, 174].

In all, the combination of various symptoms may give rise to varied and misleading clinical pictures:

— "Arthritic back pain" or intercostal neuralgia, and even pleurodynia, coronary artery disease, and a renal or large bowel affliction may be imitated.
— The combination of a nerve root syndrome and signs of subjacent spinal cord involvement evoke spinal cord compression. Nevertheless, errors in level determination are frequent: a high thoracic disk herniation may lead to a misdiagnosis of cervical spinal cord compression, whereas a low thoracic herniation may result in a cauda equina syndrome.
— A thoracic disk herniation may develop without signs of spinal involvement and appear as a pseudomyelitic spinal cord syndrome evocative of multiple sclerosis, a posterior cord syndrome, or a Brown-Séquard syndrome.

Magnetic resonance imaging is also a very effective means for evaluating the position of the herniation relative to the spinal cord, which does not necessitate the intrathecal injection of contrast medium. The absence of artifacts from the shoulders or of restrictions secondary to CSF blockage favor its use. On a sagittal MR image, the concerned level shows evident signs of disk degeneration (i. e., a disk with a low signal intensity on T2-weighted images). The amputation of the subarachnoid space can be implied from late echoes of T2-weighted sequences. Perilesional scar tissue may be visible above and below the herniation as retrovertebral soft tissue with a high signal intensity, comparable to that of fat. Axial sections are essential for detemining if the herniation is lateralized. Nevertheless, lateralization is best evaluated on axial CT scans, which have better resolution. Thus, it is essential that the MRI employ surface coils and thin slice thickness. Nevertheless, only CT is regularly capable of properly imaging disk calcifications [55, 68–74].

Spinal cord arteriography is no longer performed; it is not devoid of risk and is presently of limited interest, given the advances in surgery making possible microscope-aided examination of spinal cord arteries.

Surgery

Exposure of a thoracic disk herniation is facilitated by the use of a posterolateral approach and transverso-arthropediculectomy. A simple laminectomy should be discouraged, since it gives rise to postoperative complications in one out of two cases. An anterior approach is onerous; this is especially true in low herniations, which call for a thoracophrenolaparotomy [39]. An intermediate approach, using transverso-arthropediculectomy, reaches the disk space tangentially. The vascular and neural structures are identified thanks to a preliminary enlargement of the intervertebral foramen. The intercostal neurovascular bundle and the arteries supplying the cord and nerve roots are dissected with the aid of a microscope. Osteotomy of the next two cephalad and next two caudad vertebral bodies prevents movement of the thecal sac and nerve roots, but requires a short-term posterolateral osteosynthesis using Harrington's rods [173, 174].

CT Scans and MRI (Figs. 44–47)

If the possibility of a thoracic disk herniation has been considered, *plain radiographs* may sometimes reveal a disk calcification of great diagnostic value. The rare form found in infants bears mentioning. It is a rare condition, in which trauma of a debilitated disk may be implicated. The calcification would then be indicative of a vascular disk disorder of infectious or mechanical origin. This complication occurs in children between 7 and 13 years of age, at a time when idiopathic disk calcifications take place. The most frequent sites are the lower cervical spine and, to a lesser extent, the upper thoracic spine. Studies of disk calcifications in children have shown that the cervical locations are the most symptomatic. There may also be multiple sites (i. e., cervical and dorsal).

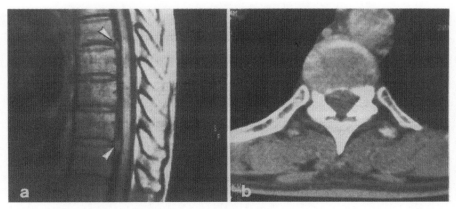

Fig. 44 a, b. A 65-year-old woman with monoparesis of sudden onset involving the right lower extremity. Exaggerated reflexes on neurologic examination. No intercostal radicularlgia. **a** MRI examination (T1-weighted sequence; TR 500 ms, TE 16 ms, 4 excitations). Median and paramedian sagittal sections show a T7-T8 herniation associated with a second T10-T11 herniation *(white arrowhead)*. **b** CT scans at T10-T11; common type of posteromedian herniation. *Comment:* Dorsal herniations are more frequent in the lower dorsal segments; they usually give rise to signs of cord compression

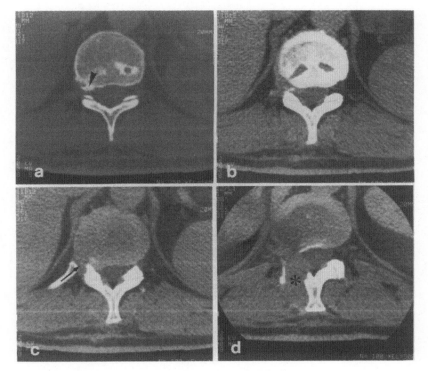

Fig. 45 a-d. A 46-year-old man suddenly experienced right paravertebral pain at T9-T10 associated with paresthesiae and a right paravertebral burning sensation irradiating towards the axillary line (T8-T12). It was resistant to medical treatment for 2 months. Neurological examination did not reveal a cord syndrome. **a-c** CT scans of the lower dorsal segments, particularly T11-T12. **a, b** Presence of a single calcification in contact with the external margin of the cartilage and located in the midportion of the T11-T12 intervertebral foramen *(arrowhead)*. **c** This calcification is associated with a subjacent lateral herniation outside the spinal canal (→). **d** Postoperative CT scan. A lateral surgical approach is more demanding at the lumbar level. Both a laminectomy and arthrectomy are required to adequate exposure of the intervertebral foramen. Scar tissue lining the surgical approach (✱). *Comment:* Since the very lateral approaches imply more extensive surgery than simple fenestration, they are not frequently employed at the lumbar level

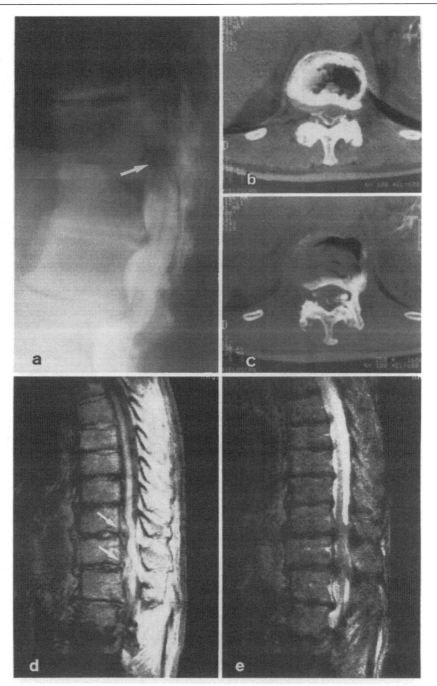

Fig. 46 a–e. A 76-year-old patient with spastic paraparesia of 3 months duration. Spastic signs at clinical examination. **a** Myelography shows a narrow lumbar canal, with a "stop" at the level of the medullary cone (—►) (T12–L1). **b, c** CT myelogram: T12–L1 level: secondary narrowing of spinal canal, associated with significant osteophytes within the canal. **d** MRI at lower thoracic level (T1-weighted sequence: TR 500, TE 16 ms) the cord is correctly identified and severely compressed by a double disko-osteophytic lesion at T11–T12 and T12–L1 (—►). **e** Similar T2-weighted sequence (TR 1800, TE 40, 4 echos): anterior and posterior subarachnoid spaces are obliterated. *Comment:* Axial CT myelography is superior to MRI in demonstrating severe diskoosteophytic lesions associated with a narrow lumbar canal. On the other hand, the MRI findings alone indicate a combined neurosurgical intervention at the lower thoracic cord

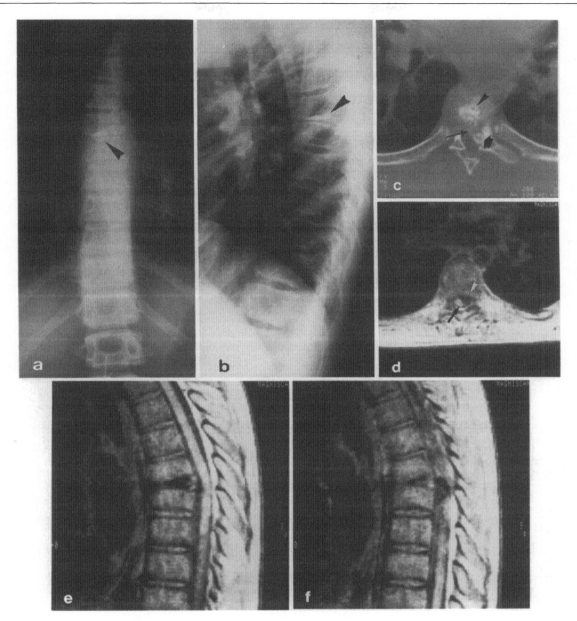

Fig. 47 a–f. (By courtesy of Dr. Christmann) A 15-year-old boy with interscapular pain of several weeks duration, associated with left intercostal radiculalgia (T6–T7 distribution). Neurological examination revealed bilateral spasticity predominating on the left, Babinski's reflex and hypoesthesia of left T7 distribution. **a, b** Routine plain films (frontal and lateral projections) of the thoracic spine. Significant calcification of the cartilaginous plates at T6–T7 *(arrowhead).* **c** CT scan. Significant calcification of the T6–T7 intervertebral disk *(arrowhead)* with diskal substance migration into the spinal canal (➡), and accumulation lateral to the spinal cord. Note the track linking the two calcified structures (→). **d** MRI.

T1-weighted axial section (TR 450 ms, TE 14 ms, 4 excitations). Narrowing of the left intervertebral foramen accounts for the intercostal radiculalgia *(white arrowhead).* Displacement of spinal cord on the right side (→). **e, f** MRI. T1-weighted median and paramedian sagittal sections (TR 450 ms, TE 14 ms, 4 excitations). Hyposignal due to the calcifications is clearly seen between the cartilaginous plates. Adjacent section: hyposignal due to the larger calcification within the spinal canal. *Comment:* The exact mechanism of disk calcification and associated herniation in young patients is poorly understood. They may be due to a disturbed microvascularization

All authors agree upon the global differences between cervical and thoracic disk herniations, with the former being symptomatic but eventually disappearing, and the latter often being asymptomatic, discovered on chest X-rays, and remaining visible much longer.

One should also keep in mind that vertebral deformities are almost always found in association with calcifications. These include the posterior cuneiformation of thoracic vertebrae, and the anteroposterior flattening and elongation of cervical vertebrae. The observed differences in the evolution of symptomatic cervical sites and rather asymptomatic thoracic ones may be related to differences in segmental vertebral mobility between the cervical and thoracic levels. In any case, the evolution is often towards a spontaneous regression and disappearance of the calcifications, just as with uncomplicated idiopathic disk calcifications [213].

Myelography combined with tomography enables one to detect a lateralized disk protrusion which may have gone unnoticed or been minimized on routine myelography. However, at present only *CT scans* are capable of determining the volume, density, and exact location of the herniations; furthermore, they are essential for deciding upon the side for a surgical approach when the herniation is lateralized. Performing such CT scans may be a delicate task because of the physiological curvature of the thoracic spine (i. e., whence the value of lateral scout views). Combining these scans with myelography (i. e., *CT myeloscans*) permits a precise evaluation of the hernia's position with respect to the spinal cord and the thoracic nerve roots.

Lumbar Disk Herniations

Clinical Findings

A lumbosacral disk herniation may give rise to a rich variety of symptoms: acute lumbar pain, radicular pain of a crural (L 3 or L 4 nerve roots) or sciatic [L 5 or S 1 (S 2)] nature. Ordinary sciatica is a monoradicular pain of vertebral origin due to nerve root compression of diskal origin at the L 4–L 5 or L 5–S 1 level and involving a mechanical or degenerative process.

The most frequent cause of sciatica is a soft disk herniation, in which the nucleus pulposus is extruded through the peripheral anulus fibrosus. Slowly evolving degenerative lesions affect the vertebrae and lateral recesses, and hypertrophic changes predominate. In such a predisposed subject, global disk protrusion or disk bulging is more frequently responsible than true herniation. The clinical examination, the patient's age, and the type of sciatica (i. e., monoradicular, incomplete, atypical) are of great importance: the examination of a young subject with monoradicular sciatica is very different to that of a 70-year-old patient with multilevel hypertrophic changes of the lumbar spine.

The compression preferentially affects the sensory nerve root. Clinical examination is still essential in the diagnosis of sciatica, since it is often very informative. Recognition of both the diagnosis and (very often) the causative factor depend upon the thoroughness with which it is carried out. On the basis of the clinical findings, a radiodiagnostician should be able to predict the location of the herniation and thus select appropriate imaging procedures and define the indications for a neuroradiologic work-up.

Medical History

The patient's past medical history [43, 152, 272] should be scrutinized for episodes of acute and recurrent *lumbago,* chronic lumbar pain, or sciatica. Lumbar pain reflects nerve root involvement of diskal or vertebral origin; it is closely linked to the symptoms and evolution of the sciatica. The *initial episode* is often one of acute lumbar pain (straining of posterior longitudinal ligament?), with the sciatica only appearing a few days later. A *provoking factor* is often found (lifting a heavy load, sudden movement).

The pain is monoradicular and of a constant *mechanical type:* it is more severe on standing or walking, and generally less intense in the supine position. In one of five cases, though, pain is worse in the supine position. The pain is diurnal.

Triggering and aggravation of the lumbar pain and/or sciatica by *coughing and defecation* suggests disk herniation.

The patient interview seeks to establish the pain distribution (Fig. 48). Monoradicular pain has a vertebral origin and is referred to the lower

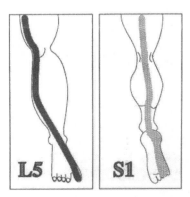

Fig. 48. Clinical signs 1. L5 and S1 sciatic irradiations

extremity along a specific path. The topography differs according to whether the sciatica is due to irritation of the fifth lumbar nerve root (L 5 sciatica) or the first sacral root (S 1 sciatica):

- *L 5 root involvement* results in pain originating in the lumbar region and referred to the buttocks, the posterior aspect of the thigh down to the popliteal fossa, the anterolateral aspect of the leg, the lateral malleolus or the region just anterior to it, the dorsum of the foot, and the first toe.
- *S 1 root involvement* results in pain having the same distribution as far as the popliteal fossa; it is then referred to the posterior aspect of the leg, the zone posterior to the lateral malleolus, and the lateral margin of the sole of the foot as far as the fifth toe.

Knowledge of the pain distribution at the level of the foot is essential for identifying the nerve root involved. The actual pain often ends at the ankle, giving way in the foot to paresthesiae of a pins-and-needles or burning nature with the same diagnostic orientational value, in all cases, one should ascertain how the pain has evolved and whether there are any sphincter or genital disturbances which might have a direct bearing on the therapeutic approach.

Physical Examination [43, 140, 152, 272]

In the case of unilateral lumbosciatic nerve root pain (nerve root irritation syndrome) of diskal origin (i. e., disk herniation in the axilla of the L 5 or S 1 root), the clinical examination first explores the state of the vertebrae, and then searches for objective signs of nerve root involvement:

On such sign, in the *standing* patient, is a pain-avoidance posture, either naturally occurring or elicited by the anterior flexion of the trunk. Such a position is more characteristic of L 4–L 5 herniation (two thirds of cases) than for L 5–S 1 herniation (half the cases): The pain is often crossed for the L 5 root and direct for the S 1 root. When it is limited to the vertebral segment affected by the disk herniation, the spinal movements, lose their rhythm and become discontinuous.

In *ventral decubitus,* examination of the lumbar and lumbosacral regions may reveal [140]:

- painful cellular infiltration opposite the intervertebal segment involved;
- contracture of the paraspinal muscles;
- tenderness elicited by palpation of the spinous processes, the interspinous ligament, and the posterior articular processes.

Radicular pain and its characteristic referral may be elicited by [140]:

- paraspinal pressure (doorbell sign);
- pressure on the peripheral nerves (femoral or sciatic) at particular sites (Valleix's points);
- stretching of the root in the supine position by means of the classic Lasègue's maneuver (passive raising of the limb with the extended knee). This maneuver seldom fails to elicit the radicular pain and its L 5 or S 1 radiation and should be performed on both sides, the healthy side first. A positive Lasègue's sign confirms the diagnosis of sciatica, quantifies the severity of the nerve root involvement, and helps monitor its evolution. There may be an associated contralateral Lasègue's sign, often less intense but of great value. One should differentiate Lasègue's sign in sciatica from the lumbar Lasègue's sign eliciting of spinal column pain in cases of banal pain, without discal origin.

A systematic neurological examination of the lower extremity is then carried out:

- *Muscle hypotonia* (with no accompanying motor deficit) may indicate clearly which spinal level is involved. In the case of L 5 involvement, the muscles of the anterolateral aspect of the leg are affected, with S 1 involvement, the muscles of the calf and the gluteus maximus muscle.
- Impairment of the *deep tendon reflexes* should be systematically sought. Essentially, the Achilles reflex and plantar reflex are impaired in the case of S 1 involvement, and, less frequently, the flexion reflex of the leg is impaired with L 5 involvement.

— *Sensory disturbances* such as localized dysesthesias or paresthesiae are limited to the affected dermatome. The most frequent disturbance is cutaneous hyperesthesia, the topography of which varies according to the nerve root involved:

L 5: dorsum of foot and medial margin of forefoot

S 1: lateral margin of foot.

In common lumbosciatic pain occurring as a single acute episode in subjects between 30 and 50 years of age (1.5 males for every female), which is favored by trauma of the lumbosacral spine, the neurological signs of root involvement are minimal and regressive. In most common or "medical" sciaticas, rest and treatment bring about healing in a few weeks. Residual lumbar pain is sometimes found.

Atypical Sciatica [43, 70, 140, 152, 272]

Hyperalgesic Sciatica

The clinical picture in hyperalgesic sciatica is identical to that in typical sciatica, but the pain is excruciating and leads to complete insomnia. The patient remains motionless (in a pain-avoidance posture) and cannot stand or walk, making clinical examination difficult. Three to six days of corticosteroid therapy may obtain clear-cut improvement (of the nerve root edema), but sometimes no benefit is obtained (large disk herniation), and the hyperalgesia may sometimes necessitate surgery.

Recurrent Alternating Sciatica

Recurrent alternating sciatica features chronic lumbar pain accompanied by episodes of radicular (especially lumbosciatic) pain at variable intervals. The repeated occurrence of radicular pain (especially lumbosciatic pain with the same topography each time) should prompt one to search for a disk herniation. The same holds true for radicular (especially lumbosciatic) pain which alternates between the left and right sides or tends to become bilateral [140]. In such cases the possibility of a median L 4–L 5 disk herniation should be considered.

Cauda Equina Syndrome

Cauda equina syndrome or hemisyndrome refers to bilateral or unilateral involvement of the sacral (S 1–S 5) or lumbosacral (L 2–S 5) nerve roots, distal to the lower end of the spinal cord. The cause of compression varies; in some cases a large lumbar disk herniation which is median or free (not posterolateral, as in ordinary sciatica) may compress the cauda equina, resulting in pluriradicular and bilateral sciatic pain with loss of bladder and rectal sphincter control as well as loss of sensation in the saddle (sella) area. In certain cases, the symptoms may be strictly unilateral (cauda equina hemisyndrome).

Cauda equina syndrome may manifest itself acutely or progressively [141]. In the case of *sudden onset* (often due to acute compression by a free disk herniation) an initial short-lived episode features:

— sudden weakness of the lower extremities
— parasthesias of the lower extremities and perineum
— retention of urine (due to bladder atony) and constipation (due to rectal atony)
— sexual impotence

This episode is followed by severe lumbocrural, lumbosciatic, and perineal pain. The diagnosis is confirmed by the existence of (a) a sensorimotor peripheral paralysis, which may be unilateral or bilateral and is usually incomplete, in the distribution of the sacral or lumbosacral roots, and (b) parasympathetic fiber involvement, with decreased bladder, rectal, and sexual motoricity and sensitivity. The arguments in favor of a disk herniation being responsible are the suddenness of onset, following a lifting movement or straightening or torsion of the trunk, and the lack of any other detectable cause. Emergency ablation of the disk herniation responsible is justified; the results are excellent if this is done sufficiently early. If the ablation is performed too late, genital and sphincter disorders may persist.

In cauda equina syndrome of *progressive onset,* the multiradicular deficit manifests as alternating sciaticas for a certain period, and there is overflow urinary incontinence. The clinical picture mainly involves the L 5 roots, regardless of whether the disk herniation, generally large, originates at L3-L4, L4-L5, or L5-S1. It should be noted that L3-L4 disk herniations usually result in multiradicular involvement, especially since the lumbar spinal canal is narrower at this level [9].

Sciatica with a Motor Deficit

Sciatica with a motor deficit is indicative of a lesional radicular syndrome, and is often found if one systematically searches for a motor deficit by routine precise testing of muscle strength. There are two basic modes of onset [140].

In the *acute mono- or biradicular unilateral form,* an initial episode of particularly violent radicular pain of short duration (a few hours or days) is followed by a partial, more or less marked, sensorimotor deficit of the lower extremity, which coincides with the disappearance of the spontaneous radicular pain and may even go unnoticed by the patient. The sciatica is usually of the L5 type with a motor deficit of the anterolateral muscles of the leg (along with a steppage gait), the internal hamstring muscles, and the thigh adductors. One sometimes observes a decreased tibial adductor reflex. There are often associated sensory symptoms, consisting of hypoesthesia of the dorsum of the foot, the internal

margin of the forefoot, and the first toe. The sciatica may exceptionally be of the S1 type, with a motor deficit of the posterior leg muscles and the inability to stand tiptoe. In a high proportion of these cases the Achilles tendon and medioplantar reflexes are abolished and there is hypoesthesia of the lateral border of the foot (Table 2). In practice, the involvement is likely to be biradicular, with L5 and S1 signs (i. e., an L5-S1 herniation which has migrated into the intervertebral foramen of the L5 root) [9, 152]. Associated S1 and S2 involvement may also be encountered and results in a significant and extensive deficit affecting the calf and plantar muscles, the lateral hamstring muscles (biceps muscle of thigh) and the thigh extensors (gluteus maximus muscle).

Spinal nerve signs are minimal, and may be associated with trophic disturbance, cyanosis, and decreased skin temperature, as well as edema of the foot and sometimes the calf. Wasting may be observed even at an early stage.

Electrical examinations furnish diagnostic and prognostic information in forms of sciatica with a motor deficit, even though they are less commonly performed that at the cervical level [140]. On *stimulation electrodiagnosis* performed during the 3rd week, the affected muscles are hypoexcitable to a faradic current and slow down

Table 2. Myotomes and dermatomes of the lumbar and sacral roots

Level of lesion	Topography of the motor deficit (myotome)	Decrease or abolition of reflexes	Topography of the sensory deficit (dermatome)
(L1)	– Hip flexors	– Patellar reflex	– Anterior aspect of thigh
L2	– Quadriceps		
L3	– Adductors	– Adductor reflex	
L4	– Quadriceps – Tibialis anterior	– Patellar reflex	– Anteromedial aspect of leg
L5	– Anterolateral musles of the leg (the tibialis anterior to a lesser degree) – Medial hamstring muscles – Gluteus medius muscle	– Tibio-adductor reflex	– Anterolateral aspect of the leg, dorsum of foot and first toe
S1	– Plantar muscles	– Medioplantar and plantar reflexes	– S1: lateral border of foot, sole of foot and posterior aspect of leg
S2	– Calf muscles – Lateral hamstring muscles – Stookey reflex – Gluteus maximus muscle	– Achilles tendon reflex	– S2: posterior aspect of thigh
S3 to S5	– Anal and urethral striated muscle sphincters	– Anal reflex – Bulbocavernous reflex	– Anal and perineal region (hypoesthesia or anesthesia in the saddle area)

somewhat in respond rather slowly to galvanic stimulation. Upon *electromyography* (EMG) one first observes, in the affected muscles, either desynchronization of muscle activity, with alternating polyphasic groups and irregular, jagged, interfering oscillations, or clear-cut denervation, with decreased muscle activity and the predominance of high frequency potentials (about 25 cycles/s). If the EMG is performed during the 3rd week, it may also reveal spontaneous denervation activity in the paralyzed muscles. There is frequently a discordance between the severity of the motor deficit and the minimal EMG signs of denervation; this is a positive prognostic factor.

These acute, paralytic forms of sciatica are very probably due to sudden compression of the nerve root by the disk herniation, resulting in a more or less rapidly reversible blockage of conduction. The prognosis following ablation of the disk herniation is usually favorable, with complete sensorimotor recovery in a few months. Some authors also invoke a mechanism of lesional ischemia of the root due to damage of the radicular artery by the disk herniation.

Paralytic sciatica, which is infrequent, involves complete or nearly complete paralysis of the leg and foot. Most surgeons consider it to be grounds for emergency surgery within a few hours after its onset [9].

The very rare *mono- or biradicular type of sciatica with a secondary deficit* [140] is most often found in the wake of recurrent lumbosciatic pain. After a final episode of radiculalgia of mild to moderate intensity, there is a significant sensorimotor deficit together with atrophy of the paralyzed muscles; for certain muscles, the motor deficit is almost complete.

Upon *stimulation electrodiagnosis,* the muscles are hypoexcitable; there may be a global slowing down in response to a galvanic current. *Electromyography* may show complete muscle atrophy, with only minimal, spontaneous, denervation activity detectable in the muscle. If the atrophy is incomplete, the minimal residual muscle activity consists of high-amplitude, irregularly shaped potentials which pulse at a high frequency.

In these progressively paralyzing types of sciatica, the clinical and EMG findings are indicative of chronic compression of one or more roots by the disk herniation, provoking successive denervation episodes. At the stage of significant muscle atrophy, the motor recovery possible is at best minor, even after surgical ablation of the herniation.

Sciatica with Lumbar Spinal Stenosis

Lumbar spinal stenosis [9, 70, 114] comprises varied anatomical and nosological types. Constitutional and acquired forms of stenosis exist, often in association; a moderate constitutional stenosis becomes pathogenic when hypertrophic bone lesions narrow the spinal canal still further. One should be wary when confronted with a disk lesion in a narrow lumbar canal; even a moderate disk lesion which would be well tolerated in a normal spinal canal has marked clinical repercussions in the presence of stenosis.

Clinically, one can be guided by other signs:

— The early stage is dominated by common painful symptoms such as lumbar pain and bilateral or alternating sciatica of a few years' duration. There are few objective signs at this time (i. e., segmental lumbar stiffness, uni- or bilateral Lasègue's signs, and signs of neurologic deficit are absent).
— Later, the most frequent (94%) and most suggestive sign is intermittent neurogenic claudication arising from the cauda equina. In 6% of cases the pain is purely radicular in origin [9]. The pain occurs in the territory of L 5 or S 1 and appears on walking a few tens or hundreds of meters. It disappears remarkably quickly at rest, but recurs with the resumption of walking. It must be distinguished from arterial claudication (cramps in the calf region in the presence of occlusive arterial disease of the lower limbs).

Sciatica with lumbar spinal stenosis may express itself as numbness (63%) or a sensation of muscular weakness (43%); these symptoms are often associated. The sciatica is bilateral in 69% of cases, though often clearly asymmetrical. The pain may involve the entire lower extremity

(78%), only the part below the knee (7%), or only the thigh and buttock (15%). One should search for:

— provoking factors: walking or prolonged standing;
— a pain-avoidance posture: flexion of the lumbosacral spine;
— signs of deficit which appear with walking and did not exist previously, especially in the territory of L 5;
— signs of bilateral or multiradicular involvement;
— minimal vertebral signs: relatively uninformative clinical findings.

In terms of intensity, the pain never equals that of a disk herniation. True radicular deficits may appear, but they remain moderate for a long time; nevertheless, they sometimes constitute a true chronic cauda equina syndrome.

Sciatica with a Narrow Lateral Recess

Nerve root compression is not always due to disk herniation; the lateral recess may be narrowed either by diskal degenerative changes or by hypertrophic changes of the articular surfaces or of the lateral third of the laminae near the articular surfaces [9, 70]. The resulting symptoms may simulate radiculitis caused by disk herniation, except that the pain often increases on walking or prolonged standing. Objective radicular signs are infrequently found. This condition often involves the L 4 and L 5 roots, since their lateral recesses are especially long and narrow. An associated disk abnormality may be present; this is most often a simple bulging or protrusion without an actual herniation, which may exacerbate the narrowness of the lateral recess.

Femoral Sciatica

Femoral sciatica leads one to suspect a large L 4–L 5 herniaton ascending towards the L 4 vertebral body. The clinical findings alone are sometimes insufficient for a precise etiological or topographic diagnosis.

Incomplete Sciatica

In some cases the sciatic pain is felt only in the proximal portion of the lower limbs (gluteal and inguinal pain), making clinical topography diagnosis impossible, or only in the distal portion of the ankle or the foot, with no other signs of radicular pain. One should remember the possibility of a sciatic radiculalgia and avoid the pitfall of paying attention only to the painful region.

Mild Sciatic Pain

Mild sciatica is found especially in elderly subjects; the pain radiation is inconsistent. Associated hypertrophic degenerative lesions are frequently present.

Radiculalgias at Other Sites

Femoral Neuralgia of Diskal Origin

Femoral neuralgia of diskal origin [43, 272], more properly termed crural radiculalgia, is much less frequent than the commoner forms of sciatica. It results either from irritation of the L 4 root by an L 3–L 4 or (more frequently) L 4–L 5 disk herniation which has migrated slightly into the L 4 intervertebral foramen [9], or, very infrequently, from irritation of the L 3 root by an L 2–L 3 disk herniation. The clinical findings do not permit accurate identification of the disk in question. The condition is observed especially in men between 45 and 60 years of age. It is usually abrupt or very rapid in onset, often in the wake of a lifting action or a sudden movement of the lumbar spine. The lumbocrural pain is usually very sharp and paroxysmal, occurring especially at night. The pain radiates from the lumbar spine to the inguinal region and the anterior aspect of the tigh as far as the knee, where there are frequently associated paresthesias; it may, in the case of L 4 root irritation, continue over the anteromedial aspect of the leg down to the medial malleolus. The pain is aggravated by hyperextension of the lower limb in the prone position (inverted Lasègue's sign). Lumbar stiffness is common; pain-avoidance postures are infrequent. The pain is often accompanied by anterior thigh hypoesthesia, a decreased or abolished patellar reflex, and decreased strength, then wasting, of the quadriceps and (to a lesser degree) the anterior tibiali muscle.

Although some crural neuralgias result from disk herniations, the etiology often remains unclear. In numerous cases of lumbocrural pain, myelography or surgery have not revealed a disk herniation. At surgery, the involved root has an inflamed edematous, and congested appearance. When confronted with this common radiculalgia, one should systematically search for signs of diabetes.

Meralgia Paresthetica

Meralgia paresthetica [43], also termed neuralgia of the lateral cutaneous nerve of the thigh, corresponds to the radicular involvement of L2 or L3. The condition is characterized by paresthesia in the sensory territory of the lateral cutaneous nerve of the thigh (oval area with vertical long axis on lateral aspect of thigh), manifesting itself as pins-and-needles, numbness, or a burning sensation (Fig. 49). The only additional sign uncovered by clinical examination is a painful tactile hyperesthesia which is in contrast with the hypoesthesia to temperature and pain. Meralgia paresthetica is an infrequent condition, usually without an obvious cause, whose pathogenesis is not clearly understood. Compression of the nerve at the level of the osteofibrous ring below the anterior superior spine of the ilium has been postulated. The condition usually persists for months or years.

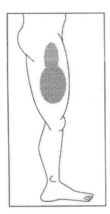

Fig. 49. Clinical signs 2. Meralgesic irradiation

Refractory Sciatica

The large majority of sciaticas (80%) regress spontaneously; it is probable that in most cases the disk herniation is small and the radicular inflammation is the dominant factor. Nevertheless, the herniation, whether extruded or not, is sometimes large, and then remains a source of radicular irritation for a very long time.

"Symptomatic" Sciatica

Although the great majority of cases of lumbosciatic pain are due to disk herniation, spinal stenosis, spondylolysis, or spondylolisthesis, one should always keep in mind other possible etiologies. These "symptomatic" sciaticas [70] give rise to a clinical picture which is not clear-cut:

— There is no activating factor of a mechanical nature; the onset is insidious.
— There is no context of mechanical or degenerative diskopathy.
— The pain is continuous, persistent, and worsens rather than regressing. It is worse in the supine position.
— The involvement tends to be multiradicular and bilateral.
— Other associated signs are present: neurological, visceral, infectious, impaired general health, etc.

The major etiologies are laid out in Fig. 50. The variety of etiologies underscores the importance of a thorough patient interview (medical history) and a complete clinical examination.

Concerning a patient sciatica the decision on whether to perform a neuroradiological workup depends upon:

— the patient's history (previous sciatica, refractoriness to classical treatments, socioprofessional repercussions, etc);
— the mechanical nature of the disturbance;
— the presence or absence of objective neurological disturbances whose onset, progressive or sudden, is unexplained;
— the appearance on standard plain films.

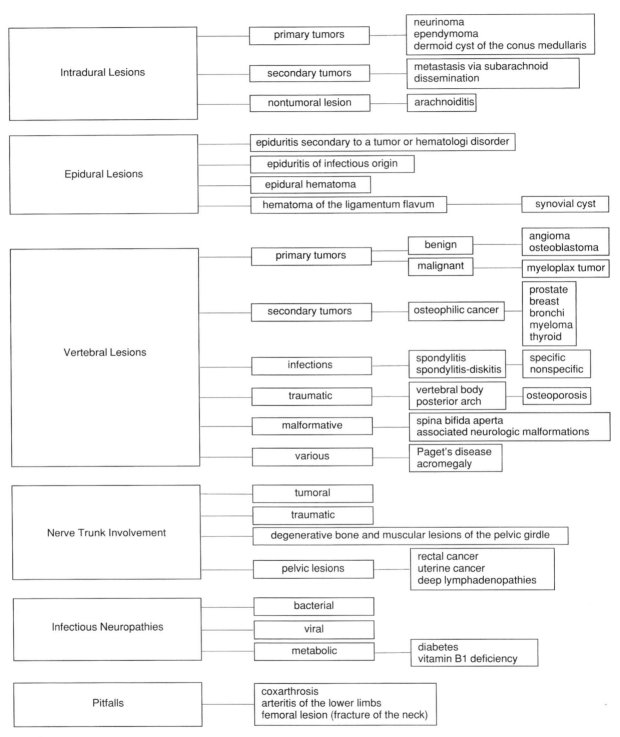

Fig. 50

Whether the pain is femoral or sciatic, only 15%–20% of cases will be referred to the radiologist. These are [29]:

— refractory disease resistant to properly conducted medical treatment comprising at least 2 weeks of absolute bed-rest and 4–6 weeks of treatment with anti-inflammatory agents and analgesics;
— hyperalgesic sciatica refractory to corticosteroid therapy;
— recent paralytic sciatica;
— sciatica with disturbances of sphincter control;
— sciatica with true radicular claudication causing definite dysfunctional discomfort;
— repetitive forms of disease, each episode identical, with detrimental socioprofessional repercussions;
— femoral pain not responding to corticosteroids (excluding diabetes);
— sciatica of uncertain etiology ("symptomatic" sciatica);
— sciatic or femoral pain presenting a medicolegal problem (e. g., disk herniation following an accident at work).

Radiological examination techniques (including CT) are not aimed at determining whether to operate, but rather where to operate and which procedure to employ.

The decision whether to operate, and if so when, should always be based on the clinical signs. Emergency surgery is indicated in patients with loss of bladder sphincter control or nonregressive neurogenic pain with a neurologic deficit. Other patients are treated surgically after failure of properly conducted medical treatment. However, the recent spread of CT and the ease and widespread use of radiological techniques for examining the spine have widened the selection criteria. Numerous patients now consult a specialist having already undergone CT examination well before the classic time limits of medical treatment. Although CT provides images of remarkable quality in cases of nerve root compression of diskal origin, one should not succumb to the temptation to operate simply because the disk is clearly visualized, but always adhere to rigorous, clinical selection criteria.

Pathogenesis

The factors engendering herniation of lumbar intervertebral disks are alteration of the physiochemical characteristics of the intervertebral disk, as well as modifications resulting from repeated mechanical stresses, and the anatomical structure of the lumbar spine itself. In this section, we shall examine the structure of the intervertebral disk, its biomechanics, and the genesis of disk herniation. The anatomy of the lumbar spine will be elaborated on the following section.

Development of Lumbar Disks

The intervertebral disk is a connective tissue structure which firmly unites the vertebral bodies, confers mobility upon the spine, and absorbs the loads to which it is subjected. It is the key component of the intervertebral junction [58, 235, 241].

Embryo and Fetus

Development of the spine begins during the 3rd week of gestation. It results from the condensation of mesodermal tissue on both sides of the notochord. This precursor of the spine undergoes a first segmentation, resulting in the formation of sclerotomes. The notochord induces the formation of the vertebral bodies, the neural tube that of the neural arch. Each vertebral body results from the combination of the caudal portion of one sclerotome with the cephalad portion of the next caudal sclerotome. A second segmentation occurs in the 6th week: arteries derived from the primitive aorta penetrate the developing vertebral bodies, chondrifying them and leaving the intermediate mesenchymal tissue to evolve toward a diskal structure.

The intervertebral disk is therefore composed of two portions: hyaline cartilage is arranged in a ring around notochord remnants. These two formations soon differentiate; the ring of hyaline cartilage undergoes fibrous transformation, thus becoming the *anulus fibrosus,* which is bound by both surfaces to the cartilaginous plates of the opposing vertebral surfaces. The notochordal tissue undergoes cellular multiplication and forms a mucoid substance which is the *nucleus pulposus*.

From the start, the disk develops in an environment poor in blood vessels and limited by a perichondrial band whose continuity foreshadows that of the longitudinal ligaments. The disk is vascularized by perforating arteries originating in the opposing surfaces of the vertebral bodies and by a few direct dorsal and lateral arteries [241].

Child

Shortly after birth, the disk is biconcave. It is composed of a small, free-moving, mucoid nucleus which is richly hydrated (88% water) and still contains numerous cells of notochordal origin, and a thick, lamellar, fibrocartilaginous anulus whose deepest layers have fibers which interlace with the nucleus.

During growth, the *nucleus* develops and increases in size, and almost all the notochordal cells disappear. It becomes more gelatinous and less fluid. The *anulus* progressively acquires its fibrillary structure, while remaining hydrated (78%). The thick cartilaginous plate of the vertebral body decreases in thickness centrally and bulges anteriorly, posteriorly, and laterally, forming the *anular epiphysis*. This structure is initially cartilaginous, but becomes bony at the age of 8 years. The peripheral fibers of the anulus are firmly anchored to it.

At the end of growth, the disk is slightly biconvex.

Until 10-12 years of age, a child's disk is vascularized. Some blood vessels originate in the adjacent vertebral body and pass through its cartilaginous plate; the radiate vessels derived from the periosteum at the periphery of the vertebral body penetrate the disk at its periphery, where the disk meets the vertebral surface. The vascular channels of the vertebral cartilaginous plates remain patent in adults, constituting a pathway for nutritional exchanges with the disk [58, 295].

Anatomy of Adult Disk

The two essential components of the intervertebral disk, the nucleus pulposus and the anulus fibrosus, are in close contact with the cartilaginous plates of the overlying and underlying vertebrae. The thickness of the lumbar disks increases from L 1-L 2 to L 4-L 5. The L 5-S 1 disk varies in thickness.

Nucleus Pulposus

The nucleus pulposus is an oval, shiny, gelatinous, homogeneous structure located at the junction of the middle and posterior thirds of the disk. Its boundary with the lamellar anulus fibrosus is not always distinct, since it is penetrated by a few deep fibers from the annulus. Thus, there exists a zone between the nucleus and the annulus which exhibits intermediate physiological behavior. At the lumbar level, the nucleus pulposus represents about one fourth to one third of the disk's volume [58, 118, 241].

Anulus Fibrosus

The anulus fibrosus is composed of concentric fibrous lamellae which surround the nucleus and are attached by their edges to the cartilaginous plates of the adjacent cartilaginous plates. It is wider anteriorly and laterally than posteriorly; it is also thicker anteriorly, helping to explain the normal lumbar lordosis and the off-center posterior shift of the nucleus pulposus [71, 299]. The fibrous lamellae are 200-400 μm thick, increasing in thickness toward the periphery of the disk. Each lamella is composed of dense, closely spaced, parallel fibers having an oblique orientation. The orientation of the fibers reverses itself somewhat (by a maximum of 60°) from one lamella to the next [235]. This alternating fiber arrangement provides the lamellae with a certain sliding capacity with respect to each other, thus increasing the elesticity of the whole. The fibers of the anulus are inserted into the cartilaginous plates. Anteriorly and laterally, they penetrate deeply into the bony annular epiphysis and somewhat less firmly into the anterior portion of the cartilaginous plate. The least resistant fiber insertions into the plate are found posteriorly.

Vertebral Cartilaginous Plates

The opposing vertebral surfaces are composed of a wide central cartilaginous plate surrounded by a thin bony rim: the annular epiphysis. The cartilaginous plate is thicker peripherally than centrally, with a thickness ranging from 1 to 1.5 mm; it marks the anatomic limits of the disk [235].

Vascularization and Innervation

The normal adult disk is not vascularized.

Only the posterior portion of the disk is superficially innervated by the sinuvertebral nerve (which corresponds to the recurrent meningeal branches of the cranial nerves). The latter is supplied by a posterior nerve root immediately distal to the root ganglion, and then has a recurrent path, receiving sympathetic fibers; it not only innervates the dura mater, but also the posterior surface of the first two disks caudal to its origin. Certain authors have also reported sparse nerve fibers on the lateral and even anterior disk surfaces [71, 235].

Histology

Like all other connective tissues, the fibrocartilaginous disk is composed of cells, collagen fibers, and a ground substance essentially made up of proteoglycans [16, 19].

The adult intervertebral disk contains few cells (chondrocytes and fibrocytes), which are more numerous at the periphery of the anulus fibrosus and close to the cartilaginous plates [18, 19]. These cells help elaborate the matrix of the disk and play an active part in its metabolic exchanges. The cells of the nucleus pulposus have a greater capacity for proteoglycan synthesis than those of the anulus fibrosus. Only a few notochordal cells are found in the adult nucleus [231].

The extracellular matrix of the nucleus is exclusively composed of randomly distributed, thin type II (30 nm) collagen fibers, which make up a three-dimensional lattice with a wide mesh and are embedded in a richly hydrated gel. On the other hand, the collagenfibers of the anulus are thicker, especially peripherally, where the type I fibers (60 nm) predominate. These are rigorously aligned and parallel to one another [231]. There is no definite or uniform boundary between the central area and the peripheral fibrous wall. There is a marked interrelationship of both components, so that the nucleus is not just a very round sphere [233]. Starting with the second or third decade of life, the anulus emits lamellar extensions toward the central portion of the nucleus; on sagittal T2-weighted MRI sections of the disks, this results in an image evoking an intranuclear defect. Finally, elastic fibers have been demonstrated in both the anulus and the nucleus [35, 105]. They presumably help the disk return to its initial form after mechanical deformation, but their contribution is modest compared to that of the viscoelasticity of the nucleus-anulus system.

Biochemistry

The essential chemical components of the disk substance are collagen and the proteoglycan gels, which account for the disk's mechanical properties of resistance to stress and compression. With the recent development of chemonucleolysis, particularly using chymopapain, the importance of a detailed knowledge of this complex structure has become more evident [105, 211, 231, 241, 278].

Collagen

This is the essential constituent fibrillary structure of the disk and the one responsible for its elasticity. It accounts for 50% of the disk's dry weight and is three times more abundant in the anulus than in the nucleus. It is more abundant in the anterior and lateral portions of the peripheral lamellae; on the other hand, there are lesser amounts in the posterolateral portions, which are the preferential sites for the passage of disk herniations. Collagen fibers are only minimally synthesized in adults. Once deposited, they undergo a "maturation" making them insoluble, due to the creation of numerous cross-links at two levels: at the substrand level, between the three polypeptide chains making up the tropocollagen molecule, and at the subfibrillary level, between tropocollagen molecules.

In addition to this very coherent structure, collagen is deeply embedded in a proteoglycan gel. Nevertheless, chondrocytes in adults still produce small amounts of collagen and proteoglycans. Proteoglycan turnover takes about 500 days, and collagen turnover is even longer. Furthermore, minimal histological repair remains possible over several years, as is shown by possible disk reexpansion following the initial post-chemonucleolysis collapse [144, 214].

Proteoglycans

Proteoglycans [16, 18, 19, 71] account for 50% of the dry weight of the nucleus and for only 10% of that of the anulus. The basic unit consists of a protein axis to which are attached linear lateral chains of polysaccharides or glycosaminoglycans (GAGS): keratan sulfate (KS) and chondroitin sulfate (CS). These clearly differ from cartilage proteoglycans in the shortness of the protein axis and the relative abundance of keratan sulfate in comparison to chondroitin sulfate. Nevertheless, there is a heterogeneous distribution of keratan sulfate and chondroitin sulfate on the protein chain. Within a disk, the length of the protein chain varies widely, as does the molecular weight and the keratan sulfate: chondroitin sulfate ratio.

Glycosaminoglycans are sulfated disaccharide chains bearing negative charges: two negative charges in the case of CS, and one for KS. This concentration of negative charges is responsible for ionic equilibrium and also, for the strongly hydrophilic nature of the disk. The greater their concentration, the greater the internal tension of the disk.

Hyaluronic acid is responsible for the aggregation of proteoglycan molecules. It is found in high concentrations in the disk. The percentage of aggregated proteoglycans is approximately 30% in the nucleus and 60% in the anulus.

Glycoproteins are abundant in the disk, compared to other cartilaginous structures. They favor very strong links between proteoglycans and collagen and help stabilize bonds between proteoglycans and hyaluronic acid.

Water and Solutes

Water is an essential disk constituent (65 to 90% by volume). It predominates in the nucleus (88% versus 78% in the anulus), and decreases with age. Most of this water is extracellular and fixed to the hydrophilic groups of the proteoglycans. A small portion is fixed to type II collagen fibers [16, 19, 71].

Ions: their presence is explained by the electric charge previously described. Cations (sodium) are more numerous than anions (Gibbs-Donnan equilibrium). The greater concentration of ions in the disk than in the plasma creates a greater osmotic pressure within the disk, thus favoring its hydrophilic character. The major mechanism of solute transport within the disk is passive diffusion [295].

Enzymes

Poorly understood enzymatic reactions assure the turnover of collagen and other proteins. The disk contains proteolytic enzymes (i. e., collagenase, elastase, gelatinase) which seem to exist as proenzymes capable of being activated by various factors, such as inflammatory phenomena [16, 18, 19, 273].

Disk Aging

With age, the disk undergoes biochemical and histological changes. Although widespread after the age of 30, these degenerative changes begin earlier, although to a different degree in different individuals [235, 241].

After the third decade of life, the disk changes gradually. The nucleus slowly loses its turgescent, gelatinous and elastic aspect, becoming firmer and more fibrous. It becomes less distinguishable from the deeper layers of the anulus. The lamellar arrangement of the anulus becomes less evident; it takes on a more homogeneous appearance than in young subjects.

Histochemically, there are few cellular modifications. The collagen content of the disk is unchanged, but the collagen fibers of the anulus increase in size. There is a decreased water content, especially in the nucleus, which is invaded by type I collagen fibers. In particular there is a decrease in the hydrophilic nature of the nucleus, secondary to a decrease in the osmotic potential of the nuclear constituents (reduced proteoglycan content) and thus in the negative charge of the nucleus [231, 278]. Since these histochemical changes occur slowly, the mechanical properties of a nondeteriorated disk are preserved until about the age of 60.

Biomechanics of the Lumbar Disk

The intervertebral disk is part of the mobile segment of Junghans, together with the articular processes, ligaments, etc. We shall first describe the physiological role of each disk component and then that of the disk as a whole, as a functional unit [223, 235, 241, 25].

Individual Physiological Roles
of Disk Components

The cartilaginous plates play a double role:

— Stress resistance is very great (a load of about 400 to 500 kg is necessary to break the end-plate of a lumbar vertebra removed at autopsy). The underlying cancellous bone and its adjacent cortex contribute to the resistance of the end-plate. Metabolic exchanges, as well as the nutrition of the nucleus and the deeper part of the anulus, occur through the cartilaginous plate, which retains in its central portion small channels left by vascular pathways dating from childhood.

The nucleus pulposus also plays a double role:

— It is a load distributor on "hydraulic chamber," thanks to its high water content. Obeying the laws of hydraulics, it distributes loads applied to it equally, in a centrifugal manner, over its entire surface (Fig. 51).

Uniform load distribution by the nucleus. Transmission of forces to the lamellae of the anulus, whose elasticity dampens and absorbs them.

It is a shock absorber for loads applied to the disk, by virtue of its internal pressure which is closely related to that of the anulus. The internal pressure is linked to the markedly hydrophilic nature of the nucleus. This avidity for water de-

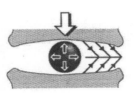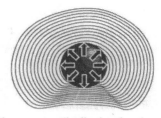

Fig. 51. Pathogenesis 1. Uniform stress distribution by the nucleus pulposus. Transmission of stresses to the lamellae of the anulus, whose elasticity dampens and absorbs them

rives from its strong osmolarity, which is due to the high negative charge of the proteoglycans. Within the disk, the nucleus is in a prestressed state; its internal pressure is in equilibrium with the resistance to distension exhibited by the anulus fibrosus. The stressing or destressing of a disk is therefore accompanied by a new equilibrium obtained by an increase or decrease of the disk pressure equal to that of the applied force. The disk slowly loses its water, or, conversely, becomes saturated with water. The hydraulic permeability of the disk is inversely proportional to the proteoglycan concentration.

The anulus fibrosus has three properties:

— It is a powerful link between two adjacent vertebra, by virtue of the insertion of peripheral fibers in the ring apophyses, and of its closely woven structure..
— It is the agent of discal prestress. Its closely-knit structure and oblique fibers strongly enclose the nucleus and maintain its internal pressure.
— It is an effective shock absorber for loads, functioning by stretching of its lamellae. When loads are dampened, the fibers become elongated while at the same time becoming slightly more oblique (Fig. 52).

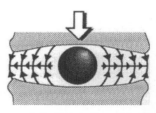

Fig. 52. Pathogenesis 2. Role of anular fibers. Stretching forces on the anular lamellae are transformed into traction forces on their constituent fibers, which are anchored at their extremities in the cartilaginous plates

The stretching forces of the anular lamellae become traction forces on their constituent fibers, where these are anchored to the cartilage plate (Fig. 52).

Physiological Role of Disk as Functional Unit

The mechanical functions of the disk are related to vertebral stability, spinal mobility and the absorption of shocks and loads.

Vertebral Stability

The disk plays a fundamental part in vertebral stability. It does not permit any translational movement of one vertebra with respect to another. This is ensured by the prestressed state of the nucleus-anulus complex, the tight lattice of anular lamellae and the crossed obliquity of the fibers.

Other factors involved in vertebral stability, though to a lesser degree, are the articular pillar (via the facet joints); the lumbar muscular mass; the posterior longitudinal ligament, ligamenta flava and interspinous ligament.

Spinal Mobility

Since it is deformable in nature, the disk confers mobility upon the spine. The thicker the disk, the greater the range of movement. This mobility is limited by the neural arches and their attachments, the oblique orientation of the inferior articular facets, and the wedging of the lumbosacral disk between the iliac crests. Coordinated activity of the agonist and antagonist muscles permits harmonious movements.

Three basic types of movement may be distinguished:

Flexion-extension. In flexion, the nucleus is decentered posteriorly and becomes ovoid; the posterior fibers of the anulus are tensed, whereas its anterior portion narrows and bulges sligthly. The opposite occurs during extension. In each cases, there is an increased intranuclear pressure.

The transverse axis of the movement does not seem to pass through the nucleus, as previously thought, but just anterior or caudad to it, according to the range of movements. For most of the

overall range of flexion-extension, movement occurs at the last 3 lumbar disks.

Lateral flexion. In lateral flexion, the changes in shape and the mechanical stresses at the disk are comparable to those produced by flexion, with the addition of an automatic axial rotation of the vertebral bodies. The anular fibers and the intertransverse ligaments limit lateral flexion and/or rotation.

Rotation. Rotational movement is slight (2° to 3° per disk). The center of rotation is posterior to the disk. The peripheral lamellar fibers, particularly the anterior and anterolateral fibers, are subjected to the strongest traction forces.

Absorption

Absorption of Loads. Load absorption occurs by a compression-stretching mechanism.

The load distributed by the nucleus is dampened by stretching of the anular fibers. The tensing of these fibers creates increased traction on their cartilaginous plate attachments, although direct compression of the peripheral anular fibers occurs to a lesser degree. Due to the effects of the load, the disk tends to collapse and to bulge, rapidly at first and then more slowly. A return to the initial volume is rapid for a load of less then 130 kg applied less than 5 minutes, but it may take longer (a few hours) for greater and more prolonged loading.

Load absorption also depends on two other factors:

1. *The articular pillar formed by the facet joints,* which plays a greater part in a subject leaning forward than in one standing up. Depending on the position, the joint system of the normal lumbar spine transmits from 3% to 25% of the applied load, in contrast to an arthritic spine, which transmits up to 40% of the load [214].
2. *The thoracoabdominal caisson,* which is comparable to a "hydropneumatic damper".

The load applied to the disk may be decomposed into 2 forces: one of compression, perpendicular to the disk, and one of shearing, which increases with the obliquity of the disk. The disk is more resistant to compression than to shearing strains, which explaining the major value of the posterior abutments of the articular processes.

The pressures to which lumbar disks are subjected may be measured using two different methods: mathematically, by calculating the force vectors, and by direct measurement of the intradiskal pressure, through the insertion of a pressure transducer into the disk.

The pressures measured are twice as high in a sitting as in a standing subject. Man is much less adapted to sitting than to standing. The intradiskal pressure during walking is little more than the standing pressure. The load is greatest when standing and leaning forward, with the body overhanging the lower part of the spine. Lifting a load is made possible only by the powerful contraction of the posterior spinal muscles and the help provided by the thoracoabdominal caisson and the articular pillar of the facet joints.

Shock Absorption. Shock, whether due to an accident or an awkward movement, results in a sudden increase in the load on the disk load. The effects have been studied in autopsy specimens, by dropping a heavy load on a spinal segment. The shock sets off rapid oscillatory phenomena at the disk level, conditioned by the internal pressure and elasticity of the anulus. The disk first collapses by stretching of the lamellae; this provokes a recoil inducing reexpansion of the disk with a return of fiber stretching which is now vertical instead of horizontal. These compression-rebound phenomena are repeated rapidly (a dozen times in less than a second) with decreasing amplitude until a new disk equilibrium is attained. The great viscosity of the nucleus slows the oscillations and reduces their amplitude. Nevertheless, in case of violent shock, the initial fiber stretching may exceed resistance limits, provoking the rupture of certain fibers.

There are thus two circumstances under which the high resistance limits of the disk may be surpassed: certain straightening-up efforts with a heavy load and the effects of a violent shock.

Structural Deterioration of Lumbar Disk

It permits nuclear sagging and limits mobility. It cannot be equated with simple aging, even if certain biochemical and histochemical abnormalities of degeneration somewhat resemble those of aging: connective tissues have only a limited range of expression.

Mechanisms of Onset

The mechanisms of onset of disk herniation may be traumatic, degenerative, and often combined.

Traumatic
The cause may be an accident (fall) or a violent effort (lifting heavy load) or making an awkward movement. The mechanical resistance of the anulus fibrosus is exceeded, resulting in a rupture of the fibers of the anulus which takes on the appearance of a deep slit or a radiate fissure. In general, only one disk gives way, but sometimes two are affected. In addition to major acute traumata, the microtraumata of the kind associated with driving an automobile, an tractor – and also with a prolonged sitting position are other factors in the genesis of structural disk deterioration.

It should be noted that lateral, functional, mechanical overload of a disk adjacent to a transitional anomaly or vertebral ankylosis may also lead to structural deterioration of the disk.

Degenerative
In some cases, structural disk deterioration occurs without an obvious specific causal factor. A familial tendency may sometimes be found. The anatomic changes are comparable to those of normal aging, but are accelerated. This idiopathie presentation of the deterioration may conceal metabolic or tissue disturbances of the cartilage plate or of the other disk components. Hydrocortisone administration seems to accelerate the degenerative process in the nucleus level in mice [86, 103, 129, 238, 253].

It has been suggested that the etiology may be that of an autoimmune process [211] (Fig. 53). This implies formation of antibodies against the nuclear constituents, which would alter its physicochemical properties. The nucleus would then

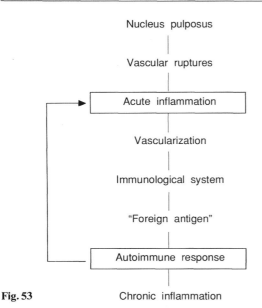

Nucleus pulposus

|

Vascular ruptures

|

Acute inflammation

|

Vascularization

|

Immunological system

|

"Foreign antigen"

|

Autoimmune response

|

Fig. 53   Chronic inflammation

no longer play a part in pressure distribution. Modifications of the anulus fibrosus would be secondary to a poor distribution of mechanical stresses. This hypothesis is still debated. It has been supported by studies of cellular immunity, using proteoglycans or isolated nuclear cells as antigens, but other studies have not confirmed it [103, 104, 211].

Anatomic Alterations:
Genesis of Disk Herniation

Nucleus
The nucleus first loses its gelatinous appearance and homogeneity; its volume decreases due to a reduction in proteoglycans and proteins other than collagen (whose concentration increases proportionately). It no longer completely occupies the center of the disk, and no longer transmits stresses to the anulus in uniform fashion. At a more advanced stage, the nucleus becomes fibrotic and may fragment [105, 241, 253, 278].

Anulus
At the earliest stage, small foci of amorphous hyalinization appear, which disrupt the fibrillary structure. These foci tend to multiply and coalesce. They predominate in the deeper layers of the posterior portion of the anulus.

Subsequently, small fissures appear at these sites, making the anulus fragile. Actual cracks may form as a result of trauma, and violent or repeated physical exertion. These cracks play an important part in disk pathology and may be divided into two types:

Radiate Cracks or Ruptures. Radiate lesions are the most frequent and extend from the center to the periphery, like the spokes of a wheel [86]. They may be incomplete, being limited to the deeper layers, or complete and reaching the peripheral layers. Recent cracks are narrow and sometimes sinuous, whereas old cracks are wider and lined by clumps of cartilaginous cells or even by chondrometaplastic tissue. Although often solitary at first, there may later be several cracks with different orientations in the same disk. They are preferentially posterolateral, less often lateral or anterior (Fig. 54).

Concentric Cracks. These are less frequent and occur later. They are crevasses like circular arcs, which are parallel to the lamellae in the peripheral anular layers. They are usually found anteriorly or anterolaterally and promote discal bulging [241].

Intradiskal Migration
Under normal conditions, the fissures or cracks are functionally closed because of the pressures exerted on the disk. With certain movements (eg. flexion or rotation of the trunk), they may open to permit the entry and then the in situ blockage

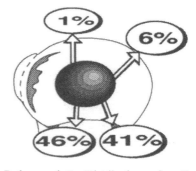

Fig. 54. Pathogenesis 3. Distribution of radiate fissures (Lindblom). Percentage orientations of 393 radiate fissures. Anterior and lateral herniations provoke the formation of localized osteophytes. Usual location and appearance of a concentric fissure responsible for a ringshaped osteophytosis

of a nuclear fragment. At rest, small fragments may make their way back to the center of the disk bed; others may remain jammed in the narrow fissures, resulting in lumbar pain. It is common for a large nuclear fragment to carry with it a few deep anular lamellae. This blockage may occur at any site, but the most important lesions from a pathological viewpoint are posterior, since only the superficial posterior fibroligamentous plane of the disk is innervated.

All radiate ruptures may create conditions for recurrent blockage of nuclear fragments, thus explaining the recurrent nature of attacks of lumbar pain.

Nevertheless, in certain cases radiate cracks are capable of at least partial repair. If a complete crack extends to the subligamentous space and permits the passage of a small nuclear fragment, a localized inflammatory reaction may develop with proliferation of connective tissue and blood vessels. This reaction tends to resorb the small nuclear fragment, and also to fill in part of the disk gap by entering the anular crevice and laying down fibrous scar tissue from the periphery towards the center. In the case of a wide or old crack with cartilaginous metaplasia, repair is usually no longer possible.

Disk Herniation

A degenerate disk may bulge beyond its normal anatomic boundaries. Two conditions should be distinguished [73, 206, 253, 299]:

— disk protrusion, or rather a simple outward bulging of the disk, which is especially marked when it is submitted to stress. It usually corresponds to stretching of the peripheral lamellae or even a concentric rupture (Fig. 55);
— disk herniation, which corresponds to extrusion of part of the nucleus pulposus through a ruptured anulus fibrosus, toward the spinal canal or intervertebral foramen. The fact that anulus involvement is an essential feature accounts for the classical rarity of lumbar disk herniations in adolescents and children.

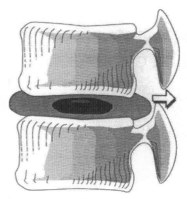

Fig. 55. Pathogenesis 4. Disk protrusion or bulging

Posterolateral or posterior disk herniations are the most frequent. Their size varies: every intermediate form may be observed, ranging from the extrusion of a small nuclear fragment to the massive expulsion of the entire nucleus as well as of deeper anular layers (Fig. 56).

When the herniation is small or lateral it compresses, only the homolateral nerve root sheath; if sufficiently large, it compresses also the anterolateral aspect of the thecal sac.

The nature of the herniation also varies. The disk herniation of young adults are essentially composed of nuclear substance, while those of elderly subjects, which are rarer because of nuclear involution, are composed of degenerate disks and particularly, of anulus fibrosus fragments detached from the cartilage plates. These compress the nerve roots at their emergence from the thecal sac.

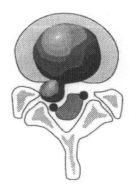

Fig. 56. Pathogenesis 5. Posterolateral disk herniation

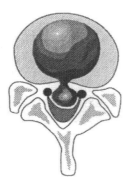

Fig. 57. Pathogenesis 6. Posteromedian disk herniation

More seldom, a herniation may be median and remain asymptomatic, or give rise to lumbar pain and intermittent blockage episodes when it is small, compressing the anterior aspect of the thecal sac but sparing the nerve root sheaths. When large, it may compress the roots on both sides and give rise to bilateral clinical signs (Fig. 57).

Several types of disk herniation may be distinguished in terms of their relation to the posterior longitudinal ligament:

— *Direct sub- or preligamentous:* the extruded fragment remains opposite the fissure. The herniation usually remains attached to the disk by a predicle composed of a few deep anular layers (Fig. 58 a). However, it may become completely detached, thus forming a "free subligamentous herniation," which is now a free fragment (Fig. 58 b).

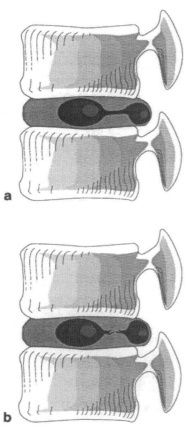

Fig. 58 a, b. Pathogenesis 7. Subligamentous disk herniation **a** still in contact with the nucleus **b** subligamentous free fragment

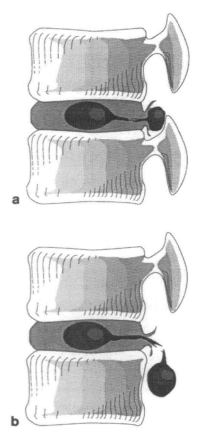

Fig. 59 a, b. Pathogenesis 8. Transligamentous disk herniation **a** buttonhole herniation **b** transligamentous or extruded migratory free fragment

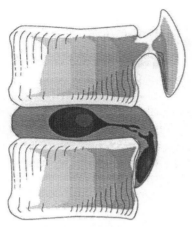

Fig. 60. Pathogenesis 9. Subligamentous migratory free fragment

— *Transligamentous:* the plane of the posterior longitudinal ligament has been breached, and the fragment is either opposite the disk ("buttonhole" herniation) (Fig. 59 a) or has migrated caudad or cephalad (transligamentous migratory free fragment) (Fig. 59 b). This may also be described as an extruded fragment. Migration may occur toward the axilla of a nerve root at an upper level, giving rise to deceptive clinical signs.

— *Migratory:* as stated, transligamentous migration is by far the most frequent; the fragment may also glide behind the next cephalad or caudad vertebral body and into the subligamentous space, after having detached the posterior longitudinal ligament from its anchorage to the ring apophysis (Fig. 60).

The following table groups the different types of herniation:

Subligamentous Herniation	• Large predicle
	• Free fragment
	   – Opposite the intervertebral space
	   – Migratory

Transligamentous Herniation (Free Fragment)	• Opposite the intervertebral space ("buttonhole") • Migratory (extruded)

A disk herniation need not produce painful symptoms, especially if there is a wide spinal canal, as at the L 5–S 1 level. The herniation usually causes sciatica or femoral pain, which varies in severity according to the degree of root compression and the anatomic space available. The importance of assessing the herniation: nerve root: osteodiscal canal ratio emphasizes the indispensable role of CT.

A natural history of posterior or posterolateral disk herniations must be appreciated. A minority of disk herniations are reducible, either spontaneously or by a reduction movement (e. g. hyperflexion), or with rest and treatment. However, the anular fissure remains and obviously entails the risk of recurrence. It is possible to directly demonstrate this reduction size of the herniation on follow-up CT scans. The posterior margin of the herniation remains well-defined. A partial reintegration of the hernia through the fissure in the anulus seems to be most probable, together with dehydration and contraction of the disk material [112, 283].

In our experience, most herniations (i. e., disk herniations which are extruded, migratory or large) are not reducible. Some are partially resorbed by a localized inflammatory reaction; others migrate into a silent zone, at a distance from neural elements. Other herniations remain compressive and poorly tolerated, thus justifying their surgical excision.

Lateral disk herniations (Fig. 61) may result in nerve root compression in the intervertebral foramen, or in compression of the root above extraspinally, at the foraminal entrance [233].

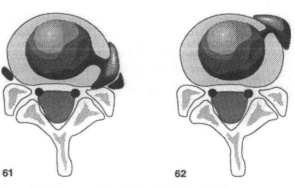

Fig. 61. Pathogenesis 10. Lateral disk herniation

Fig. 62. Pathogenesis 11. Anterior disk herniation

Anterior disk herniations (Fig. 62) do not compress any neural elements, but displace the anterior longitudinal ligament, separating it from the ring apophysis. They extend into the zone of easy cleavage [90, 143].

In conclusion, the spatial relationship between the herniation and the nerve root are determined by the emergence level of the lumbar roots with respect to the disk, the transverse location of the herniation, and possible ascending or descending migration.

At a Subsequent Stage

Structural degeneration of the disk increases with time and may result in actual anatomic disorganization of the disk. The nucleus continues to fragment and to degenerate. The lamellae of the anulus are separated by arciform fissures, and become fragmented, separated from the cartilage plates in certain places, and frayed. At the end of this evolution, the disk has a disorganized appearance, and there is even stripping of the cartilage plates in places and the presence of intradiscal gas. A ring of osteophytes may form under the influence of anulus fragments extruded anteriorly or laterally, the condition of arthrotic discopathy.

Biomechanical Consequences of Disk Degeneration

A posterior radiate fissure, as an isolated lesion and with an apparently normal nucleus, may be observed in subjects suffering from recurrent episodes of lumbago without intermediate lumbar pain. The spinal stability, lower lumbar mobility, and the resistance to loads are normal. Nevertheless, such a disk is vulnerable under two circumstances: during straightening-up efforts with a flexed trunk, when (as we have seen) there is a great load on the posterior portion of the anulus and the radiate fissure may open further; and during efforts involving trunk rotation, which may also open the fissure and favor the entry of a nuclear fragment.

Selective involution of the nucleus is observed in patients with radiographic signs of disk collapse and without a previous history of lumbago or sciatica. The nucleus is too small and no longer fulfills its role. It no longer "permanently tenses" the anulus fibers, nor does it function as a uniform distributor of applied loads, and it has lost hydrophilic properties. This results in diskovertebral instability responsible for small vertebral gaps; increased disk malleability, which often somewhat increases the mobility of the overlying vertebra; and poor loads absorption. The anulus fibers no longer function by stretching traction at their insertions, but there is a direct compression of the anulus between the two cartilaginous plates, resulting in degenerative lesions. The diskovertebral instability and direct compression of the anulus facilitate the detachment of anulus fibers and the formation of horizontal arciform fissures. Thus the loss of nuclear function leads to deterioration of the anulus.

Combined degeneration of the anulus and nucleus provokes even greater diskovertebral instability which may result in spondylolisthesis, retrospondylolisthesis or lateral spondylolisthesis; intradiskal migration of nuclear or even anular fragments; and direct compression during the absorption of loads, with progressively decreasing resistance.

At a late stage the disk has collapsed; osteophytosis has developed; and both the nucleus and anulus are profoundly altered. The disk has lost all its functional capability. The diskovertebral instability and increased mobility of the overlying vertebra have disappeared. Load absorption now takes place by compression of a fibrocartilaginous disk, or between the ring apophyses and the osteophytes.

The nucleus thus plays a fundamental role in the physiology of the disk; although a radiate fissure of the anulus may be compatible for several years with a normal nucleus, any nuclear alteration has rapid repercussions on the anulus because it greatly modifies the functional aspects.

Radiologic Examinations

Although CT is the first noninvasive examination capable of directly showing a disk herniation, any radiologic investigation of lumbosciatic pain should begin with a conventional examination. Obviously, the latter will provide very few arguments in favor of a diskal etiology, but it can exclude other causes such as spondylolisthesis, bone tumors, spondylitis with diskitis, etc.

Routine Radiographs

Radicular pain is investigated using three radiographs:

— a large frontal view in the standing position using a large format, permitting an analysis from the 11th intercostal space down to the hip joints;
— a large lateral view in the standing position, extending from T12 to the sacrum;
— a focussed frontal view centered on the clinically suspect disk.

Sometimes additional radiographs (specially focussed lateral projections) are necessary for more detailed analysis of a vertebral body or disk.

The radiographs permit an evaluation of:

— the general appearance of the lumbosacral spine, which is normally rectilinear in frontal views and shows a lordosis in lateral views;
— the disk heights, the thickest disk in the body being the L4-L5 disk, whereas the L5-S1 disk varies in height. A lateralized collapse was traditionally considered as good evidence of a disk herniation. In fact, this sign is very inconstant and sometimes misleading, since the herniation may be contralateral. The existence of an irreducible posterior bulge in lateral views is a good sign of a median disk herniation, but is only exceptionally found [50, 53, 70, 71, 73].

Functional radiographic methods are of little aid in confirming the pathologic nature of disk bulging or collapse. The radiographic work-up usually only reveals a normal intervertebral space in young subjects, or a markedly collapsed disk accompanied by osteophytes and indicative of advanced disk degeneration in older subjects. Elements to be considered are:

— the bony structure, when searching for tumoral or other pathologies
— the adjacent soft tissues
— a narrow spinal canal, spondylolisthesis or spondylolysis
— the presence of apophyseal joint arthropathy, which calls for caution during subsequent CT evaluation and for the use of a bone window setting

Finally, it is essential to search routinely for a transitional abnormality, as this influences the conduct and interpretation of the CT examination.

Nevertheless, the chief value of conventional radiographic examination lies in its *negative findings*.

Myelography

Since myelography requires the subarachnoid injection of contrast medium and hospitalization it is often dreaded by patients. The use of new iodinated nonionic contrast media (i. e., Amipaque and, more recently, Iopamiron, Iohexol, etc.) makes this examination much less invasive [109, 120, 122].

The available contrast media permit a systematic study of the medullary cone, which should always be investigated if the examination is negative and does not show a disk herniation, since the symptoms may be due to a tumor at this level. It is worth underlining the value of positional myelograms in the standing position, possibly associated with functional myelograms, which sometimes visualize soft disk herniations that are not very evident in the supine position (the position used in CT studies) [198]. This capacity for functional examinations is undoubtedly the only major advantage of myelography, since CT and MRI cannot provide such information.

Myelography is very sensitive in detecting posterolateral and median herniations, but only provides indirect signs [44, 153, 184, 299]:

— A small posterolateral herniation appears only as an amputation (lack of opacification of a nerve root sheath), sometimes associated with a widening of the compressed nerve root ("blunderbuss" sign). This is seen in the frontal and especially the oblique views; the lateral view appears normal.

— A large posterolateral herniation manifests itself as an anterolateral compression of the thecal sac, which is visible on all three projections.

— A median herniation results in compression of the anterior aspect of the thecal sac, well shown in the lateral views: the nerve root sheaths are not usually compressed.

— A herniation associated with lumbar spinal stenosis may result in complete obstruction to the passage of contrast medium.

The performances of myelography and computed tomography are almost identical as regards reliability (slightly greater than 90%). On the other hand, the successes and failures are very different, so that the two examinations are actually complementary [26, 44, 76, 109, 159, 172, 206, 229, 236, 276, 314].

CT may be performed following myelography (postmyelography CT scans), thus permitting good visualization of the disk compression of the opacified root and thecal sac [5, 13, 77, 88]. We now rarely use this technique in cases of disk pathology because it requires lumbar puncture. On the other hand, we used it widely in cases of traumatic or tumoral pathology before the advent of MRI (Table 3).

Lumbar Phlebography

With the advent of CT, this onerous and lengthy examination no longer has any indications in disk pathology. Nevertheless, it bears witness to the importance of the epidural venous network, and to its value, when opacified, in making CT sections easier to interpret [75, 102, 279, 288, 299].

Table 3. Comparative table of the advantages and disadvantages of myelography and CT in the investigation of sciatica

Disadvantages		Advantages	
Myelography	CT	Myelography	CT
Disagreeable examination + + + Requires hospitalization Slight neurotoxicity Risk of infection and hematomas	Few devices Reliability varies with experience Uninterpretable if not perfect + + + Obligatory supine position Segmental study of spine Weight, scoliosis and hyperlordosis perturb the examination	Easily performed examination Familiar tested technique Mediocre myelograms are interpretable Myelograms possible in the upright position	Noninvasive examination + + + Outpatient examination + + + (less cost)
Only indirectly studies lesions which deform the subarachnoid space + + + (at L5–S1, less informative than CT if the thecal sac is narrowed Does not visualize extraspinal lateral herniations Posterior arch and lateral recesses are poorly investigated Poor postoperative specificity	Presentation dependent on epidural fat. False-negatives due to the absence (narrow lumbar canal) or disappearance (postoperative) of the fat + + + Existence of false-positives No visualization of contents of subarachnoid space	Wide investigation of the subarachnoid space, down to the conus medullaris + + + Visualization of nerve root edema ("blunderbuss" sign) Good evaluation of the height of the narrow lumbar canal; demonstration of deviation of compressed roots at a distance from the hernia	Direct visualization of the herniation, whatever its location, and even if the subarachnoid spaces are not deformed + + + Good investigation of the posterior arch and the lateral recesses Permits very accurate measurements Good examination of the perispinal space, sacrum and pelvis.

Epidurography

Like lumbar phlebography, epidurography is now largely inrelevant to the investigation of disk herniations [96, 245]. Also termed peridurography or canalography, it consists of the extradural injection of a contrast medium, following catheterization of this space via a sacrococcygeal approach (sacral hiatus, first sacral foramen, injection between the median sacral crests).

Diskography

Before the advent of MRI, diskography was the only examination capable of showing the normal and pathologic anatomy of the intervertebral disk [49, 50, 190, 193]. The increasingly widespread use of chemonucleolysis, in which diskography constitutes a preliminary procedure, has revived interest in this old technique. CT may be performed immediately following diskography (Postdiskography CT), in order to better visualize the intradiskal injection site.

Normal Diskogram

In a normal disk, the injection of contrast medium is made against great intranuclear pressure and the volume injected does not exceed 1 ml or 2 ml. The normal nucleus is uniformly dense, with clear-cut and regular limits. Seen frontally, it appears median; seen laterally, it appears to be slightly posterior, its center being located at the junction of the middle and posterior thirds of the disk. It remains separated from the cartilaginous endplates. The longest diameter of the nucleus, whether seen frontally or laterally, is always less than half the length of the intervertebral space. Normal nuclei vary in shape: the two most frequent appearances are rounded-ovoid and bilobar.

The injection of contrast medium into a normal disk is entirely asymptomatic.

Disk Herniation

If there is a disk herniation, and regardless of the structural appearance of the disk, the injectable volume is increased, exceeding 1 ml. The herniation is easily recognized when it involves an un-degenerated disk. The nucleus has an apparently normal shape and preserves its clear-cut limits. Apart from the nucleus, the contrast medium opacifies a localized anular rupture (which may be posterior, median or lateral) as a channel through which a certain amount of disk substance escapes to bulge into the spinal canal, and visualizes the herniation by enhancing or opacifying it.

This herniation image may be found opposite the intervertebral space, or it may be displaced cephalad or caudad. If the posterior longitudinal ligament is perforated, contrast medium diffuses toward the epidural space. The injection of contrast medium may elicit pain identical to that usually experienced by the patient.

Degenerate Disks

There is an increase in the volume of contrast medium that may be injected into the disk. The contrast medium opacifies a flattened extensive cavity, with irregular and fringed contours, which occupies more than half the intervertebral space. At a more advanced stage of degeneration, the contrast medium spreads throughout the intervertebral space and the disk has a more or less lamellar and irregular appearance. This degenerated disk appearance may be associated with disk herniation; contrast medium then enhances the hernia within the spinal canal or opacifies it.

CT

The use of CT to detect a disk herniation requires both a precise clinical examination to identify the distribution of the radiculalgia, and a rigorous technique. Given the present increase in the number of CT scans and the shortened examination waiting times, it is logical to start the investigation of a lumbar disk herniation with CT. A clear CT abnormality which is consistent with the clinical findings may lead directly to surgery. On the other hand, a negative or doubtful CT scan, or one inconsistent with the clinical findings, should indicate a secondary myelography. It is necessary to differentiate between lumbar pain which seldom has a sciatic irradiation and typical sciatica, which is a stronger indication for CT examination [28, 76, 159, 191, 194, 199].

Magnetic Resonance Imaging (MRI)

MRI is a very attractive technique. Through the use of adapted sequences, it enables one to differentiate between the anulus and the nucleus, to evaluate the degree of disk degeneration, and to visualize the disk herniation. Adapted oblique sections are best capable of demonstrating nerve root compression of diskal origin [73, 271]. This promising technique is discussed later (cf chapter: Magnetic Resonance Imaging, p. 163).

Postdiskography CT

The widespread performance of diskography during chemonucleolysis at the lumbar level has led to the creation of a new type of CT investigation: postdiskography CT [1, 106, 262]. This refers to CT examination of a given lumbar segment at which contrast medium has been injected into the disk (Iopamiron 300: usually 1–1.5 ml). This investigation is usually made within one or two hours after chemonucleolysis (Figs. 63, 64).

This is a valuable investigation for several reasons.

The symptomatology of lumbar disk herniations varies widely and is sometimes complex. In

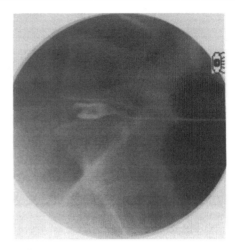

Fig. 64. Sagittal L5–S1 normal; Diskography. The nucleus is slightly posterior and appears bilobar

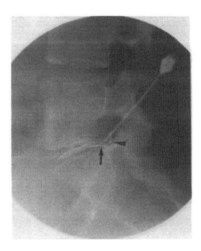

Fig. 65. Sagittal L5–S1 diskography – Diskal herniation. The nucleus has a normal appearance with clear-cut limits. Posterior localized anular rupture (→) and opacification of the herniation *(arrowhead)*

a young patient with a herniation migrating below the disk plane or upwards toward the next foraminal entrance, enzyme action on a fragment remote from the disk may appear uncertain, since the chymopapain is injected into the intervertebral space. Diskography alone, using anteroposterior and sagittal projections, is a poor indicator of contrast medium uptake by the disk. In contrast, the sensitivity of postdiskography CT is 100 times that of plain films and almost always demonstrates uptake by both the disk and the herniated fragment. Given the good opacifica-

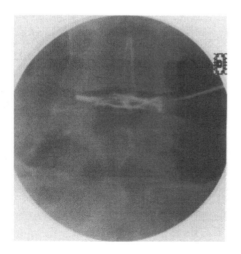

Fig. 63. L4–L5 normal; A-P diskography. The nucleus appears median, at a distance from the cartilaginous plates

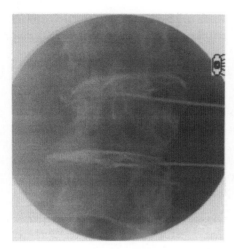

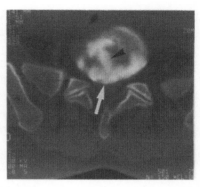

Fig. 68. Postdiskography CT scan of a degenerate L5-S1 disk. Filling of the median part corresponding to the nucleus *(arrowhead),* and of the peripheral anulus (—►)

Fig. 66. L3-L4 and L4-L5 diskography: degenerated disk. Filling of both disks by contrast; the contrast spreads throughout the entire intervertebral spaces, with irregular fringed contours

tion of the hernia as evidenced by postdiskography CT, a good uptake of the enzyme by the fragment, can be assumed (Figs. 65-68).

Postdiskography CT is evidently capable of providing direct images of almost all the types of herniation that we will subsequently consider: common herniations, migratory herniations and lateral-foraminal herniations.

The routine performance of postdiskography CT, usually after chemonucleolysis, has let to the following conclusions:

— The herniation almost always becomes saturated with contrast medium, given the hydrophilic nature of the nuclear substance.
— Disk herniations, though commonplace, include varieties which are barely suspected from standard CT findings. Postdiskography CT may show images of narrow orifices permitting the passage of a nuclear fragment through the anulus fibrosus, as well as totally unexpected signs of disk degeneration.
— By disk degeneration (as seen on postdiskography CT), we refer to the localized or global absence of differentiation between the nucleus pulposus and the anulus fibrosus. Disk degeneration in young subjects is often partial, particularly involving the posteromedian region of the disk.
— Postdiskography CT enables one to detect a possible ligamentous perforation associated with the herniation, by showing epidural leakage of contrast medium around the herniated fragment. This obviously indicates the intraspinal leakage of contrast medium during diskography.

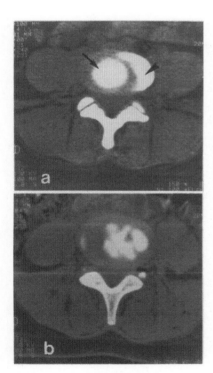

Fig. 67 a, b. Normal postdiskography CT at L4-L5 after intradiskal injection of 1 ml of Iopamiron 300. Two types of opacification are shown: **a** Homogeneous opacification of the nucleus pulposus, which has an even contour (—►). Adjacent cartilaginous plate *(arrowhead).* **b** In another case, the nucleus appears fragmented

— Using postdiskography CT, the sub- or trans-ligamentous location of a hernia may be precisely defined.

— In cases of femoral pain due to a lateral extraspinal herniation, postdiskography CT shows that the mechanisms are identical for posteromedian and posterolateral herniations (extrusion orifice, opacification of fragments in contact with a nerve root or ganglion).

— In very specific postoperative situations with clinical recurrence of sciatica, standard CT scans may prove inadequate, since they may be incapable of differentiating between scar tissue and a residual or recurrent fragment. Postdiskography CT may then be of great value, showing the existence of a fragment within the scar tissue.

— Finally, on a purely technical level, postdiskography CT shows partial peripheral annular opacification which is often barely hinted at in standard diskography.

In conclusion, the recent technique of postdiskography CT, usually performed after diskography and chemonucleolysis, confirms the signs on standard CT by showing the anular rupture or disk degeneration associated with the hernia. It also shows that the herniated fragment is accessible to both the contrast medium and the enzyme.

CT: Anatomic Aspects

The lumbar vertebral canal ensures the protection of the nervous structures. It is formed by 5 lumbar vertebrae, each of which is made up of a vertebral body anteriorly, a neural arch posteriorly, and two pedicles which unite the above.

In this chapter, we describe the normal CT appearance of the specific anatomic structures affected in pathologic conditions of the cauda equina nerve roots. CT studies rely on axial sections oriented according to the inclination of the disk. With other authors, we distinguish four basic section levels necessary for the examination of each dermatomal segment of the spine [59].

Section Through the Disk

The anterior wall of the lumbar vertebral canal is composed of the stacked intervertebral disks and vertebral bodies, lined posteriorly by the posterior longitudinal ligament [76, 123, 296] (Figs. 69–71).

The disk appears homogeneous, with a density of approximately 70 HU; it may be denser peripherally, because of a higher collagen content or a partial volume effect. However, it is not possible to differentiate between the nucleus and the anulus, as can be done using sagittal images on MRI. Disk degeneration is easily identified by disk collapse and the vacuum disk phenomenon. The posterior margin of a normal disk is well defined and even; it is usually concave at L2–L3 and L3–L4, horizontal and rectilinear at L4–L5, and slightly convex at L5–S1 [51].

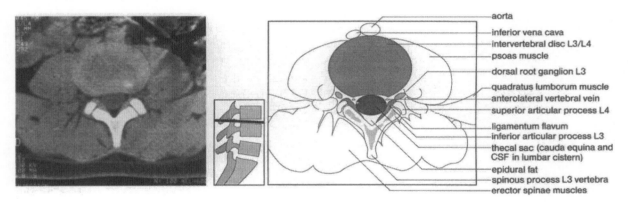

aorta
inferior vena cava
intervertebral disc L3/L4
psoas muscle
dorsal root ganglion L3
quadratus lumborum muscle
anterolateral vertebral vein
superior articular process L4
ligamentum flavum
inferior articular process L3
thecal sac (cauda equina and CSF in lumbar cistern)
epidural fat
spinous process L3 vertebra
erector spinae muscles

Fig. 69. Section through the L3–L4 disk. The L3 nerve roots exit via the L3–L4 intervertebral foramina; the posterior disk margin is slightly concave posteriorly

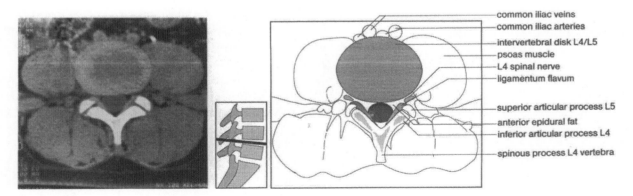

common iliac veins
common iliac arteries
intervertebral disk L4/L5
psoas muscle
L4 spinal nerve
ligamentum flavum
superior articular process L5
anterior epidural fat
inferior articular process L4
spinous process L4 vertebra

Fig. 70. Section through the L4–L5 disk. L4 roots are clearly visible laterally, within the foramen. It is at this level that one should search for a lateral foraminal herniation (responsible for femoral pain). The posterior disk margin is rectilinear. There is usually no epidural fat between the thecal sac and the disk

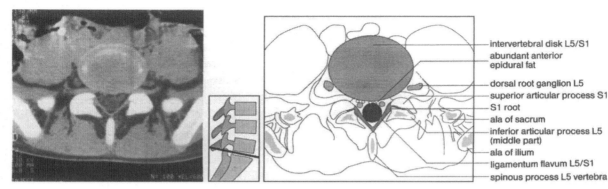

Labels in figure:
- intervertebral disk L5/S1
- abundant anterior epidural fat
- dorsal root ganglion L5
- superior articular process S1
- S1 root
- ala of sacrum
- inferior articular process L5 (middle part)
- ala of ilium
- ligamentum flavum L5/S1
- spinous process L5 vertebra

Fig. 71. Section through the L5–S1 disk. The disk is sometimes difficult to align, given its inclination. The S1 roots are free from the thecal sac and very well silhouetted by the epidural fat, which is usually abundant at this level. The poste-rior disk margin is slightly convex posteriorly. The L5 nerve roots follow the lateral margin of the disk after leaving the intervertebral foramina

The posterior longitudinal ligament is primarily composed of vertical fibers; it has a characteristic scalloped appearance, since it is wide opposite the disks and narrow behind the vertebral bodies. Its median portion is the most resistant, but its width gradually decreases in a caudal direction. It adheres to the posterior aspect of the disk [241]. Its hourglass shape, together with its disk insertions and centrally-located point of maximum resistance, resist median deformation of the disk and explain the preferential occurrence of disk herniations towards the intervertebral foramina [73]. Its transverse fibers may join the posterior extensions of the anterior longitudinal ligament to form protective girdle around the disk. Certain authors have reported the existence of an epidural membrane covering its entire posterior surface, whose role would be to protect the anterior aspect of the thecal sac [16, 19, 124]. The posterior longitudinal ligament has pain nerve-endings derived from the sinu-vertebral nerve where the ligament is adherent to the anulus. Ligamentous stretching may be responsible for lumbar pain of distal origin [299]. The resolution obtained by CT does not permit clear differentiation between the posterior disk margin, the posterior longitudinal ligament, the epidural veins and the dura mater.

Posteriorly, the *ligamenta flava,* which are approximately 3 mm thick, line the interlaminar intervals. Caudad, they are attached to the superior edge and posterior surface of the subjacent lamina, whereas cephalad, they are attached slightly anterior and superior to the lower edge of the overlying lamina; this facilitates flexion of the spine [72, 241]. The ligamenta flava join medially and posteriorly at the level of the spinous process of the subjacent vertebra. They take part in the formation of the capsule of the small articulations, lining them very laterally. During surgical fenestration, the lateral ligamentous excision should be limited to preserve the joint capsule [152]. The ligamenta flava are always clearly seen on CT, and any hypertrophy is evident. Although very elastic in young subjects, they progressively lose this property, tending to bulge anteriorly with lumbar spine extension and to thicken in reaction to hypertrophic changes of the neural arch (i. e., spinal stenosis) [72]. They may be the site of calcification [111].

Laterally, the articular processes (the superior process in front and the inferior process behind) make up the posterior wall of the next-cephalad intervertebral foramen. The nerve root ganglion lies close to the posterolateral disk margin, surrounded by the extraspinal fat.

The *epidural space,* which is occupied by fat and venous plexuses, lies between the disk and the nervous structures. The fat is particularly prominent at L5–S1; it is also a protective agent, filling the interstices and surrounding the thecal sac and nerve roots. The amount of fat depends on the size of the thecal sac and of the lumbar spinal canal. By virtue of its hypodensity (of about – 50 HU), it is a natural contrast medium, making an essential contribution to lumbar CT presentation.

The veins are intertwined with the posterior longitudinal ligament, fixed by the large basivertebral veins, and divided into anteromedial and anterolateral longitudinal plexuses which are very widely cross-anastomosed (rather like the rungs of a ladder). At the level of the lumbosacral junction, the lateral anterior epidural veins are found directly posterior to the medial anterior epidural veins, and join the network of sacral veins. The intricate relationship between these veins and the posterior longitudinal ligament favors the routine injection of Iopamidol prior to CT, in order to obtain excellent definition of the posterior disk margin (Fig. 72).

A disk herniation occupies the epidural space locally, constituting a CT sign [73] comparable in importance to the images of venous network lamination, displacement or amputation obtained with lumbar phlebography [233]. Obliteration of the epidural fat located posterior to the thecal sac is an indirect sign of anterior compression and backward displacement of the thecal sac. The veins of the anterior plexuses with a diameter greater than 2 or 3 mm are frequently visible in the anterior epidural fat, posterior to the L5-S1 disk [72, 196, 247, 258].

In cases of major thrombosis of the pelvic and abdominal veins, the veins of the plexuses participate in shunt formation and have increased diameters. They may then simulate a disk herniation on CT [72].

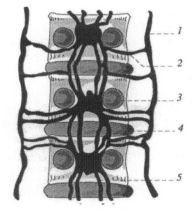

Fig. 72. Anterior epidural venous plexus. *1*, Ascending lumbar vein; *2*, Intervertebral veins; *3*, Basivertebral vein; *4*, Lateral anterior epidural vein; *5*, Medial anterior epidural vein

The thecal sac is located at the center of the epidural space. It constitutes the dura mater sheath for the cauda equina roots and extends from the T12-L1 intervertebral space down to S2 or the S1-S2 junction. It comprises two membranes: the arachnoid and the dura mater [72]. It has an oval shape at the level of L1 and becomes triangular midway down the lumbar spinal canal, adapting itself to the internal configuration of the canal. Below this level, its anteroposterior diameter and shape vary. The thecal sac sometimes retains its triangular shape as far as the lumbosacral level, or it may become cylindrical, tapered, narrow and detached from the walls of the canal [209].

The Cauda Equina Nerve Roots [141, 235, 237] include:

— The ventral motor rami from L2 to S5, which are responsible for mobility of the lower limbs, the perineum, and especially the striated-muscle sphincters.
— The dorsal sensory rami from L2 to S5, which carry superficial and deep sensory impulses from the lower limbs and perineum.
— The parasympathetic fibers, whose efferent elements are responsible for bladder, rectal and sexual activity (eg erection, ejaculation) and accompany the sacral motor rami from S2 to S4, and whose afferent elements accompany the sensory rami to the filum terminale (visceral, bladder and rectal sensation).

The *filum terminale* originates at the mid-portion of the cauda equina, and links the distal extremity of the medullary cone to the base of the thecal cul-de-sac; it prolongs the pia mater, is composed of primitive spongioblasts and is covered by ependymal cells. It is not visible on CT [72].

The nerve roots of the cauda equina are arranged in an arc which is concave anteriorly, and within the thecal sac. At each end of this arc, there are situated the right and left roots which will emerge at the next-caudad segment. At the center of the arc are the most caudal nerve roots. In contrast to the MRI appearances, the nerve roots are not usually visible within the thecal sac, having a homogeneous density of about 20 HU. They can be visualized only by an intrathecal injection of an iodinated contrast medium. Only the S1 roots are distinguishable in the discal plane, since they emerge from the thecal sac at the level of the L5-S1 intervertebral space or slightly above it, in contrast to the other roots, which emerge below the levels of the disks. As has been demonstrated by MRI, their initial course is a vertical descent over a considerable distance; the nerve roots appear as two antero-laterally-located cylindrical cross sections in relation to the thecal sac.

This section plane is fundamental, given the position of the two major factors involved in lumbar spine pathology: the disk and the posterior articular processes. Measurement of the diameter of the vertebral canal at this level would be interesting, but it is nevertheless difficult to perform, since there are no lateral boundaries (i. e. intervertebral foramina), the anterior and posterior limits are composed of soft tissues (the disk anteriorly and the ligamenta flava posteriorly) which vary according to the subject's position, and the posterior dihedron, located between the ligamenta flava, contains epidural fat and is seldom occupied by the thecal sac.

Only a measurement of the size is of the thecal sac possible, and even this varies according to the position (i.e., flexion-extension movements during myelography).

At this level, the thecal sac is often compressed anteriorly by the disk, and posterolaterally by the articular pillars and the ligamenta flava [206].

Section Through the Upper Portion of the Vertebral Body

This section passes through the upper third of the vertebra, and displays the nerve root sheath at the level of the upper portion of the bony groove of the lateral recess. The lateral recess effectively exists only at the level of the last two or three lumbar segments. Above these levels, the roots are much more horizontal and this anatomic concept is of no value [76, 123, 166, 168, 206, 235] (Figs. 73, 74).

The lateral recess is an anatomic-surgical concept. It is traversed by the extrathecal portion of the nerve root. Thus, it starts where the enveloped nerve root leaves the thecal sac and ends in continuity with the intervertebral opening. The lumbar spinal nerve emerges at this point.

Its posterosuperior wall is composed of the ligamentum flavum and the superior articular process. The latter is located anterior and medial to the inferior process of the vertebra above. The uniform facet joint space is 2 to 4 mm wide and has a more sagittal orientation in the upper lumbar vertebrae. Even in the absence of a pathologic condition, the joint space may appear empty [151].

Its anterior wall is composed of the posterior surface of the vertebral bodies covered by the posterior longitudinal ligament.

Its internal wall consists of the lateral aspect of the thecal sac.

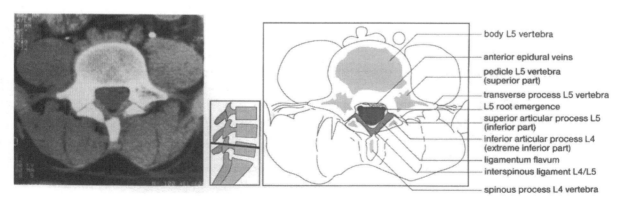

body L5 vertebra

anterior epidural veins

pedicle L5 vertebra (superior part)

transverse process L5 vertebra

L5 root emergence

superior articular process L5 (inferior part)

inferior articular process L4 (extreme inferior part)

ligamentum flavum

interspinous ligament L4/L5

spinous process L4 vertebra

Fig. 73. Section through the upper portion of the body of L5. The L5 nerve roots leaving the thecal sac appear as lateral mounds. The L4 roots are no longer visible within the psoas muscle

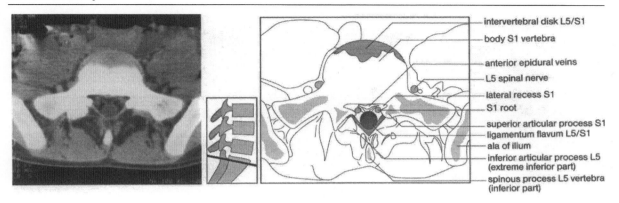

Fig. 74. Section through the upper portion of S1. The L5 roots course anterior to the alae of the sacrum, and medial to the sacroiliac joints. The lateral recesses here are quite distinct

Its external wall consists of the upper portion of the corresponding pedicle.

Vertically, the lateral recess extends from a horizontal line passing through the superior border of the pedicle to a horizontal line through its inferior border. The overall posterior and downward inclination of the posterior articular pillars results in the lateral recess becoming wider in its lower part. The critical zone for the nerve root is in the upper portion of the recess, where it is narrowest. It is this section level that should be used to measure the lateral recess. The normal anteroposterior diameter exceeds 5 mm; the recess is considered to be borderline in size, if between 3 and 5 mm and narrow if less than 3 mm [206]. However, these measurements are not very reliable: 13% of vertebrae are asymmetric, making orientation of the section plane the prime source of error. There is no significant relationship between the median sagittal diameter of the vertebral canal and the diameter of the lateral recess [168, 205].

Each root is numbered, as is the pedicle to which it is anatomically related. The lateral recesses at L4 and especially at L5 are particularly long and narrow, exposing the nerve roots to anterior disk compression, or to posterior bony compression.

On each side of every intervertebral segment, a pair of nerve roots consisting of a sensory dorsal root and a motor ventral root passes through the thecal sac toward the intervertebral foramen (the roots being enveloped by their dural sheaths) and form the spinal nerve roots. If the thecal sac ends at the level of the S1–S2 junction, the emergence level of each nerve root is constant. The emergence levels are as follows:

— the midsection of the L2 vertebral body for the L2 spinal roots (section through the midportion of the vertebral body);
— the upper third of the L3 vertebra for the L3 spinal roots (section through the upper portion of the vertebral body);
— the upper fourth of the L4 vertebra for the L4 spinal roots (section through the upper portion of the vertebral body);
— the upper fifth of the L5 vertebra for the L5 spinal roots (section through the upper portion of the vertebral body);
— the L5–S1 intervertebral space for the S1 spinal roots.

However, if the thecal sac ends at a lower level, each pair of roots emerges lower; the opposite applies if the thecal sac ends at a higher level.

Certain authors have used the term "root collar" to refer to the fibrous and rather rigid dural orifice corresponding to the emergence of the nerve root from the thecal sac, and to which the root is attached by a few connective tissue fibers. The external portion of each sheath, which is made up of dura mater, is also attached to the external margins of the intervertebral foramen by connective tissue fibers. Because of this, the nerve root is hardly mobile during its short epidural course of 3 to 4 cm, between the two attachments represented by the "root collar" and the intervertebral foramen [241]. This meningeal

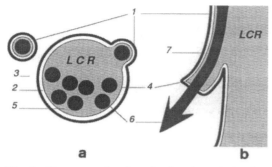

Fig. 75 a, b. Nerve root sheath. **a** Section through the thecal sac and nerve roots (the right root is free of the thecal sac; the left root is about to emerge). **b** The radicular sheath varies greatly in length: *1,* Dura mater; *2,* Subdural space (potential but cleavable between the dura mater and the arachnoid membrane); *3,* epidural space; *4,* arachnoid membrane; *5,* subarachnoid space; *6,* nerve root (covered by the pia mater); *7,* root sheath

arachno-dural sheath has a very variable length; it contains little CSF capable of being opacified by myelography [206] (Fig. 75).

At the level of its emergence, the nerve root may be compressed anteriorly by a disk herniation or a simple protrusion. The root involvement will be greater if its displacement backwards is hindered by a hypertrophied posterior arch and/ or ligamentum flavum occurring within the context of a spinal stenosis. Compression at this level may also occur posteriorly, at the level of the facet joint, as by an osteophyte or degenerative hypertrophy of the superior articular process [151, 158, 206].

The nerve root is even more vulnerable if the lateral recess through which it passes is deep and

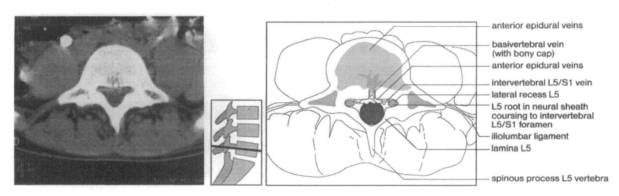

Fig. 76. Section through the midportion of the body of L5. The lateral recesses are distinguishable. The L5 roots are pressed against the internal aspect of the pedicles; their anteroposterior diameter may be measured at this level. This is where one should search for spinal stenosis with a trefoil appearance and pinched lateral recesses. The basivertebral vein is clearly seen

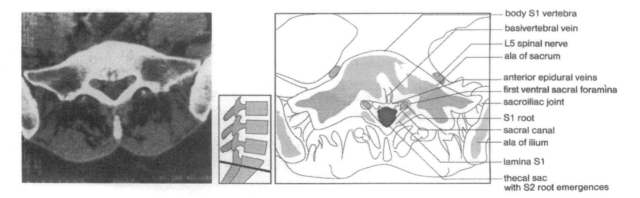

Fig. 77. Section through the midportion of S1. The S1 roots are about to enter the first sacral foramina. The S2 roots start to emerge from the thecal sac. The L5 roots still descend, anterior to the sacrum; they join the S1 roots after the latter emerge from the first sacral foramina. The sacroiliac joints are clearly seen

of borderline dimensions. In extreme cases, major narrowing of the lateral recess may itself be pathogenic, resulting in radicular claudication. Hypertrophy of the superior articular process is the major cause of lateral recess stenosis. At this level, it is often impossible to visualize the root by myelography since it is no longer enveloped by its arachno-dural sheath. The lateral recess is one of the preferential sites for disk fragment migration. A narrowed lateral recess is usually considered to be a contraindication to chemonucleolysis [166, 178, 206].

Section Through the Midportion of the Vertebral Body

This section passes though the middle third of the vertebra. It displays the inferior portion of the lateral recess, and the nerve roots which course obliquely outward and downward to exit from the spine via the intervertebral foramen. The roots may also be subjected to disk compression at this level, although (as we have seen) the lateral recess is wider in its lower portion [73, 76, 166] (Figs. 76, 77).

The vertebral canal appears as an intact ring containing the thecal sac posterior to the retrovertebral plexus. The basivertebral vein may give rise to a hypodense Y-shaped image within the vertebral body, with a posteromedian rupture of the cortical layer [72]. At the point where the basivertebral vein flows into the transverse anastomoses of the anterior internal vertebral plexus, there may exist a small bony spur or "cap bone" (to use Haughton's term), which should not be mistaken for an osteophyte or a calcified extruded herniation. The posterior longitudinal ligament is firmly attached to the posterior vertebral margins and bridges the nutrient foramen of the vertebral body posteriorly, adhering only slightly to the adjacent portions of the posterior vertebral surface [241, 258].

The groove-shaped posterior, wall of the canal is formed by the laminae; the deepest part of this groove corresponds to the junction of the laminae and the anterior cortical layer of the spinous process. There are no posterior longitudinal veins which are clearly identifiable throughout the extent of the lumbosacral spine, but certain levels there are small posteriorly-located veins [246, 247].

The facet joint and lamina make up the posterior wall of the epidural space, and the pedicle the lateral wall. The vertebral canal is shaped like an isosceles triangle at L1 and becomes an equilateral triangle by L5. This zone is usually compact and easily measured, since it is surrounded by an unbroken ring of bone. Several authors have studied the variations in the anteroposterior, interpedicular, and interarticular diameters of the canal in relation to individual lumbar segments.

The normal anteroposterior diameter at the narrowest segments exceeds 15 mm. A vertebral canal between 13 and 15 mm may be considered to be borderline, one between 12 and 13 mm as narrow, and below this as very narrow. However, the shape of the vertebral canal is more important than any numerical values. The progressive decrease in pedicular length accounts for the change in the shape of the canal, which is oval above and becomes triangular or trifoliate in the lower lumbar region. This level is virtually spared by degenerative lesions, being narrowed only in cases of constitutional stenosis, which are rare; it is of much less surgical interest than the disk region [205, 206].

The sections routinely made at this level are mainly aimed at searching for a possible migratory free disk fragment, especially if a subjacent herniation is present.

Section Through the Intervertebral Foramen

This section passes though the inferior third of the vertebra. It displays the exit of the nerve root from the lateral recess to the foraminal fat via the intervertebral foramen. The nerve root courses obliquely forward and outward, passes below the pedicle, and swells to form the spinal ganglion or dorsal root ganglion [76] (Figs. 78, 79).

The anterior limit of the section is formed by the overlying vertebral body above and by the disk below. The posterior limit is formed by the anterior aspect of the pedicle above and by the superior articular process of the subjacent vertebra below. Since the articular processes are almost sagittal in orientation the facet joint space

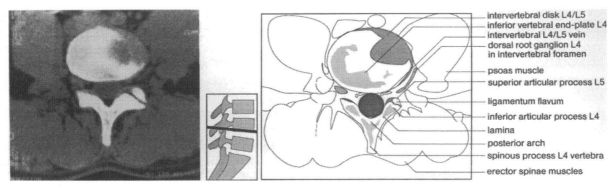

Fig. 78. Section through the L4–L5 intervertebral foramen. It contains the L4 nerve roots; the anteroposterior diameter of the spinal canal can be measured

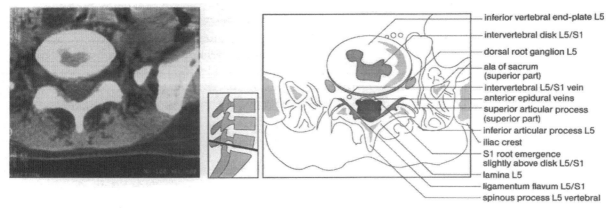

Fig. 79. Section through the L5–S1 intervertebral foramen. The L5 root accompanied by veins passes below the L5 pedicle and gives rise to the dorsal root ganglion within the L5–S1 intervertebral foramen, at the level of the extremities of the S1 superior articular processes. The origins of the S1 nerve roots on both sides of the thecal sac are visible as two small lateral protuberances

lies on the same plane as the intervertebral foramen.

The intervertebral foramen has the bilobed shape of an ear, with a superior portion formed by the vertebra above, and an inferior portion formed by the vertebra below. The transverse axis of each intervertebral foramen lies on the same horizontal plane as the spinous process of the superior vertebra. The diameter of the foramen increases progressively from one segment to the next-caudad one, except for the L5 foramina, which are the smallest of all, even though the largest roots pass through them. The L5 foramina are also the farthest from the median plane. The nerve root or spinal ganglion may be observed in the upper portion of the intervertebral foramen; it occupies only 35% to 50% of the to-

tal area, the rest being filled by fatty tissue, radicular vessels and the sinuvertebral nerve [73].

The epidural venous plexuses communicate with the extraspinal system (i.e. ascending lumbar veins) by means of the intervertebral vein; this system, which is of metameric origin, accompanies the root as a vascular sleeve which is sometimes recognizable [233, 235]. Shortly beyond the spinal ganglion, the nerve root divides into a ventral and a dorsal ramus. The dorsal ramus is not visible on CT [72].

In 1% to 3% of cases, two lumbar roots may arise conjointly from the thecal sac. The lower portion of the lateral recess and the intervertebral foramen are then filled with tissue having densities close to or greater than those of the thecal sac. A careful study of successive CT sections enables one to recognize the anomalous emergence of the two nerve roots, but sometimes only myelography is capable of confirming the diagnosis [72].

At the level of the intervertebral foramen, the nerve root may be compressed by an ascending disk fragment originating in the subjacent disk. A double radicular compression may be observed at this level: involvement of the nerve root originating at the same level as the disk, together with involvement of the upper root exiting via its intervertebral foramen.

There are two other possible causes of root compression at the intervertebral foramen:

— compression by the superior articular process of the underlying vertebra; this is often due to degenerative changes secondary to spontaneous or postoperative disk collapse (Crock's syndrome);
— compression by fibrous callus surrounding a zone of isthmic spondylolisthesis and by the slipping of the upper vertebra [206].

The Paraspinal Region

CT investigation of the lumbar spine permits examination not only of the lumbar vertebral canal, but also of the paraspinal region. The study of this region has become more important with the increasing indications for chemonucleolysis. The need for an extradural approach (usually posterolateral), implies passage of the needle through certain anatomic structures under normal conditions, and through others in case of technical error [299].

Paravertebral Muscles

The lumbar spine is framed by four muscular columns, formed on each side by the psoas major anteriorly, with attachments to the transverse processes, the disks and the cartilaginous plates of all the lumbar vertebrae [246], and by the lumbosacral muscle masses posteriorly. Between the above are the aponeurosis of the transversus abdominis muscle and the quadratus lumborum, which extends transversely between the transverse processes.

The existence of a coagulopathy is a contraindication to chemonucleolysis, as there is a risk of creating a hematoma in the psoas.

The Extraspinal Course
of the Lumbosacral Roots

Since the course of the L5 nerve root passes anterior to the sacroiliac joint, this explains its possible involvement in cases of sacroiliac tumors or trauma.

The intrasacral course of S1 is also noteworthy, by virtue of its distance and strictly vertical direction (as demonstrated by frontal MRI views). Given this anatomic situation, compression by a distant descending migratory disk fragment is possible.

The posterior fourth of the psoas muscle is crossed by the rami of the lumbar plexus which form the femoral nerve. During the posterolateral approach to the disk in chemonucleolysis, puncture of the anterior branch of a nerve roots which has just left the intervertebral foramen (i.e. L4 at L4–L5, and L5 at L5–S1) may provoke homolateral pain. Such a puncture close to the intervertebral foramen should be avoided in

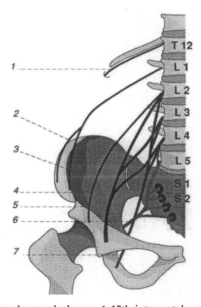

Fig. 80. Lumbosacral plexus; *1*, 12th intercostal nerve; *2*, Iliohypogastric nerve; *3*, Ilioinguinal nerve; *4*, Lateral cutaneous nerve of thigh; *5*, Femoral nerve; *6*, Sciatic nerve; *7*, Obturator nerve

view of the risk of enzyme diffusion towards the subarachnoid space, especially since neural cysts may occur at this level (Fig. 80).

The Ascending Lumbar Veins [247]

These are two large, irregular venous channels which originate in the posterosuperior aspect of the common iliac veins. After a short course directed upward and posteriorly, they ascend vertically along the anterior margin of the transverse processes of the lumbar vertebrae. At the thoracolumbar junction, they flow into the azygos vein on the right side and into the hemiazygos vein on the left side. They receive numerous veins from the paravertebral muscles, the vertebrae themselves, and the intervertebral veins. They are in communication with the inferior vena cava via the segmental lumbar veins, which course around the vertebral bodies. The physiology of this venous network is poorly understood; it is difficult to specify in which direction blood flows within a given segment.

An ascending lumbar vein, radicular artery, or even radiculomedullary artery may be punctured during chemonucleolysis, with exceptional opacification of the epidural veins at diskography. If the puncture is too medial, the needle will tend to glide along the lateral disk margin, ending up near the iliac vessels, and particularly the vein, which is more posteriorly located. Although this does not entail a risk of hemorrhage, thromboembolic complications are possible because of chymopapain-induced alterations of the vascular endothelium. Neurologic complications due to ischemia of the medullary cone have been reported [299].

Bowel

If the puncture is too lateral, the ascending colon and especially the cecum (the most posteriorly fixed structure) on the right, and the descending and sigmoid colon on the left, may be pierced. Such a transcolonic puncture may result in peritonitis, but more particularly in a combined spondylitis and discitis due to gramnegative microorganisms, and in a lesser degree, to staphylococci [286, 299].

Kidneys and Ureters

The kidneys and ureters are difficult to evaluate with limited exploration fields of 13 cm. In the performance of L3–L4 chemonucleolysis, or if there is renal displacement, there is a risk of damage to the renal parenchyma. Finally, if the needle goes beyond the anterior disk margin, there may be exceptional involvement of the ureter [299].

Consequences for the Nervous Structures

The dimensions and shape of the vertebral canal should be carefully studied. Three types of anatomic conditions may have pathologic consequences:

— a *discrepancy* between a particularly wide thecal sac and a normal or slightly narrow vertebral canal;
— a *definite narrowness* of the vertebral canal, which exposes the contained nervous structures to compression of diskal origin;
— an *abnormal* shape of the vertebral canal giving it a trifoliate aspect, especially when the lateral recess becomes very narrow as a result of hypertrophy of the posterior articular pillars and shortened vertebral pedicles. This abnormality is mainly found at the last two lumbar segments; it particularly exposes the nerve root to posterolateral compression from a simple bulging of the anulus fibrosus, which would be entirely asymptomatic with a normal vertebral canal.

Disk herniations, whether posterolateral or posterior, are of considerable pathogenetic importance, since they may compress to various degrees and according to their site:

— a nerve root in its extradural course;
— two nerve roots, close to the emergence of one of them;
— all or part of the cauda equina nerve roots.

In most cases, the disk herniation involves only one nerve root. All the intermediate forms may be observed between a simple nerve root irritation occurring only with certain spinal positions, and a severe persistent compression of the nerve

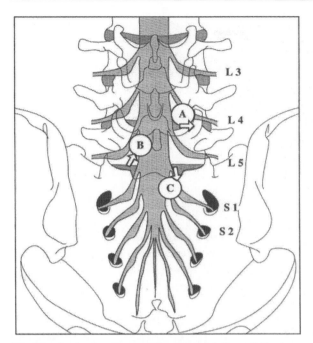

Fig. 81. Anatomico-topographic representation of the lumbosacral thecal sac and the cauda equina nerve roots. Shows the relationship between the thecal sac and nerve roots, and the intervertebral disks and foramina. *A,* an L4–L5 foraminal herniation which laterally compresses the L4 nerve root. *B,* an ascending L5–S1 disk herniation which may compress the L5 and S1 nerve roots. *C,* a descending L5–S1 migratory disk herniation compressing the S1 and S2 nerve roots

If the herniation is more medially located and sufficiently large, it compresses the nerve root which has just left the thecal sac as well as the border of the sac, and through the latter, one or more nerve roots within (Fig. 81).

Persistent tissue involvement of mechanical origin may elicit a local reaction resulting in the formation of various degrees of adhesion between the nerve root and the herniation, or between the herniation and the thecal sac; in certain cases, there is actual localized inflammation of the epidural space. Surgeons are well-acquainted with these adherent herniations, whose excision is always difficult. Such herniations respond poorly to conservative treatment.

If the nerve root compression of diskal origin is severe, it may evoke an acute inflammation of the root, which becomes red, congested and swollen (a condition which corresponds to hyperalgesic sciatica). In such cases, there may be significant secondary fibrosis around the nerve root, resulting in perineural thickening, adhesion of the root to its sheath, and of the whole structure to the disk and thecal sac.

A nerve root which has become so inflamed remains sensitive for several years; the slightest traction during movement and even the physico-chemical modifications due to atmospheric changes are sufficient to re-evoke the so-called residual sciatic pain [233].

By permitting an optimal investigation of the relationship between the enclosing structures and their contents, CT has proved an exceptionally valuable technique for investigating nerve root lesions of diskal origin. It is currently the examination of choice in sciatica, visualizing both the disk abnormalities and associated conditions such as degenerative changes of the lateral recess or of the lumbar vertebral canal itself. This detailed CT anatomy accounts for the superiority of CT in the detailed study of a pathologic segment over the indirect evidence furnished by myelography.

root by the herniation. Whether root compression occurs depends not only on the size, site and reducibility of the herniation, but also on the shape and dimensions of the vertebral canal. A small, irreducible herniation located just in front of the root collar in a subject with a narrow or trifoliate lumbar vertebral canal may result in more severe root compression than a larger herniation occurring away from the root collar, at a site where the root is more mobile, and in a subject with a wide lumbar vertebral canal. This explains the lack of a consistent correlation between the radiographic and the clinical findings.

Computed Tomography Technique

This chapter deals with our CT technique, our methodology and our imaging approach to lumbar disk herniations.

CT Examination Technique

The CT diagnosis of disk herniation requires an image of the utmost quality, which is achieved only with the most rigorous technique. Experience also plays an important part in the final quality of the examination. The machine should be a scanner having a high resolution and the capability of locating sections on lateral digital radiographs (scout view). The ability to perform thin sections (1 to 1.5 mm) is also necessary. Finally, total patient cooperation is indispensable (i.e., absolute stillness); it can be obtained through a good understanding of the examination procedure.

The Patient

An intravenous catheter is routinely inserted just prior to the examination and an injection of 100 ml of an iodinated water-soluble contrast medium is given in the fasting patient, in order to opacify the richly developed epidural venous network and thus obtain a better definition of the posterior margin of the intervertebral disk. This injection is all the more useful in elderly patients, who have a lumbar spinal canal of borderline dimensions (almost a narrowed canal). In patients with an atopic background or known allergies, medical preparation is carried out during the three days prior to the examination. A contrast medium is required which has a high iodine concentration, is well tolerated by the venous system, and provokes a minimum of nausea. We currently use nonionic substances, especially Iopamiron 300, a nonionic triiodinated contrast medium with a 30% iodine content (Schering Laboratories, Lys-lez-Lannoy, France).

The injection is not given as a bolus but over about 30 seconds. Untoward incidents due to intolerance of the contrast medium are infrequent; the treatment is the same as for other incidents involving hypersensitivity to iodine.

The routine use of intravenous contrast medium is accepted in studies of the cervical spine; however, many authors perform the injection at the lumbar level only for postoperative evaluation. We believe that the improved contrast quality of the injection image and its informative value justify routine injection [27, 38, 74, 76, 88, 93, 109, 249].

The patient is positioned as comfortably as possible in the supine position on an inclined plane, with both hips and knees flexed, so as to reduce the lumbosacral lordosis as much as possible [88, 109].

The arms are placed behind the head in order to avoid the artifacts created at the abdominal and pelvic levels when they remain alongside the body. It is not necessary for the patient to hold his breath during sections through the last lumbar segments; calm and rhythmic breathing does not provoke movement of the spine at this level.

Sections

The apparatus we use is a CGR CE 10000 CT scanner. Its technical specifications are as follows: 130 kv, 100 mA, and an acquisition time of 6.8 seconds.

The localization of sections by a profile scout view is essential. If the patient is correctly positioned and not scoliotic, then all the intervertebral disks are perfectly aligned, since the radiation is not divergent as in conventional radiographs [206]. Section planes are oriented so as to be parallel to the plane of the intervertebral disk (a bisector of the angle formed by the two adjacent cartilaginous end-plates) [131]. The use of an inclined plane beneath the patient's back usually allows correct alignment of the L5–S1 disk, with a maximum gantry angling of −20°. If tilting is too pronounced, certain authors advocate the performance of overlapping sections of the last disk followed by reconstruction of this last intervertebral space in the sagittal and coronal planes [88]. We perform only axial sections, since the quality of the three-dimensional reconstruction available to us is not sufficiently informative. Sections are numbered in order to facilitate localization during their interpretation. The selection of the study site obviously depends on the region of clinical interest; thus, the region usually selected in sciatica is that of the last two disks. These should be routinely investigated, even if the clinical signs are typical of the isolated involvement of one segment; this is necessary because of possible discordance between the anatomic lesion and the clinical signs [152] or of a double herniation affecting both levels.

These two segments are explored by means of thin, parallel axial sections 1,5 mm thick performed at 2 mm intervals. The first section passes through the uppermost portion of the intervertebral disk; the penultimate section shows the radicular emergences in the plane passing through the midportion of the vertebral body; a final section is performed 5 or 6 mm caudad in order to rule out a possible free fragment. Each level is therefore explored with about 7 sections. The entire examination (about 14 sections) thus lasts about 6 to 8 min. In case of small herniations, intermediate contiguous sections may be helpful. Migratory disk herniations call for supplementary sections, either cephalad in the intervertebral foramen (ascending herniation) or caudad in the case of a migratory free fragment (descending herniation). In cases with femoral pain, in addition to the study of the last two levels, a study of the L3–L4 disk and L4 intervertebral foramen must be routine. Certain authors even recommend the routine performance of a so-called "safety" section at the level of the L3–L4 disk. In cases of sciatica with clinical signs suggesting S1 root compression but negative upon exploration, the performance of more caudad sections may be useful in searching for a lesion of the sacrum or sacral canal [206].

All sections are reconstructed on a 131 mm field with a 512 × 512 matrix and an F2 convolution filter. The window setting (100 Hounsfield units or HU) and its width (600 HU) are always the same; they permit a good study of the soft tissues, and disk material in particular, as well as an evaluation of the bony lumbar canal. Nevertheless, if there is associated bone pathology

(i. e., spinal stenosis or facet joint disease) a bony window with a setting of 250 HU and a width of 1600 HU may be helpful. The views are recorded on multiformat films, with enlargement of pathologic sections.

Qualitative Criteria of CT Images

The quality of a CT image depends on [109] its contrast resolution, its spatial resolution, and possible artifacts.

Contrast Resolution is the ability to distinguish structures having a density which differs little from that of their environment. It is limited by the "background noise" due to signals showing interference. Background noise is inversely proportional to the amount of X-ray radiation picked up by the detectors, and therefore, to the thickness of the section. The thicker the section, the better the contrast resolution [191].

Our experience has shown that there are low densities at the level of the spinal column (densities close to those of disk material and epidural veins, and densities intermediate between a recurrent herniation and a postoperative fibrosis). We do not perform 5 mm-thick sections at this level, as advocated by numerous authors, but attach greater importance to the features of lesions seen on thin sections [88, 109, 135].

Spatial Resolution is the ability to distinguish one high-contrast small detail from another. It depends on the specification of the CT scanner and is inversely proportional to the section thickness.

Artifacts are more or less structured interfering elements found in the reconstructed image, but which do not exist in the actual subject. Their elimination or identification is necessary for a correct interpretation of disk images [191].

Artifacts due to movement

Involuntary patient movements during the examination, especially in hyperalgesic sciatica, may be avoided with good patient cooperation and comfortable patient positioning (it is seldom impossible to maintain the inclined position because of pain). These artifacts are responsible for streaks and blurred contours.

Bowel gas motion during image acquisition may also interfere with the image.

Artifacts due to sudden density variations

The presence of very dense material in the region under examination, whether it be exogenous (eg metallic objects, lipiodol droplets or opacified ureters) or endogenous (eg calcified atheromatous plaques, or thickened cortical bone, especially at the posterior articular processes), may result in linear or star artifacts. Contrast resolution errors may occur along certain axes. On the other hand, the very low density of the air within bowel structures may create linear artifacts, especially if there is associated movement.

Artifacts due to beam hardening

The hardening of an incident polychromatic beam during its passage through very opaque structures ("facet joint artifacts" of the posterior articular facet) results in contrast resolution problems involving streaks of different widths.

Artifacts due to partial volume effect

A unit volume ("voxel") may contain two adjacent structures having very different densities; the resulting image ("pixel") takes on an intermediate density which does not correspond to either structure. This effect can be reduced to a minimum by performing thin millimetric sections. Nevertheless, the effect may appear on sections tangential to a bony structure (pedicle, ring apophysis, joint facet, etc).

Circular artifacts due to calibration

These appear at the center of rotation of the machine, in the form of concentric rings. They are the result of faulty calibration of certain detectors, and give rise to disordered spatial and contrast resolution. Nevertheless, they are quite rare in the lumbar spine, in comparison to the cervical spine and especially the skull.

Artifacts due to the patient's weight

Overweight remains a handicap even with the most modern scanners. The image acquires a "granite-like" grainy appearance which also seriously disrupts spatial and contrast resolution at the level of the lumbar spinal canal.

Artifacts due to a faulty section plane

Scoliosis with an asymmetric section plane results in a deformed, asymmetric image with false protrusion images capable of leading to false-positive diagnoses.

An insufficiently inclined section plane, particularly at the L5–S1 level, complicates the analysis of the posterior disk magin. The latter appears on every section as a short segment enclosed by two bony segments.

Irradiation and Cost [80, 99]

High-resolution axial CT scan sections of 1 mm may result in radiation doses ranging from 2.5 to 4.2 rads (0.025 to 0.042 Gy), according to the milliamperage chosen [65, 80, 99]. This irradiation remains very localized because of the strong collimation of the incident beam. The examination may thus be repeated without risk of radiation overdose, especially since there are no sensitive organs in the section planes (as in the case of the lens of the eye in axial hypophyseal sections). However, the radiographic mode (scout view) delivers a radiation dose to the ovaries which is by no means negligible (0.325 rads); it is therefore recommended that only one such section be performed during the examination. The radiation dose delivered during myelography is greater (6 to 7 rads at skin level) and is much more variable according to the settings used. These are affected by factors such as obesity.

The official cost assignment of the examinations is artificial and does not correspond to the real cost. The price differences between hospital and private outpatient procedures are questionable. The French listing does not reflect economic realities. Thus, the cost of a CT examination is underestimated in France (Z 90, or about 900 FF = $ 150); its exact price is difficult to determine but is usually estimated at double the official figure. Moreover, it is undoubtedly the least expensive examination. Myelography is never performed on an outpatient basis but requires a 2-day hospital stay, thereby increasing its cost. It has a baseline rating of K 15 + Z 20, to which is added Z 2.5 per view.

Methodology and Approach to Herniation Imaging

This work is based on four years of experience (from 1984 through 1990) of CT investigation of sciatica in the Radiology III Department of the Strasbourg-Hautepierre University Hospital (using a CGR CE 10 000 scanner). In all 2500 disk herniations were studied. With few exceptions, 900 of these patients were operated on in the Neurosurgery Department after a CT scan work-up alone.

Though lumbar disk herniation, is a very common condition, the images actually relate to a number of different entities. These should be identified according to their level, extent, possible existence of a free fragment, or possible association of osteophytes with a narrowed lumbar spinal canal. At the level incriminated one must look for an associated intervertebral collapse or vacuum disk phenomenon. Whatever the findings, the other level (L4–L5 or L5–S1) is routinely investigated.

Based on the CT appearance of the herniation, we distinguish several subgroups as follows:

Common herniation. These are the ones most commonly found, are easily diagnosed, and remain close to the discal plane in a posterior position.

Calcified herniation. These are mostly herniations with disk calcification, but also those with a calcified posterior longitudinal ligament, or even a compressive retrovertebral osteophytosis.

Migratory herniation. These are herniations with migration of all or part of the nucleus pulposus away from the disk and the intervertebral space.

Foramino-lateral herniation. These are herniations which are found in the intervertebral foramen, or even extraspinally outside the foramen, thus requiring the performance of supplementary CT sections.

Double herniations. The association of two herniations simultaneously involving two disk levels.

Difficult herniations or diagnostic error. These are herniations presenting CT interpretation problems, as well as false-positives and false-negatives.

Postoperative herniation. These are postoperative failures in which, after follow-up CT examination, the patients are reoperated. Related to these are the Postchemonucleolysis herniations, which will be subsequently considered.

This classification is quite arbitrary, and interrelations between the different subgroups exist (eg a calcified migratory herniation).

The CT-surgical correlations in our series were distributed as follows (Fig. 82).

Common herniations are the most frequent (41%), with migratory herniations second (18%), and then equal numbers of postoperative herniations and herniations presenting CT interpretation problems (14% each). Double herniations (6%), foramino-lateral herniations (4%) and calcified herniations (3%) are much less frequent.

The factors to be routinely noted include:

— the *location* of the lesion at the affected level: posterolateral (isolated unilateral overlap of the posterior disk margin), posteromedian, simple bulging or posterior protrusion (symmetrical and even overlap), or foraminal (within the intervertebral foramen) lateral (extraspinal)
— its *size*: small, medium, or large
— the *existence of a hypodense zone* within the herniation image, indicative of nuclear substance
— its *mode of presentation:* above the disk, directly in the plane of the disk, or better seen below the disk plane

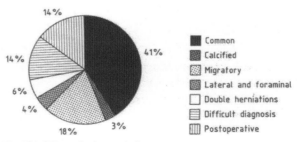

Fig. 82. CT-surgical correlations

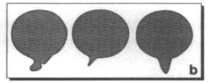

Fig. 83 a, b. Method 1. Varieties of posterior diskprotrusion. **a** smooth protrusion **b** abrupt protrusions

— the *existence of a rupture* of the posterior disk margin, indicative of a localized rupture of the anulus fibrosus fibers
— the *structure* of the herniation; we distinguish two structural types (Fig. 83): *regular* (smoothly sloping, and without violent rupture of the posterior disk margin) and *abrupt* (with breaking-off of the posterior margin)
— the *vertebral extension*: ascending or descending. The distance of ascending herniations from the superior disk margin and of descending ones from the inferior disk margin is then assessed in mm. There may be image discontinuity in successive sections involving the herniation.
— *signs of nerve root involvement:* nerve root visible or not
— *signs of diskal root compression:* displacement, swelling, deformation, dense root, possible root emergence abnormalities (e. g. conjoined roots)
— *epidural fat abnormalities:* simple asymmetry, filling-in, obliteration
— *thecal sac deviation*
— the *existence of calcification:* disk, ligamentous, ring apophysis, osteophyte
— *diagnostic difficulty,* usually due to a narrow lumbar spinal canal
— in postoperative CT, the possible *existence of scar tissue or fibrosis*

If there has been an operation, the following should be noted:

— level
— surgical approach: fenestration (the most frequent), hemilaminectomy, or possibly facetectomy and foraminotomy
— appearance of nerve root (e. g. stretched or edematous) and its position

— herniation: posterior longitudinal ligament is torn or not, existence of free fragments, migration
— possible presence of a narrow lumbar spinal canal or of narrow lateral recesses
— associated calcification or degenerative lesions
— in secondary operations, the relative contributions to the pathology of fibrosis and recurrent herniation

All the images shown in this work are the correlations of the CT and surgical findings, save for certain cases of femoral pain due to very lateral herniations, where the current treatment of choice is chemonucleolysis or intradiscal injection of corticosteroids.

Before examining each subgroup, it is useful to consider the principal clinical features.

Radiation of lumbosciatic pain
All patients exhibited radiation of sciatic pain into the L4, L5 or S1 dermatomes, or incomplete radiation (eg to the leg) hindering an accurate topographic diagnosis, or a combined radiation (essentially L5 and S1). The typical L4 and L5 radiations clearly predominate (79% in one series of 160 CT-surgical correlations) (Fig. 84).

Femoral pain seldom leads to surgery (4%); it is due in most cases to an L4–L5 foramino-lateral herniation or, less frequently, to an L3–L4 herniation within the vertebral canal. In routine practice, the CT investigation of femoral pain begins at the L4–L5 level, with sections centered on the subjacent foramen, which is where the L4 root emerges. If the results are negative, the

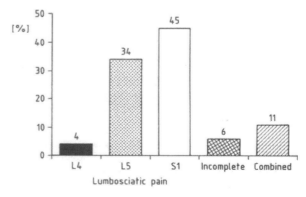

Fig. 84. Distribution of lumbosciatic pain

L3-L4 level is then investigated paying detailed attention to the foramen in order to explore the extraspinal course of L3.

There is always the possibility of an anatomic-clinical discrepancy, which is more frequent in cases of L5 sciatica; an L5-S1 disk herniation results in L5 sciatica in 15% of cases, and an L4-L5 herniation results in S1 sciatica in 3% of cases.

Incomplete pain radiations occurs mainly in L5-S1 disk herniations (80%), and to a lesser degree in L4-L5 herniations (20%).

Combined L5 and S1 radiations is secondary to herniation at both L4-L5 (55%) and L5-S1 (45%). It occurs in about 10% of cases.

The value of accurate CT diagnosis of the lesional level is evident, given the imperfect correlation between the clinical features and the location of the herniation, and the existence of poorly systematized pain radiation.

The medical history refers to preceding trauma or violent exertion in only 6% of cases. On the other hand, chronic lumbago or recurrent episodes of sciatic pain is reported in 30% of cases.

Duration of Clinical Signs. The mean duration of the clinical features, from the onset of pain until surgery is performed, is 4.1 months.

Distribution according to different herniation levels. The distribution according to the levels involved is as follows (Fig. 85).

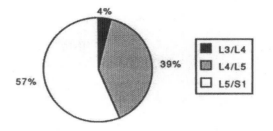

Fig. 85. Distribution according to different herniation levels

Reliability of CT
(in 160 CT-Surgical Correlations)

As stated, there were 6 false-positives in our series (3 during our first few months of using CT) as well as 2 false-negatives: a total of 8 incorrect CT interpretations. The reliability is thus estimated at 95%. This figure is somewhat better than those given in the literature (85% to 90%), which may be explained by the routine performance of millimetric sections every 2 mm and of intravenous injection of contrast medium [15, 38, 48, 76, 88, 109, 207].

False-positives and false-negatives were infrequent during the last 18 months of the study; for a total of 900 herniations operated on out of 2500 herniations diagnosed on CT, the reliability was undoubtedly somewhat greater than the 95% obtained in our series of CT-surgical correlations.

Common Herniations

A disk herniation is defined as the passage of all or part of the nucleus through a gap in the anulus fibrosus. The herniated portion of the nucleus elevates or even perforates that portion of the posterior longitudinal ligament opposite the gap [206]. This subgroup of "common" herniations comprises all disk herniations easily diagnosed on CT, which remained opposite or close to the intervertebral space and had a posterior expansion toward the spinal canal. Calcified herniations and herniations involving a previously operated disk are excluded.

Clinical Considerations

By definition, common herniations constitute the largest subgroup (41% of the entire series).

In cases eventually operated on, the preoperative duration of the clinical symptoms was lengthy (an average of 4.5 months), underlining the resistance to medical treatment.

The neurologic findings were usually slightly abnormal; sciatica with a motor deficit was rare, less frequent than in the series as a whole. The deficit varied in severity, but was usually slight. There were no paralytic sciaticas, but a cauda equina syndrome necessitated emergency operation immediately after CT study.

A sensory deficit (hypoesthesia of the corresponding dermatome) was either an isolated finding or occurred in conjunction with a motor deficit.

On the other hand, impairment of the Achilles tendon reflex was common, comparable in frequency to that of herniations as a whole. The quadriceps reflex was not affected.

CT Features

The CT findings should provide a good idea of the anatomic nature of the disk lesion. However, there is a problem here, since, contrary to MRI, the posterior longitudinal ligament is not directly seen [109, 113, 116], and indirect evidence must be used to determine its integrity or perforation. Moreover, this subgroup of herniations is heterogeneous, and does not correspond to a specific anatomic variety.

The CT diagnosis of a disk herniation relies on direct signs of an altered disk image and on *indirect signs* as regards the epidural fat, nerve roots and thecal sac.

Direct Signs of Disk Lesions
[29, 38, 74, 76, 88, 93, 98, 188, 225, 309, 314]

Focalized Deformation of the Posterior Disk Margin

This is a constant sign which is the direct expression of the passage of disk material beyond the normal limits of the anulus and into the spinal canal. The routine intravenous injection of contrast medium enhances the posterior disk margin particularly well, by opacification of the adherent anterior portion of the epidural venous plexus. This opacification is even more useful in cases of lumbar spinal stenosis (especially at L4–L5), in which the anterior epidural fat no longer closely conforms to the posterior border of the disk [109].

Two types of deformation of the disk margin may be distinguished:

— a smooth protrusion with a gentle contour and no sudden break in the disk outline; this is found in 75% of cases (Figs. 86, 87);
— a sharp, pointed protrusion with an abrupt break in the disk boundary; this sign is found in only 25% of cases (Figs. 88, 89).

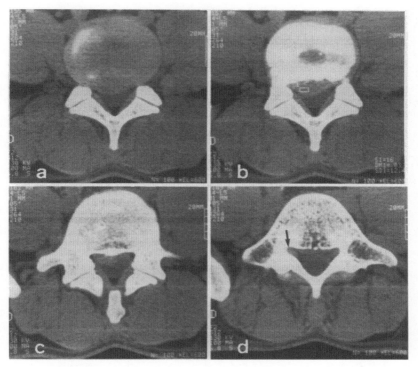

Fig. 86 a–d. 40-year-old man. Right L5 sciatica without neuro-deficit: common type of right diskal herniation at L4–L5. **a** Homogeneous, smooth diskal prolapse is well seen below the diskal plane after intravenous injection of contrast medium (as an 75% of all common herniations); in this case there is a right posterolateral herniation. **a–c** Herniation extends to the pars interarticularis in the upper part of the lateral recess.

Anterior epidural fat has been obliterated. **d** Deformed (65% of all cases), hyperdense (80% of all cases) appearance of the right L5 root in the plane of section through the midportion of L5: this is representative of radicular involvement below the compression site (→). *Operative findings:* Preligamentous disk herniation with smooth (94% of all cases) overlap

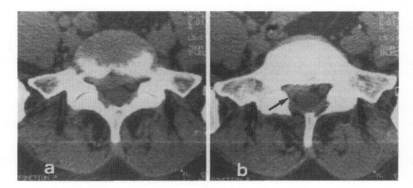

Fig. 87 a, b. 30-year-old woman. Right S1 sciatica of 2 months' duration. Common right disk herniation at L5–S1. **a** Right posterolateral disk prolapse is very even; the herniation is homogeneous. **b** Herniation descends to the axillary part of the S1 root, which is deformed and compressed against the articular pillar (→). *Operative findings:* Preligamentous disk herniation; however, the posterior longitudinal ligament is undergoing perforation (undetectable on CT)

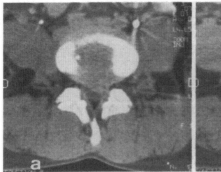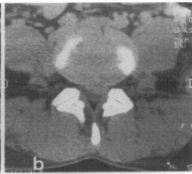

Fig. 88 a, b. 35-year-old woman. Left L5 sciatica of 3 months' duration without neuro-deficit. Common left posterolateral disk herniation at L4–L5. **a** Disk prolapse is abrupt (25% of all common herniations) and readily visible in the disk plane.

b Herniation compresses left L5 root at its emergence from the thecal sac. *Operative findings:* Ligamentous rupture with a large buttonhole herniation. An abrupt overlap is found in 40% of CT of transligamentous herniations

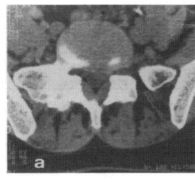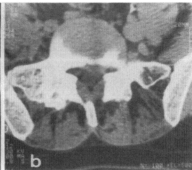

Fig. 89 a, b. 40-year-old woman. Left S1 sciatica of 3 weeks' duration. Left posterolateral disk herniation at L5–S1. **a** Very abrupt disk prolapse in lateral recess; such an overlap is associated with a transligamentous herniation in only 60% of cases. **b** Left S1 root is compressed in the upper part of the

lateral recess. Obliteration of epidural fat at this site; the root is distinguished with difficulty. *Operative findings:* Perforation of the posterior longitudinal ligament; buttonhole disk herniation located at axillary portion of S1 root

It is tempting to associate a smooth protrusion with a subligamentous herniation and an abrupt protrusion with a transligamentous herniation, and there was quite a good correlation in our series. Nevertheless, although 75% of smooth protrusions were subligamentous herniations, a ligamentous perforation was present in 25%. Again, an abrupt protrusion corresponded to a transligamentous herniation in only 60% of cases, to which can be added 17% for subligamentous free fragments. The correlation is therefore invalid in approximately 25% of cases, despite the use of optimum CT capabilities (i. e., millimetric sections and a 512 × 512 matrix).

Rupture of Posterior Disk Margin

The posterior disk margin may assume a blurred fringed appearance, and even show a loss of continuity. This represents a rupture of the anulus fibrosus fibers and the passage of nuclear material through this gap (Fig. 90). In common herniations, this is a rare (10%) sign of great value. At operation, the surgeon finds either a ligamentous rupture or a subligamentous free fragment.

Horizontal Location

According to classical descriptions, most herniations tend to occur posterolaterally, in an area of ligamentous weakness (see Fig. 86). The rest have a posterior or paramedian location, and prove to be commoner than was supposed prior to the advent of CT [109, 206, 299] (Fig. 91).

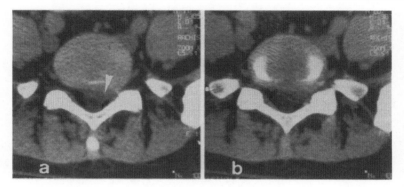

Fig. 90 a, b. 47-year-old woman. Left S1 sciatica with modest motor deficit. Left posterolateral L5–S1 herniation. **a–b** Tear of posterior margin of disk, which has an indistinct, fringed appearance (arrowhead). This infrequent finding (10%) in common herniations corresponds to either a transligamen-tous herniation or a preligamentous free fragment. *Operative findings:* Preligamentous herniation in the process of perfo-rating the posterior longitudinal ligament; excision of several free fragments. Such a rupture of the posterior disk margin is commonar in transligamentous herniations (30%)

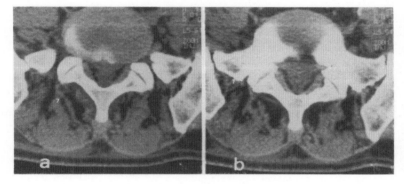

Fig. 91 a, b. 43-year-old man. Left S1 sciatica of 2 months' duration, with a modest neuro-deficit. Posteromedian L5–S1 herniation, which is less frequent than posterolateral lesions. **a** Posterior margin of the herniation is visible in diskal plane, less well below it. **b** Recession of thecal sac with disappear-ance of posterior epidural fat; the anterolateral epidural fat is less invaded and remains symmetrical. *Operative findings:* Ligamentous rupture and large free fragment. The abrupt dis-kal overlap was a feature of transligamentous herniation

CT Appearances

The herniation is visible on sections through the disk plane in 74% of cases. Nevertheless, it has a tendency to be slightly descending and to coil up in the concavity of the vertebral body, below the ring apophysis (see Fig. 86). This is even more likely if the ring apophysis of the subjacent carti-laginous plate ascends slightly. The herniation is often better seen below the disk plane, thus pos-sibly giving rise to false-negatives if the investiga-tion is limited to the disk plane (Figs. 92, 93).

Hypodense Areas [3]

No great value is to be attached to densities for differentiating between the disk and the epidural veins or fibrosis. On the other hand, the existence of hypodensities (30–50 HU) *within* the hernia-tion should always be carefully sought. These may be small, well-defined, easily detected hypo-dense nodules or, on the contrary, blurred areas which are difficult to detect unless routinely sought. Sometimes the hypodense lesion is large, almost entirely occupying the herniation; this was the case, in 30% of common herniations.

This hypodense image indicates the presence of an abnormally located nucleus and probably that of a free fragment. Such a fragment is the di-rect result of migration of disk material (in this

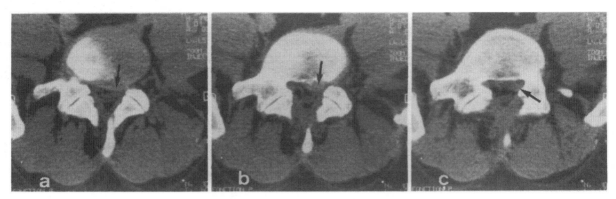

Fig. 92 a-c. 41-year-old man. Left L5 sciatica of 10 months' duration. Left posterolateral L4-L5 herniation. **a-b** Homogeneous herniation is better visualized below the diskal plane. Discontinuity of sections **a** and **b** (→). **c** Herniation assumes an oval shape at axillary portion of left S1 root. The flattened root is deviated posteriorly and compressed against the articular pillar (→). *Operative findings:* Free fragment adjacent to nucleus pulposus. Such a discontinuity in CT is always indicative of a free fragment, most often transligamentous (80% of cases)

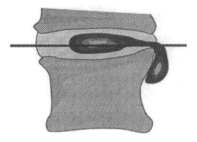

Fig. 93. Common herniations 1. Inclination of the section plane. The herniation has a tendency to collect beneath the ring apophysis and in the concavity of the vertebral body, especially since the ring apophysis of the caudad end-plate ascends slightly. Caudad extension of the herniation may appear to be greater, because of the elevated position of the ring apophysis

case the nucleus pulposus). It has lost its attachments to the nucleus but may remain contiguous with the anulus fibrosus, whether the free fragment be subligamentous or, as is more usually the case transligamentous (Fig. 94).

Such cases are not absolute contraindications to chemonucleolysis, since the chymopapain can still reach the free fragment, as shown by postdiskography CT. On the other hand, the fragment may migrate to some distance from the intervertebral space, a classical contraindication to chemonucleolysis. The migratory herniation is considered later.

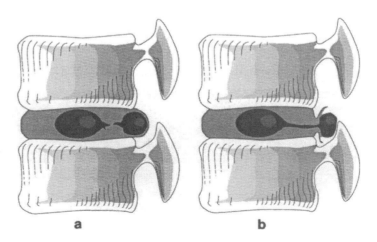

Fig. 94 a, b. Common herniations 2. Free disk fragments **a** Subligamentous **b** Transligamentous

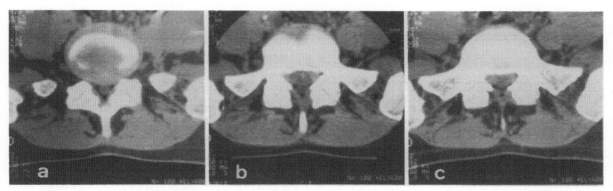

Fig. 95 a–c. 25-year-old woman. Right S1 sciatica. Postero-median disk herniation. **a–b** Herniation more visible below diskal plane. Wide, hypodense area (this is found in 30% of all common herniations and is indicative of a free fragment in two-thirds of cases, of which one quarter are preligamen-tous). Posterior margin of disk is even and bulging, indicating integrity of the posterior longitudinal ligament. **c** Displacement of thecal sac. *Operative findings:* Large, preligamentous free fragment. 75% of preligamentous free fragments are visible as hypodensities on CT

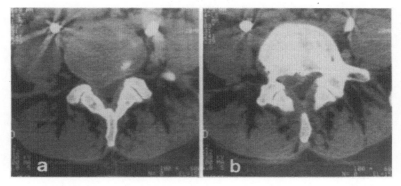

Fig. 96 a, b. 44-year-old woman. Right L5 sciatica of 3 weeks' duration with a modest neuro-deficit. Right posterolateral L4–L5 herniation. **a** A hypodense area at the level of the herniation is well outlined by the injected contrast medium. **b** Herniation descends into the upper part of the lateral recess. *Operative findings:* Perforation of the posterior longitudinal ligament; protrusion of a relatively median herniation. 75% of all free fragments appearing as hypodensities on CT are transligamentous

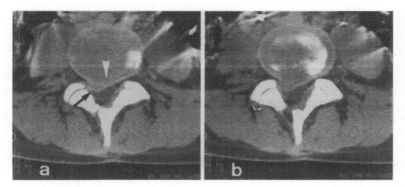

Fig. 97 a, b. 21-year-old woman. Right L5 sciatica of 4 weeks' duration. Right posterolateral L4–L5 disk herniation. **a** Herniation shows a right, paramedian constriction at the level of the ligamentous perforation *(white arrowhead)*. Retroligamentous portion lies more to the right (→). **b** Section below ligamentous perforation; herniation compresses emergence of right L5 root

The striking correlation found at the cervical level, where every hypodensity is indicative of a free fragment and ligamentous rupture, is unfortunately absent at the lumbar level [161, 162, 310]. Here, the posterior longitudinal ligament is intact in half the cases (Fig. 95) and in the other half there is a perforation (Figs. 96, 97). Nevertheless, a free fragment is found in two-thirds of cases exhibiting in a hypodensity, (in 75% of transligamentous and 25% of subligamentous lesions).

Vertical Extension

Nearly all common herniations extend slightly downwards. If we quantify the interval between the inferior margin of the disk and the plane of the last section in which the herniation is still visible, the average figure for common herniations is 4.8 mm. This limited vertical extension of less than 0.5 cm justifies performing 1 mm thick sections every 2 mm, so as to obtain at least two or three sections passing through the herniation.

Discontinuity of Section Planes

This appears as an abrupt break in the shape and size of the herniation from one section to the next. This sign is rare in common herniations and is taken to indicate the existence of a free fragment. In these cases there is indeed a free fragment with greater than average (5.8 mm) descent, corresponding to the initial stage of migration. This sign is discussed in more detail in the section on migratory herniations.

Epidural Fat Involvement

When the anterior epidural fat is of adequate volume (particularly at the L5–S1 level), it may serve as a marker for the herniation [38, 40, 93]. The fat is rarely normal, most rarely so in cases involving small median herniations, which result only in an indentation of the thecal sac (see Fig. 91). Epidural fat involvement is a valuable sign, since it is frequent (Fig. 98). The fat may show a simple lateral asymmetry, it may be invaded, or even totally obliterated in cases combining a large herniation and a narrowed lumbar spinal canal (Fig. 99). More rarely, compression of the posterior epidural fat is also a good indirect sign of thecal sac displacement by a large herniation [76, 88] (see Fig. 91).

Signs of Root Involvement

Signs of root compression by a herniation may be directly identifiable on CT sections [38, 76, 93, 98, 254]. In our series, the compressed root was invisible, because indistinguishable from the herniation responsible, in 15% of cases. A detailed analysis was therefore impossible.

The root was identifiable in the other 85% of cases. In 80% the following abnormalities were found:

— *Deviation, posterior displacement* and *deformation* were the signs most often encountered (65% of common herniations) (see Fig. 98).

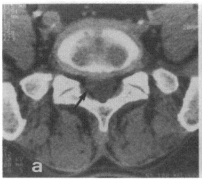 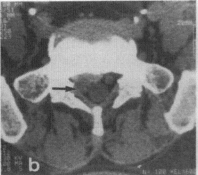 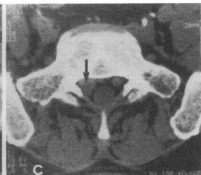

Fig. 98 a–c. 60-year-old man. Right S1 sciatica of 3 months' duration. Right posterolateral L5–S1 herniation. **a** Bulging of L5–S1. At its emergence from the thecal sac, the right S1 root is already increased in diameter and moderately deviated (—►) above the root compromised by the disk. **b** Herniation is better visualized below the diskal plane. Right S1 root is thick (50%), deformed (65%) and deviated (—►). **c** Disk herniation is immediately anterior, in contact with the S1 root (↓). *Operative findings:* Preligamentous herniation

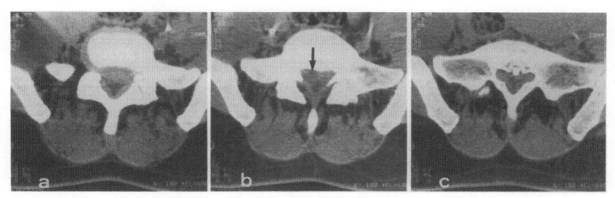

Fig. 99 a–c. 30-year-old woman. Left S1 sciatica of three months' duration. Large posteromedian L5–S1 herniation in a lumbar spinal stenosis. **a** Disappearance of anterolateral and posterior epidural fat. **b** Existence of right paramedian hypodensity within the herniation (free fragment) (→). **c** Roots are only visible at a distance from the herniation and have a normal appearance (50% of all cases). *Operative findings:* Transligamentous free fragment

— An enlarged root was the second commonest finding, present in nearly half the cases. Although physiologic asymmetry of the two roots at a given level does sometimes exist, the discovery of a large root just below the herniation is an additional argument in favor of root involvement (see Fig. 98). As we shall see, oblique MRI sections permitting good visualization of the root confirm the undue size, possible in an affected nerve root. This sign may be particularly useful if there is doubt as to the lesional level in cases with double herniations, or when a very small herniation compressing the root at its emergence from the thecal sac.

— Finally, the hyperdense appearance of the compressed root in comparison to the contralateral root, though uncommon (20% of cases), may be useful if the other signs are negative (see Fig. 98). The pathophysiologic reasons for a large hyperdense root are not well understood. There may be nerve root edema, congestion of the lateral epidural venous plexus, or venous stasis at the level of the nerve root sheath.

These indirect signs of disk herniation are especially useful when the herniation can directly visualized only with difficulty. They should attract the attention of the radiologist and possibly prompt him to make additional sections in order to obtain a direct image of the herniation.

Thecal Sac Deviation

In most cases, the thecal sac is normally located. Nevertheless, in 25% of cases, it may show a displacement accompanied by some degree of obliteration of the posterior epidural fat [76, 194, 257] (see Figs. 91, 98).

Surgical Findings

Operative exposure permits verification of the integrity (or involvement) of the posterior longitudinal ligament and the possible existence of a subligamentous free fragment. It is essential to realize that the group of common herniations, though based on CT similarities, is a heterogeneous one comprising various anatomic disk lesions. Only detailed analysis of the CT appearance of the herniation (hypodensity, posterior margin rupture, configuration, etc.) permits an approach to the structure of the lesion.

There is no typical common disk herniation. One can nevertheless try to draw a CT "profile" of the various anatomic types of herniation found at operation. We may distinguish three simplified CT images:

— Subligamentous herniations (60%) exhibit an even disk overlap (64%); they are of uniform density and have a moderate extent, averaging 5 mm, below the disk overlap (see Fig. 86).

— Transligamentous herniations (30%) also usually have a smooth overlap, although there is abrupt overlap in 40% of cases. When it is visible (30%), the rupture of the posterior disk margin is very large, and this sign is found only in this category (see Fig. 97). The presence of hypodensities indicates the existence of a free fragment (see Fig. 96). The vertical extension is the greatest of all, approaching 1 cm. Finally, image discontinuity from one section to the next is found in two out of three cases, indicating the incipient migration of a free fragment.

– Subligamentous free fragments (10%) also usually show an even overlap, but there is an abrupt overlap in 40% of cases. The presence of hypodensities within the herniation is almost indispensable, since they occur in 75% of cases (see Fig. 95). There is an intermediate vertical extent (8 mm). Image discontinuity from one section to the next occurs in half the cases (see Fig. 92).

It is useful to relate the various surgical approaches used (fenestration; hemilaminectomy or laminectomy) to the herniation group, and to necessary revision operations (foraminotomy, internal facetectomy). Fenestration was the commonest surgical approach used (80%), and virtually the only procedure for common herniations (90%). On the other hand, hemilaminectomies were rare (10%) and performed only half as often in common herniations as in the series as a whole, emphasizing the importance of an accurate preliminary CT diagnosis. The frequency of revisional surgery was identical in both series.

Even though the positive diagnosis of a disk herniation proved simple, and was never missed, it was often possible to explore the disk lesion more closely. The routine performance of millimetric sections; the intravenous injection of contrast medium (Iopamiron 300); the careful analysis of the type of disk overlap and its vertical extent; the search for a rupture of the posterior disk margin, a hypodensity, or a discontinuity of images between two disk planes: all these have revealed the presence or absence of a rupture of the posterior longitudinal ligament or of a free fragment in over 75% of cases. Such considera-

tions have practical implications; the heterogeneous nature of common herniations, which are in principle good candidates for chemonucleolysis, may explain certain failures of this therapeutic approach.

Large and Small Common Herniations

Finally, it seems necessary to distinguish two groups of common herniations based on their size. Although this may not have direct clinical correlations (a large herniation may cause less distress than a small one; a small herniation may be operated upon earlier), the size of herniations presents specific problems in CT diagnosis.

A disk herniation is considered large when it occupies three-fourths of the cross-section of the spinal canal. Small herniations remain limited to the disk plane, are difficult to distinguish and have virtually no effect on the anterior epidural fat; hence the importance in these cases of the intravenous injection of contrast medium (Iopamiron 300).

Large Herniations

Large herniations from one-sixth of all common herniations and occupy the major part of the spinal canal. They may even sometimes occupy the normal site of the thecal sac posteriorly, and then be confused with the thecal sac if they have rounded outlines and densities close to those of the CSF; this constitutes a source of interpretational error (Fig. 100).

The large size of the hernia does not necessarily imply rupture of the posterior longitudinal ligament; in fact, ligamentous rupture is found in only half the cases (Fig. 101).

The considerable size of the herniation prevents differentiation between disk substance and nerve root. The compressed root is usually seen subsequently, on sections performed below the herniation. This delayed visualization explains why the root appears normal in more than half the cases (see Fig. 99). On the other hand, the anterior epidural fat is always obliterated. The thecal sac is also deviated in virtually all cases (90%), together with obliteration of the posterior epidural fat (see Fig. 99).

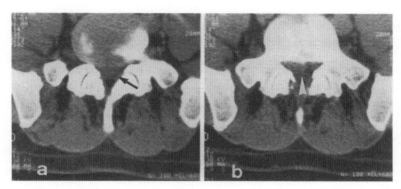

Fig. 100 a, b. 26-year-old man. Right S1 sciatica of 1 months' duration. Large, poorly visualized, right posterolateral L5-S1 herniation. **a** This typifies one-sixth of all common herniations, which occupy over three-fourths of the internal diameter of the lumbar canal. Herniation may occupy the site of the thecal sac, which is, paradoxically, only slightly displaced (→); the posterior epidural fat remains in place. **b** Boundary between herniation and thecal sac is poorly visualized, hence the use of intravenous contrast media to better delineate the outlines of the herniation *(white arrowhead). Operative findings:* Large herniation which was preligamentous (as in 50% of all large herniations), despite its size

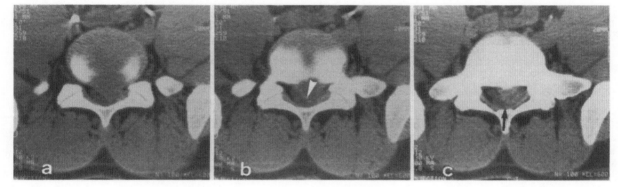

Fig. 101 a-c. 22-year-old man. Left S1 sciatica of one year's duration; significant, left posterolateral L5-S1 herniation. **a** Herniation is homogeneous with a smooth prolapse. **b** Herniation outline is enhanced after IV injection of contrast medium *(white arrowhead).* **c** Thecal sac compressed against laminae and ligamenta flava (→). Left S1 root is poorly seen at a distance from the herniation. *Operative findings:* Perforation of posterior longitudinal ligament and large free fragment. In large herniations, it is difficult to confirm the existence of a torn ligament by CT

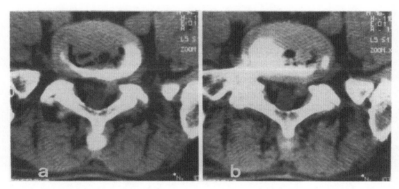

Fig. 102 a, b. 63-year-old man. Incomplete, left sciatic lesion of one months' duration. Small, left posterolateral L5-S1 herniation with buttonhole appearance. The frequency of such lesions is comparable to that of large herniations (1/6). **a-b** Very localized disk prolapse seen in only two sections (median height of 3.5 mm) opposite the displaced left S1 root. *Operative findings:* free fragment. Numerous, very hard anular fragments of lamellar appearance

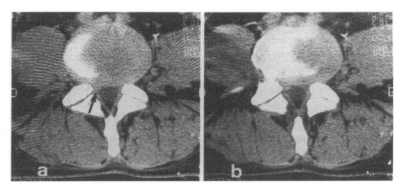

Fig. 103 a, b. 56-year-old man. Right L5 sciatica with a discrete neuro-deficit of 6 months' duration. Small, right posterolateral L4–L5 herniation. **a–b** Small, wedge-shaped prolapse of right posterolateral margin of the disk (→); numerous artefacts (target pattern). In all instances, the thecal sac is normally located. This small herniation is visible in only two sections. *Operative findings:* Ligamentous perforation

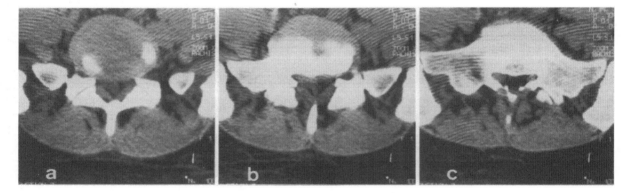

Fig. 104 a–c. 29-year-old woman. Chemonucleolysis at L4–L5 four months previously: recurrence of right sciatica two weeks later. Small, right posterolateral L4–L5 herniation. **a** Herniation poorly visible; discrete asymmetry of anterolateral epidural fat. **a–c** Indirect signs of right L5 root involvement particularly suggest the diagnosis (large root in 75% of cases). A concomitant lumbar spinal stenosis and narrow lateral recess account for the failure of chemonucleolysis in this case. *Operative findings:* Preligamentous herniation (as in 2/3 of such cases) associated with a narrow lateral recess

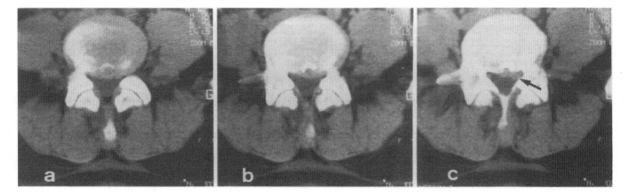

Fig. 105 a–c. 45-year-old woman. Left S1 sciatica of 2 months' duration. Small, left posterolateral L4–L5 herniation. **a** No clear-cut abnormalities at the diskal plane. **b** Discrete, localized, left disk prolapse. **c** Indirect signs are of paramount importance here: large, deformed, hyperdense root which is compressed against the articular pillar (→). *Operative findings:* Posterior longitudinal ligament thin and irregular. Small disk herniation is rendered proportionally greater by a narrow lateral recess. Large root surrounded by veins

Small Herniations

Small herniations are as frequent as large. They appear as a very localized disk overlap, often abrupt (eg the buttonhole herniation) (Figs. 102, 103). They have a small vertical extent (3.3 mm) and are most subligamentous in two-thirds of cases. Their CT diagnosis may present problems, given the difficulty in direct visualization. Even if one section is abnormal, supplementary intermediate sections should be performed. In these cases, indirect signs are of vital importance.

The compressed nerve root is always visible, because of the small size of the herniation, with evidence of deviation, displacement and deformation. Remarkably, it is quite often large (75%) and hyperdense (40%) (Figs. 104, 105). The anterior epidural fat is much less deformed than in common herniations as a whole; a simple asymmetry is observed. The thecal sac is always normal.

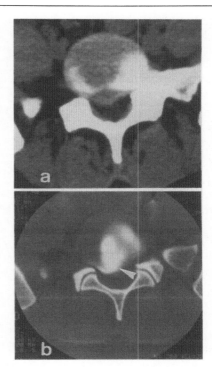

Fig. 106a, b. 20-year-old woman. Right S1 sciatica. **a** *CT:* Common type of right posterolateral L5–S1 herniation with displacement of S1 root. **b** *Postdiskography CT:* filling of herniation through a very large opening *(white arrowhead)*

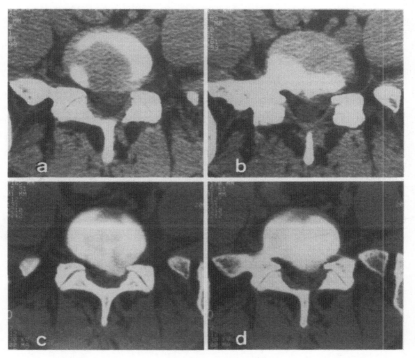

Fig. 107a–d. 25-year-old man. Left S1 sciatica. **a–b** *CT:* Left posterolateral L5–S1 with signs of left S1 root involvement. **c–d** *Postdiskography CT at L5–S1:* Impregnation of the nucleus, anulus and herniation, without signs of anular fissures. The disk is completely degenerated

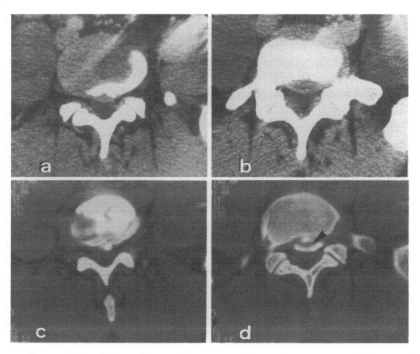

Fig. 108 a–d. Posteromedian L5–S1 herniation with a preligamentous free fragment. *CT:* **a** Small posteromedian herniation at diskal plane, compressing both S1 radicular emergences within the thecal sac. **b** Herniation is better seen below the discal plane; presence of median hypodensity.

Postdiskography CT: **c** Good injection of nucleus and opacification of posteromedian herniation. **d** Accentuated outline of a preligamentous free fragment corresponding to the observed hypodensity *(arrowhead)*

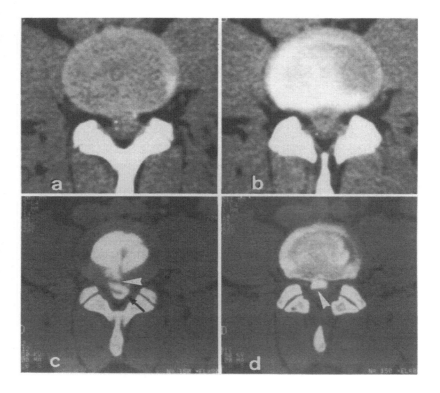

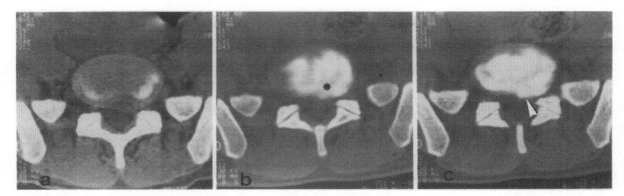

Fig. 110 a-c. Postdiskography CT. Typical left S1 sciatica resistant to medical treatment in a 27-year-old man. **a** CT: common type of left L5-S1 herniation with a displaced left S1 nerve root. **b** Postdiskography CT 1 hour after L5-S1 chemonucleolysis: there is a significant uptake of contrast medium by both the anulus and the nucleus in the left posterolateral portion of the L5-S1 disk (✳) (No differentiation). **c** Herniation shows significant contrast uptake in the next subjacent section; it is therefore probably reached by the enzyme *(white arrowhead)*. *Comment:* Postdiskography CT in young subjects for herniations with typical sciatic pain can reveal signs of disk degeneration at the level of the herniation

Postdiskography CT

The recent technique of CT following diskography shows the size of the extrusion orifice at the periphery of the anulus fibrosus, and often significant opacification of a posteromedian nuclear fragment (Fig. 106). In young subjects with an intervertebral space which is not collapsed, only postdiskography CT is capable of showing complete disk degeneration (absence of anulus-nucleus differentiation) associated with the herniation responsible for the sciatica (Fig. 107).

The subligamentous location of a disk fragment may be clearly shown (Fig. 108). The contrast medium injected into the median part of the disk spreads posteriorly to surround the hypodensity of the herniated fragment, which is clearly limited by the posterior longitudinal ligament. Similarly, the transligamentous location of a disk fragment may be perfectly evaluated, due to the presence of contrast medium on both sides of a constriction corresponding to the ligamentous rupture (Figs. 109, 110).

Fig. 109 a-d. Large, posteromedian L3-L4 herniation in a transligamentous situation. **a-b** Disk sections at L3-L4: large posteromedian herniation deforming the thecal sac. *Postdiskography CT:* **c** Median injection of the nucleus and dorsally located herniation through a small, median opening in the anulus *(white arrowhead)*. Bilobed opacification of the herniation astride the perforated ligament (→). **d** The preligamentous portion of the herniation, below the diskal plane, is well opacified; the posterior longitudinal ligament is immediately behind this portion *(white arrowhead)*

Calcified Herniations

Calcified disk herniations are easily identified on CT as hyperdensities of part of the intervertebral disk. However, the presence of osteophytes or calcified structures opposite the intervertebral foramen may create difficulties in interpretation. Calcified hernias are rare: 5% of our entire series. The interval between the first clinical signs and the time of operation is strikingly long (11 months, as opposed to 4.1 months for our entire series). This reflects the age of the herniation and the rate of development of such calcifications.

CT Features

The diagnosis of a calcification on CT scans is simple if these show structures having very high densities (more than 500 HU). It is important to have advance knowledge of the presence of a calcification, since it is a classic contraindication to chemonucleolysis and creates operating difficulties for the surgeon.

The other problem is to try to determine the exact nature of the calcified structure. This is often difficult, as may be the case for the surgeon during the operation. The performance of axial sections only is a disadvantage; reconstructed sagittal and coronal images make useful contributions; it is more sensitive than plain films and calcifications are very difficult to detect with MRI given their lack of signals.

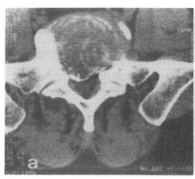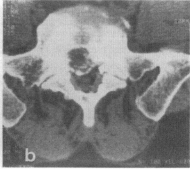

Fig. 111 a, b. 47-year-old man. Right S1 sciatica of 2 weeks' duration. Calcified right posterolateral L5–S1 herniation. **a–b** Diskal section at L5–S1. Calcifications are evident throughout the disk: they can be differentiated from possible partial volume effects due to opposing cartilaginous endplates

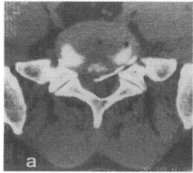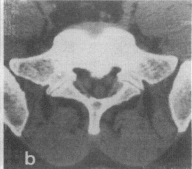

Fig. 112 a, b. 37-year-old man. Right S1 sciatica. **a** Calcification of the left posterolateral margin of the L5–S1 disk. **b** Posteromedian osteophyte below the disk

Disk Calcifications

If CT shows calcifications in the middle of an intervertebral disk, it is easy to affirm their diskal origin. However, one should beware of partial volume effects involving adjacent cartilaginous plates, especially if the disk is collapsed (Fig. 111). One may find a thin calcification of the diskal rim, whose origin will be indicated by an extension lateral to the foramen (Fig. 112).

Dorsal disk herniations are frequently calcified, but are much rarer than lumbar herniations [39, 42].

Cases involving calcified nucleus pulposus herniations in children constitute a separate entity. These are commonest at the cervical level, but sometimes occur in the dorsolumbar region. They have characteristic symptoms and generally regress spontaneously [84, 176, 183].

Calcification of the Posterior Longitudinal Ligament

This is very rare and appears as a linear calcification lining the posterior contour of the disk, within the spinal canal (Fig. 113). Two types are classically described [111]:

— the commonest type in Europe consists of ligamentous calcification associated with senile ankylosing hyperostosis of the spine. The calcification is fragmentary, circumscribed, accompanied by hyperostosis and often by posterior osteophytosis [14, 229, 242, 243];
— a type very frequent in Japan, but uncommon in Europe, which occurs after the fifth decade, especially in men. Calcification at the lumbar level is very rare, and always associated with dorsal calcification. The lesions usually involve the cervical level, appearing as variably thick calcifications (up to 5 mm) which are attacked to the posterior surface of the vertebral bodies, are often separated by a hypodense area, and bridge the disks. The histology varies from a simple amorphous calcification to a bony metaplasia with haversian ossification of the ligament. One case has been described of perforation of a calcified posterior longitudinal ligament by a herniation; this was at the cervical level (C6-C7) [130, 139, 146, 185, 219, 311].

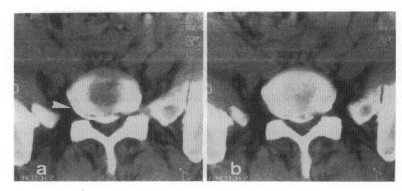

Fig. 113 a, b. 44-year-old woman. Partial left cauda aquina syndrome. Calcified L5-S1 herniation. **a-b** Calcification of the posteromedian herniation, which extends laterally to the disk margins *(white arrowhead)*. This is not due to the overlying or underlying cartilaginous endplates. *Operative findings:* Preligamentous herniation. Ablation of the calcifications

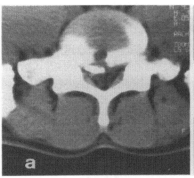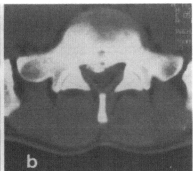

Fig. 114 a, b. 37-year-old man. Recurrent right S1 sciatica with slight neuro-deficit: detachment of ring apophysis. **a** Right posterolateral L5–S1 herniation associated with a concave posterior calcification. Disk tissue present within the concavity. **b** Subjacent end-plate: calcification forms part of the posterior aspect of the vertebral body. This is probably the same dense structure: a ring apophysis fragment which had been detached. This constitutes a classic contraindication to chemonucleolysis. *Operative findings:* calcification; preligamentous disk herniation

Tearing of the Ring Apophysis [147, 206, 270]

A bony half-ring structure which is concave anteriorly, posterior to the vertebral body, and contains tissue of disk density within its concavity may correspond to a torn ring apophysis. Instead of passing through a gap in the anulus, the disk substance exits via an unfused zone between the posterior ring apophysis and the overlying and underlying cartilaginous end-plates, displacing it posteriorly (Fig. 114). Sagittal projections using routine plain films show an avulsion of the posterior border of the vertebral body (Fig. 115).

The value of thin-section CT lies in the good differentiation between calcification of the severed ring apophysis and the herniated soft tissue which has precipitated this predisposed condition. This type of herniation constitutes a contraindication to chemonucleolysis. The same type of phenomenon may be seen with the anterior ring apophysis, but herniations at this site result only in lumbar pain.

Retrovertebral Osteophytes

A retrovertebral osteophyte may be found associated with a disk herniation within the framework of significant arthrotic diskopathy. It is then difficult to ascertain the relative contributions of the herniation and the osteophyte to nerve root compression phenomena; especially if the osteophyte develops in a lateral recess or foramen (Fig. 116).

Others

Intraspinal calcifications having other etiologies may be detected on CT, whether associated with a herniation or within a context of sciatic pain. They include the following:

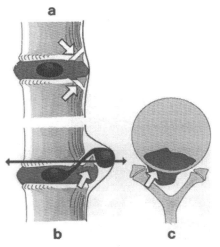

Fig. 115 a–c. Avulsed ring apophysis. **a** The ring apophyses are not fused. **b** The posterior herniation anterior to the ring apophysis, introduces itself between the vertebral body and the ring apophysis, whether cephalad or caudad. **c** Corresponding CT section

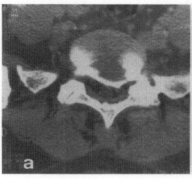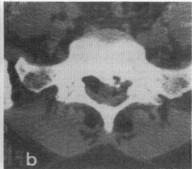

Fig. 116 a, b. 29-year-old woman. Left S1 sciatica with deficit. Left L5–S1 herniation with detached ring apophysis. **a** Common type of left posterolateral L5–S1 herniation with recession of ring apophysis on the side of the herniation. **b** Steno- sis of the left lateral recess due to retrovertebral osteophytes. At this level, the left S1 root appears to be compressed more by the osteophytes than by the herniation

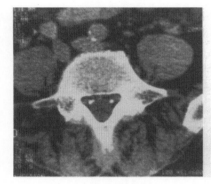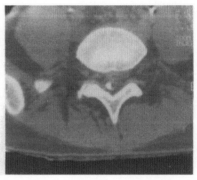

Fig. 117. Section through the midportion of the body of L5. The left and right L5 roots are clearly visible in the lateral recesses. Posterior to these two roots, one sees small, calcified hyperdense areas belonging to the thecal sac, but located just above the S1 root emergences. Calcifications of the dura mater, thecal sac or radicular sheaths

Fig. 118. Alternating S1 sciatica. No herniation is present, but there is a median calcification within the thecal sac, above the L5–S1 disk. *Operative findings:* intrathecal cholesteatoma

Calcification of the Dura Mater

One case in the lumbar spine has been reported in a patient with chronic renal failure treated by hemodialysis. There was a very fine linear calcification posterior to the vertebral surface [244]. Thecal sac calcification may also be observed at the level of the nerve root emergences [297] (Fig. 117).

Tumoral calcifications

These are located in the midportion of the spinal canal. A meningioma is the likeliest diagnosis. Less common lesions include neurinoma, primary meningeal melanoblastoma, cholesteatoma (epidermoid tumor) (Fig. 118), oligodendroglioma or osteochondroma [202].

Vascular calcifications

Vascular malformations are rarely calcified; the same applies to the intraspinal arteries [65].

Calcifications of the Ligamentum Flavum

These are frequent and asymptomatic [109, 150] and make up the vast majority of posterior calcifications. Though usually idiopathic, they may be associated with chondrocalcinosis, especially in the context of hemochromatosis. They are V-shaped, symmetric, linear calcifications which project over the interlaminar space, parallel to the internal margin of the laminae and oriented in the same direction as the fibers of the ligamentum flavum.

Arachnoidal Calcification

Ossifying arachnoiditis is rare and of disputed etiology. It results in calcified plates at the level of the arachnoid. It mainly affects the lower dorsal region, posterior to the spinal cord [81, 210].

Operative Findings

As we have seen, the neurosurgeon has as much difficulty as the radiologist in determining the exact nature of the calcification. These are most often *subligamentous* herniations (75% of our series). The distribution of surgical approaches is identical to that of our series as a whole.

Migratory Herniations

A lumbar migratory herniation may be defined as the migration of all or part of the nucleus pulposus away from the disk and the intervertebral space. This concept is further refined by the term free fragment, which is the result of the migration of disk material, in this case the nucleus pulposus. It should be stated from the start that the term "free" is inaccurate, since that part of the nucleus pulposus which has migrated need to have perforated the posterior longitudinal ligament. This fragment may be free with respect to the disk itself, while remaining subligamentous. In this specific instance, the fragment is not "free" in the spinal canal (a possibility which in any case we have found to be rather rare) [62, 76, 121, 206] (Fig. 119).

Certain authors also speak of extruded disks or disk material. For them, the term "extruded herniation" designates both a free fragment opposite the disk or in close contact with it, and a fragment that has migrated upwards or downwards and lies at a distance from the disk; in either case there is a ligamentous perforation [62, 121, 280, 306].

By a migratory herniation we refer to the migration of all or part of the nucleus away from the posterior border of the disk, either cephalad towards the intervertebral foramen or the axilla of the overlying nerve root, or caudad into the lateral recess, in contact with the root itself.

Neurosurgeons have been aware of migratory lumbar disk herniations for many years [34]. Even with the advent of modern water-soluble contrast media, their demonstration has depended on the uncertain criteria of radiculography [62]. Modern scanners are capable of providing finely detailed images of herniations. Migratory herniations are perfectly recognized, both by direct visualization of the free fragment at a distance from the intervertebral space and by the abnormalities of the affected disk. The task of the neuroradiologist is to recognize the free fragment which has migrated to a distance, and to identify the pathological disk which has expelled the nuclear fragment. The diagnosis of a migratory disk fragment is a classic contraindication to chemonucleolysis.

Migratory disk herniations make up about 20% of all operated herniations.

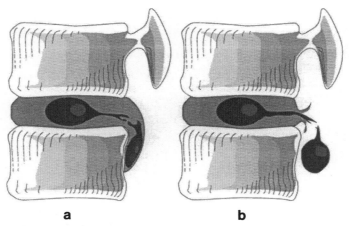

a   **b**

Fig. 119 a, b. Migratory herniations. **a** Subligamentous migratory free fragment: it is not truly free within the spinal canal, but has only lost its attachment to the disk. **b** Transligamentous migratory free fragment. The posterior longitudinal ligament is ruptured and the fragment is free within the vertebral canal

Clinical Considerations

Clinically, it is important to note the high percentage of sciaticas with a combined, biradicular topography. This reflects the frequency of compression by the migratory fragment of the roots above and below the relevant intervertebral disk. The mean duration of clinical symptoms is 1.5 months, which is much less than for the series as a whole (4.1 months). This brevity is indicative of the often florid and serious clinical picture.

Sciaticas with a motor deficit are frequent (80%), much more so than in common herniations. The motor deficit may vary in intensity. Paralytic sciaticas were present in 30% of cases, accounting for 84% of the paralytic sciaticas in our series. Cauda equina syndromes may be observed; in such cases emergency CT investigation is performed and operation is carried out immediately thereafter.

In a neurosurgical department, emergency CT is performed for hyperalgesic sciatica with a motor deficit, or for a paralytic sciatica. This is more readily observed in young subjects, who may also present a more or less complete cauda equina syndrome. However, the necessity for emergency CT does not justify the differentiation of a particular group or type of herniation. These are often large migratory herniations with a free fragment and a perforated ligament. When they are descending (the most frequent case), they reach the midportion of the underlying vertebra and even the subjacent intervertebral foramen. These are major extrusions of the nucleus pulposus into the spinal canal, with involvement of the thecal sac and the two adjacent nerve roots. Where there is a patent clinical emergency, the visualization of a large fragment usually leads to surgery, though, in our university hospital, where are 500 disk operations annually, only 25 of these are emergencies.

CT Features

In migratory lumbar disk herniations, the free fragment may be expelled upwards (ascending migration) or downwards (descending migration). Double migrations (both ascending and descending) are much less common.

Ascending Migratory Herniations

In our series, 25% of migratory herniations were ascending. The migratory free fragment originating at the posterior margin of the intervertebral disk lies above the intervertebral space and may be located in one of several places:

— It is most frequently found at the entrance to the overlying intervertebral foramen; if the fragment is large, it may be found a few mm higher, lying against the nerve root in the lowest part of the lateral recess of the overlying vertebra [76, 121, 187, 306] (Fig. 120).
— This ascending migration may also occur more remotely, in the intervertebral foramen, which constitutes a site of maximum root compression. In our experience such cases are uncommon, but their discovery on CT is a very accurately guide to neurosurgical exploration of the intervertebral foramen. The diagnosis may prove difficult in cases of lateral foraminal herniations of material directly originating in the lateral margin of the disk (Fig. 121).
— The free fragment may also be found lodged in the axilla of the overlying nerve root: on CT, there is an isolated filling of the entire lateral recess above the disk investigated. In this very specific case, the intervertebral foramen separating the two levels is normal. The posterior margin of the suspected disk is ill-defined and blurred at the site where the anulus fibrosus has ruptured and the migratory free fragment has been extruded (about 15 mm away). In rare cases, the disk of origin may appear absolutely normal [299].

In terms of distance, ascending migrations travel half as far as descending ones (6 mm versus 13 mm).

Hypodensities within lumbar disk herniations are more difficult to visualize than at the cervical level, as we have seen. They are indicative of a free fragment. Nevertheless, ascending herniations are often homogeneous.

We have considered all the varieties of ascending migratory herniations resulting from a pathological disk.

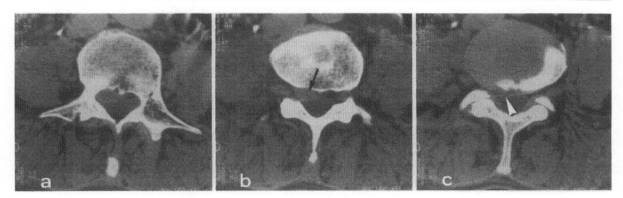

Fig. 120 a–c. 64-year-old man. Right L4 and L5 sciatica. Right L4–L5 herniation with an ascending migratory free fragment. **a** CT at level of midvertebral body (L4): Right anterolateral filling-in of lumbar spinal canal at axilla of right L4 root. (Overlying disk L3–L4 is normal.) **b** Subjacent L4–L5 foramen: ascending migratory free fragment located at the foraminal entrance (→). **c** Discal plane (L4–L5). Right posterolateral prolapse with a small hypodensity: source of the ascending migratory free fragment *(white arrowhead)*. *Operative findings:* Ligamentous perforation. Large free fragment at right foraminal entrance (L4–L5)

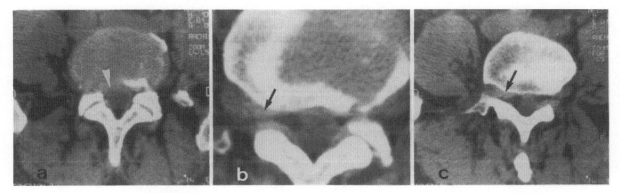

Fig. 121 a–c. 58-year-old man. Right L5 sciatica with a moderate motor deficit. Paralysis of the tibialis anterior (L4) appeared two days previously. Right L4–L5 ascending herniation. **a** L4–L5 disk: The posterior margin is irregular and fissured, suggesting a tear or defect *(white arrowhead)*.

b–c The clinical signs indicated a CT study of the overlying foramen. A migratory free fragment is clearly seen in the middle of the neural foramen, displacing and compressing the right L4 root (→). *Operative findings:* Torn ligament; foraminal free fragment above L4–L5 disk

The sign which links the ascending migratory free fragment to the disk investigated is essentially a discontinuity, with "rupture" images of the posterior disk margin which nowhere has its usual smooth and rectilinear appearance [281, 306]; this is the case for several sections. In cases of ascending migration, it is important to emphasize the difference between the appearance of the clearly identified free fragment and the posterior disk margin, which simply shows a rupture with scarring, very probably corresponding to the orifice through which the nucleus pulposus has been extruded [161].

Descending Migratory Herniations

These were the most frequent type encountered in our series (75% of cases) [74, 76, 187, 203, 206, 306]. As already noted, a herniation may be better visualized below the disk, on axial sections studying the superior cartilaginous plate of the underlying vertebra. The signs are often clearer in the upper portion of the lateral recess, close to the concavity of the vertebral body. This creates a problem: how to distinguish a descending ordinary herniation from a migratory herniation with a free fragment.

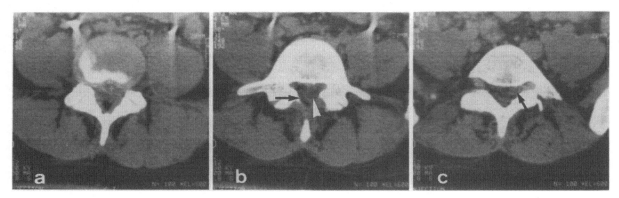

Fig. 122 a–c. 18-year-old woman. Complete L5 and S1 motor deficit. L4–L5 herniation with an underlying migratory free fragment. **a** Posteromedian herniation with a hypodensity (as in 40% of such cases). **b** Image discontinuity: herniation appears larger than in previous section *(white arrowhead)*. Thecal sac compressed against right articular pillar (→). **c** De-scending migratory fragment is wedged between the deformed thecal sac and the left L5 root; free fragment reaches the entrance to the subjacent foramen (→). *Operative findings:* Torn ligament. Extruded herniation in a lateral position between the L5 and S1 roots and still in contact with the L4–L5 intervertebral space

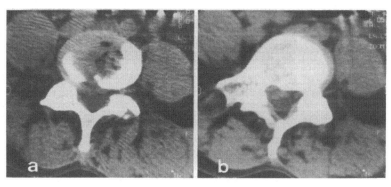

Fig. 123 a, b. 55-year-old woman; right L5 sciatica with complete neuro-deficit. **a** Diskal plane: intradiskal gas. Common type of right L4–L5 herniation. **b** Section through midportion of the body of L5, 12 mm lower down. Section discontinuity, with migratory fragment between thecal sac and L5 root. *Operative findings:* Torn ligament with right paramedian orifice. Two transligamentous free fragments in the axilla of the root, and a third, preligamentous, retrovertebral fragment. *Comment:* CT cannot individually identify all fragments

The important criterion is the *discontinuity* of images observed from one section to the next, at the level of the posterior disk margin and especially the underlying lateral recess (90%). The descending free fragment, which is very caudal to the inferior disk margin (a mean distance of 13 mm), gives rise to CT scans showing considerable obliteration of the lateral epidural fat between the nerve root and the thecal sac (Fig. 122). Nevertheless, CT has its limits, since it cannot absolutely determine the number of migratory free fragments (Fig. 123).

This free fragment almost always stops in the lower portion of the lateral recess, as though it were restricted by the nerve root blocking its mi-gration. This is no longer the case when the nucleus is entirely extruded into the spinal canal; the free fragment descends towards the intervertebral foramen and conceals the thecal sac (20%) [34, 161].

At the L5–S1 level, a free fragment may migrate farther towards the first sacral foramen, since it is no longer stopped by the underlying nerve root, which, as shown on MRI sections (sagittal oblique section derived from a frontal scout view) is very vertical (Fig. 124). Comparison with sagittal MRI sections shows that the CT scan, given the significant obliquity of the sections [43], has a tendency to exaggerate the vertical extension of the herniation, especially at

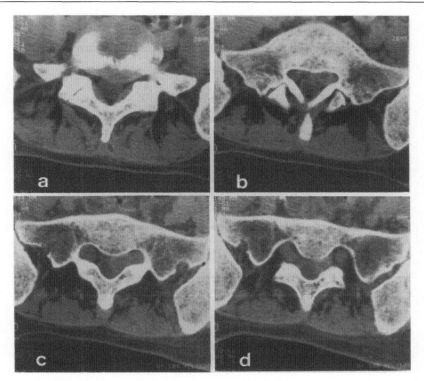

Fig. 124 a-d. 41-year-old woman. Left S1 sciatica with five weeks' neuro-deficit: L5-S1 herniation and a descending migratory fragment. **a** Moderate left L5-S1 herniation with posteromedian hypodensity. **b** Hypodense fragment visible below the disk. **c** Migratory fragment becomes larger (dis-continuity). **d** Fragment found in sacral foramen. *Operative findings:* Preligamentous free fragment, which is unusual in this type of herniation. Discordance with ordinary sections of migratory free fragments

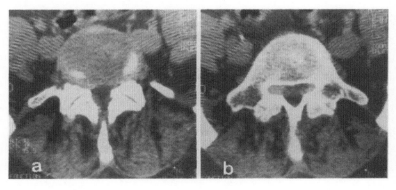

Fig. 125 a, b. 48-year-old woman. Hyperalgesic right S1 sciatica with neuro-deficit, aggravated by spinal stenosis. **a** Very small right L5-S1 herniation in a predisposed subject (spinal stenosis and lumbar facet arthropathy). **b** Isolated filling of the subjacent right lateral recess, 15 mm below the disk. Discontinuity between sections **a** and **b** (90% of all cases). *Operative findings:* Perforated ligament, free fragment. S1 foraminotomy

L5-S1. In cases with spinal stenosis, the diagnosis is obviously much more difficult, since the epidural fat is absent and one must take into account the discordance between the abnormal image of the lateral recess and the size of the overlying herniation (Fig. 125).

Descending migratory herniations seem to differ (at least in our series) from ascending herniations. Descending herniations have a remarkably high frequency of hypodense areas (40%), indicating the presence of free fragments (see Fig. 122). Also, the abnormalities of the disk margin only shows a blurring (i. e., image of a perforated anulus fibrosus) [161].

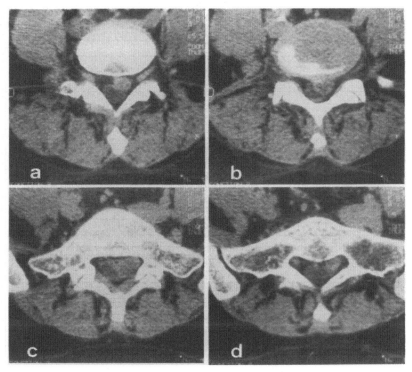

Fig. 126 a–d. 32-year-old woman. Left L5 sciatica with two-day neuro-deficit. Absence of Achilles tendon reflex. Ascending and descending L5–S1 herniation (double free fragment). **a** L5–S1 foramen: free fragment at entrance of left L5 foramen. **b** L5–S1 disk: free fragment has originated in a large left L5–S1 herniation. **c–d** A second discontinuity further down: large free fragment descending towards left sacral foramen. *Operative findings:* Perforated ligament. Very large, extruded herniation which has ascended to compress the left L5 root. S1 root displaced by a second, descending, free fragment

Double Ascending and Descending Migratory Herniations

Double migratory herniations are the most infrequent (10%) of all migratory herniations; they show all the CT signs previously described, permitting identification of the free fragments found at surgery, one at the entrance to the intervertebral foramen of the overlying level and the other lower in the spinal canal, below the disk. The ascending and descending free fragments from a given herniation are always homolateral (Fig. 126).

CT-Surgical Correlations

In a series of 30 patients with migratory free fragments clearly identified on CT and confirmed at surgery, there were 25 cases of transligamentous herniations, with a fragment still linked to the disk through the posterior longitudinal ligament in 3 cases, and 5 cases of migratory free fragments in a subligamentous position (see Fig. 124).

The types of surgical approaches to migratory herniations differ from those used for common herniations, emphasizing the importance of accurate preoperative diagnosis. Fenestration is less frequently performed, preference being given to hemilaminectomy or laminectomy, which are aimed at facilitating a more extensive investigation of the lateral recesses. Foraminotomy is also performed more often since fragments may be trapped in the intervertebral foramen.

CT Examination

A thorough clinical examination determines the segment to be explored. If the disk is normal, a CT section through the lowest portion of the lateral recess, is essential to exclude compression by a fragment from the underlying disk. Thus, an L5 sciatica can be perfectly explained by an ascending L5–S1 herniation at the entrance to the intervertebral foramen.

In cases of symptomatic disk herniation, it is important to explore the underlying lateral recess down to at least 10 mm below the last disk section, lest a descending free fragment be overlooked. Sections of 1 mm thickness are essential for the detailed analysis of such images as the scar sometimes visible on the posterior disk margin.

Nevertheless, the CT signs observed are not always pathognomonic.

In cases of *ascending migratory herniation,* two differential diagnoses should be considered [306]:

A filled-in foramen is not always indicative of a free fragment; it may be due to a *lateral herniation.* The entrance to the intervertebral foramen is normal; the lateral herniation is clearly recognizable outside the spinal canal and is often accompanied by an enlarged root or a large inflamed ganglion, as we will see in the following chapter. The fact that the posterior border of the suspected disk is absolutely normal is perhaps the best distinguishing sign [108, 142].

Double emergence, which is essentially a feature of radiculography, may present a difficult diagnostic problem in sciatica. CT shows the absence of a root in the lateral recess, and the underlying foramen is filled in by the double emergence. Thin sections demonstrate the associated herniation much better than radiculography [71, 126, 133, 306].

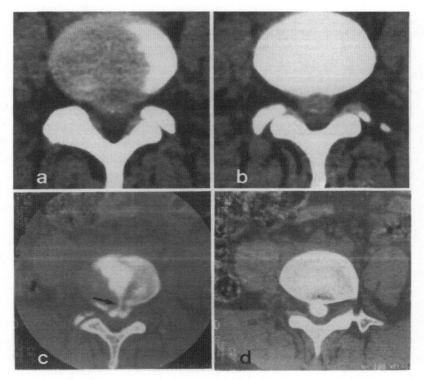

Fig. 127a–d. 24-year-old patient. Alternating L5 sciatica of 4 weeks' duration. Ascending migratory (posteromedian) L4–L5 herniation. **a–b** Median herniation with an ascending fragment in a strictly retrovertebral position. **c–d** Postdiskography CT: herniation is injected in the discal plane through a narrow orifice (→). The ascending free fragment is uniformly opacified by the contrast medium to a distance of 8 mm above the diskal plane

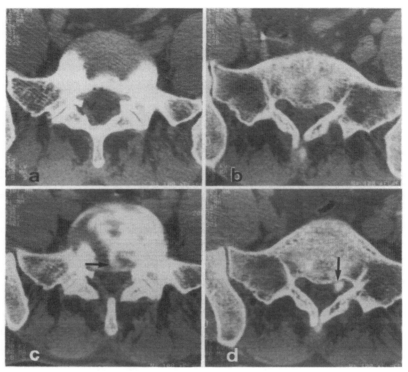

Fig. 128a-d. 35-year-old man. Typical left S1 sciatica. Descending left L5-S1 herniation. *CT:* **a** Very localized posteromedian L5-S1 herniation, with displacement of left S1 root. **b** Large left S1 root 15 mm below the diskal plane: associated free fragment or merely an enlarged root? *Postdiskography*

CT: **c** Opacification of posterior margin of the disk and of left paramedian herniation through a narrow orifice (→). **d** Descending migratory fragment is opacified remote from the disk (→). Left S1 root is readily recognizable outside the free fragment

The problem may become even more complicated when there are *"conjoined" nerve roots,* one arising or emerging from the thecal sac higher and earlier than its contralateral homolog. Two conjoined roots may perfectly simulate a free fragment.

On the other hand, the nerves follow a normal course in the lateral recess and below the corresponding pedicle.

A caudad free fragment lying at a distance should be differentiated from an ordinary posterolateral herniation. In the latter, there is no image discontinuity and above all, the herniation never reaches the midportion of the underlying vertebra.

Tumors located within the spinal canal (e. g., meningioma, neurinoma) present very different problems. The disks are not abnormal and the discrepant clinical signs necessitate radiculography as a supplementary investigation. The problem is more complicated if a concomitant herniation is present [28, 71, 206, 303].

Although CT is very useful in disk herniations, particularly when they are migratory, it is of limited value in the study of the posterior longitudinal ligament. At present, it is not possible to identify a perforation or tear associated with a free fragment, if this is strictly subligamentous. It is noteworthy that in the smaller structures of the cervical spine a perforation may be suspected when a study of the images reveals a free fragment hypodensity [160, 162, 310]. Exceptionally, CT reveals an isolated free fragment, but not the gap through which it was extruded.

Postdiskography CT

CT following diskography can show good opacification of a fragment which has migrated at a distance from the intervertebral space. An ascending migratory herniation lateral to the foraminal entrance above the pathological disk may be perfectly accessible to the contrast medium, as well as to the chymodiactin injected after diskog-

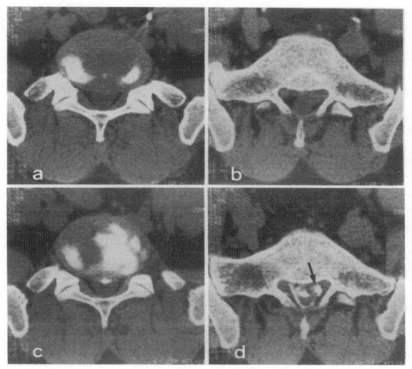

Fig. 129 a–d. 25-year-old man. Left S1 sciatica with neuro-deficit for one month. *CT:* **a** Discrete left posterolateral L5–S1 herniation. **b** Large migratory fragment lodged between thecal sac and root, 12 mm below the diskal plane (the two sections are discontinuous). *Postdiskography CT:* **c** Outlining of medially located L5–S1 herniation. **d** Contrast

opacifies the free fragment below the disk (→), as well as the entire extradural region. *Comments:* When there is a descending migratory fragment, CT cannot accurately evaluate the perforation of the posterior longitudinal ligament. Obviously, chemonucleolysis was not performed

raphy (Fig. 127). Descending migratory herniations are the most common to be so displayed. At the L5–S1 level, a migratory fragment may become wedged far from the disk, between the thecal sac and the S1 nerve root, almost at the entrance to the sacral foramen. It is noteworthy that the intradiskal injection of contrast medium also opacifies a migratory fragment 18 to 20 mm below the injected intervertebral space (Fig. 128).

Although these images of migratory fragments opacified far from the disk are impressive, one should not forget that in most cases there is an associated perforation of the posterior longitudinal ligament (Fig. 129). Extravasation of contrast medium to the epidural space accounts for the failure of chemonucleolysis in these remote fragments, which are reached by both the contrast medium and the enzyme but in insufficient quantities.

Lateral Herniations

In *lateral disk herniations* the nucleus pulposus is expelled just opposite or lateral to the posterior articular process. These herniations constitute a recent radiologic entity, having first been described in 1974 [2], when they were demonstrated using diskography. At present, CT is indispensable for their diagnosis, since the myelographic results are (by definition) negative. Both their clinical context and their treatment are quite specific. The large majority of these herniations are not operated on and heal spontaneously within 8 to 10 weeks.

Lateral herniations are frequent causes of *femoral pain*. Their incidence is variously assessed in the literature as from 1.6 to 11.7% [2, 6].

In general, one can distinguish *foraminal* herniations, which remain within the limits of the intervertebral foramen (Fig. 130), and *far lateral* herniations, which are outside the anatomic limits of the spinal canal (Fig. 131). This classification is rather arbitrary, since combined *foraminal-far lateral* forms are quite frequent.

Clinical Considerations

There is a remarkably high incidence *femoral pain* (L3 or L4 involvement). Whereas most posterolateral herniations compress the nerve root emerging at the underlying level (b), lateral herniations affect the corresponding root, which exits via the overlying intervertebral foramen (a) [2] (Fig. 132).

L4-L5 disk involvement is the most frequent, resulting in compression of the L4 nerve root. The L3-L4 disk is less frequently affected, with involvement of the L3 ganglion.

Normally, monoradicular S1 pain is never found; however, in the case of high emergence of the S1 nerve root, it may be affected by a lateral L5-S1 herniation.

Lumbar clinical signs (pain or spasm) are classically few or absent. A modified Lasègue's sign, which involves spasm of the psoas muscle, is often positive [142].

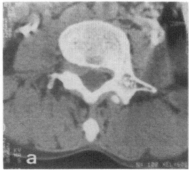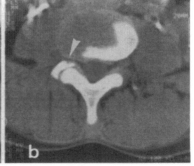

Fig. 130a, b. 40-year-old woman. Right L4 femoral pain with five days' complete neuro-deficit. Right L4-L5 foraminal herniation. Investigation of the foramen above the L4-L5 disk (in view of the clinical signs). **a** Section through L4-L5 foramen (asymmetry of section). Entire foramen is filled-in; the ganglion is no longer visible within the herniation. **b** Immediately subjacent L4-L5 disk with a small lateral protrusion *(white arrowhead)*. Posterior margin is normal. *Comments:* Slightly ascending (10 mm), strictly foraminal herniation. In contrast to ascending migratory herniations, the posterior disk margin is normal. Free fragment is very laterally located, almost extraspinal. *Operative findings:* Emergency operation: large foraminal free fragment and a perforated ligament

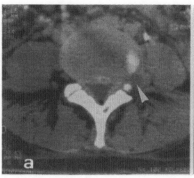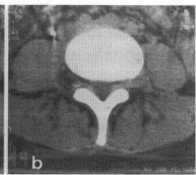

Fig. 131a, b. 34-year-old woman. Left L4 lumbocrural pain with two months' nears-deficit. Left L4–L5 lateral herniation. **a** Diskal plane. Normal posterior margin. Large extraspinal herniation with a hypodensity (nuclear fragment) *(white arrowhead)*. Disappearance of extraspinal fat. Displaced root (L4) adjacent to free fragment. **b** Ascending migration of frag-ment towards distal portion of foramen. *Operative findings:* The very lateral location of the hernia made surgery difficult. Only a moderate intraspinal bulge was found. Exploration showed that the L5 root (which originates below) was not compressed, nor the L4 root in its overlying intraspinal por-tion. No surgical improvement

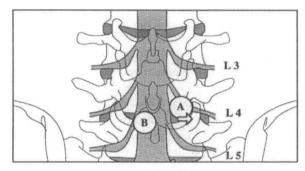

Fig. 132. Location of L4–L5 lateral herniations. *A,* Lateral herniations compress the corresponding nerve root, which ex-its via the next cephalad foramen (L4 root). *B,* Posterolateral herniations compress the nerve root exiting via the next cau-dad foramen (L5 root)

CT Features

Technique

The CT diagnosis is simple if one has taken the precaution of performing sections additional to those of the usual procedure. We have seen that, in cases of femoral pain, one should make a es-pecial search for a lateral L4–L5 herniation compressing the L4 nerve root within the inter-vertebral foramen or just outside it (extrafora-minally). In order to do so, it is first necessary to perform sections *above* the L4–L5 disk, through the corresponding intervertebral foramen. If the results are negative, one should then explore the L3–L4 disk, which may show common intrafora-minal posterolateral herniation affecting the L4 root at its emergence from the thecal sac, or a lat-eral herniation compressing the L3 root within the foramen. In case of paresthetic meralgia, a lateral L2–L3 herniation should be sought.

Elementary Signs

The elementary CT signs combine *positive signs* and negative ones [74, 94, 97, 142, 216, 218, 265, 305, 307]:

- A *localized protrusion* of the lateral disk mar-gin within or lateral to the intervertebral fora-men.
- A *soft-tissue mass* within and/or outside the foramen, and having the same density as disk tissue. These may be a hypodensity at this level, suggesting the existence of a free frag-ment composed of nuclear substance.
- A displacement or filling in of the epidural *fat* in the foramen and/or the paravertebral fat.
- A nerve root *ganglion* which is enlarged, de-formed, and displaced both laterally and pos-teriorly. It may sometimes be very difficult to distinguish between the herniation and the nerve root. MRI may prove helpful, thanks to its better discrimination between disk and root signals, and the use of oblique sections.

Two negative signs should definitely be sought:

— The *posterior margin* of the disk is normal (in contrast to an ascending migratory herniation).
— *Thecal sac deformation* is absent. It is easy to understand why these herniations do not give myelographic signs, since the nerve root sheath usually ends at the inferior margin of the pedicle, slightly cephalad to the ganglion [6, 142] (see Figs. 130, 131).

Differential Diagnosis

These herniations may become *calcified* with time, resulting in compression of diskal-osteophytic origin. Cortical defects or a sclerotic reaction may be observed [296]. The lateral portion of the ring apophysis may be torn off. It then becomes very difficult to distinguish these herniations from a bony tumoral lesion (metastasis) (see Fig. 132; Fig. 133) or a reaction associated with a *neurinoma* or an epidural lymphoma [97, 307]. In the case of a contiguous degenerated disk, a gas bubble may be found within the foramen.

A large extraspinal fragment lodged in the deeper layers of the psoas muscle may simulate a *retroperitoneal tumoral mass* [79]. The proximity of both the intervertebral foramen and space should suggest the diagnosis of a lateral herniation.

A foraminal herniation may suggest a *migratory free fragment* originating in the overlying disk. However, in such cases there is usually a posterolateral herniation of the disk or at least sequelae of the breach in the anulus fibrosus (a posterior margin which is irregular, hazy or fringed); nevertheless, it is possible that the disk of origin has a strictly normal appearance [299]. All foraminal-far lateral herniations ascend slightly, but remain close to the intervertebral foramen.

A simple diskal *bulging* (protrusion) should not be mistaken for a lateral herniation. In cases of scoliosis or improper patient positioning, this overlap may appear asymmetric. However, it is usually a question of a degenerated disk; in particular, the overlap is circumferential, with no abrupt breaks in the diskal curve.

As we have seen in the preceding chapter, an abnormal radicular emergence (conjoined roots) may simulate a migratory free fragment, as well as a foraminal herniation. In case of doubt, myelography can be used for differentiation [97]. Such an abnormal emergence may be infrequently associated with a lateral herniation.

An isolated *radiculitis* without an associated disk herniation presents a difficult problem. The existence of an apparently isolated, large inflamed ganglion is possible; these are no abnormalities of the facing diskal contour. In this case, the intravenous injection of contrast medium (Iopamiron 300) is very useful in order to better define the lateral boundaries of the disk. As we have already seen, MRI can more easily confirm the normal appearance of the disk margin; sagit-

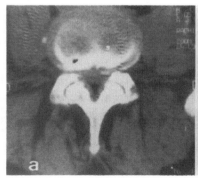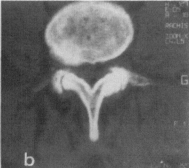

Fig. 133a, b. 49-year-old man. Resistant right femoral pain of 4 weeks' duration. Wasting of quadriceps. **a** L4–L5 disk: discrete posteromedian bulge. **b** Overlying foramen: isolated osteoblastic reaction with associated osteophytosis. *Operative findings:* Ablation of end-plate osteophytes. *Histology:* metastasis of an undifferentiated neoplasm

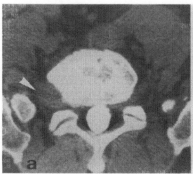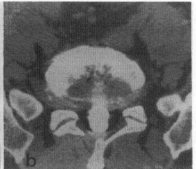

Fig. 134a, b. 59-year-old man. Metrizamide-enhanced CT. Right L5 sciatica. No explanations provided by myelogram. **a** Section through L5-S1 foramen: large right L5 ganglion *(white arrowhead).* **b** Disk: lateral extraspinal margin of the L5-S1 disk is normal. *Comments:* An inflammatory radiculitis may be manifested as a large ganglion in the neural foramen. – CT scans with 1 mm sections exclude other diskal abnormalities. – Antiinflammatory agents produce clinical regression of the radiculitis within a few weeks

tal reformatting using CT may also be useful [128, 249]. The etiology of such a radiculitis is disputed. Is it a type of healing of a lateral herniation undergoing regression? Simple mechanical strains on the nerve root (i. e., stretching in cases of spondylolisthesis, manipulations) may be sufficient causes. It is important that the diagnosis be made, since surgery is of no benefit in these cases (Fig. 134).

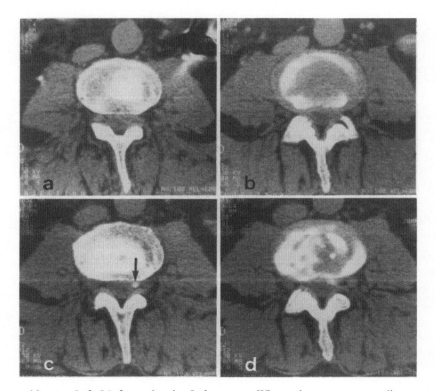

Fig. 135a–d. 60-year-old man. Left L3 femoral pain. Left L3-L4 foraminal herniation. *CT:* **a** Filling-in of left L3-L4 foramen; L3 root poorly visualized. **b** Slight asymmetry of left posterior margin of disk. *Postdiskography CT:* **c–d** Opacification of foraminal free fragment medial to root (→). *Comment:* When a large root or ganglion appears to be isolated within the foramen, postdiskography CT is quite able to demonstrate a small free fragment extruded from an apparently normal disk

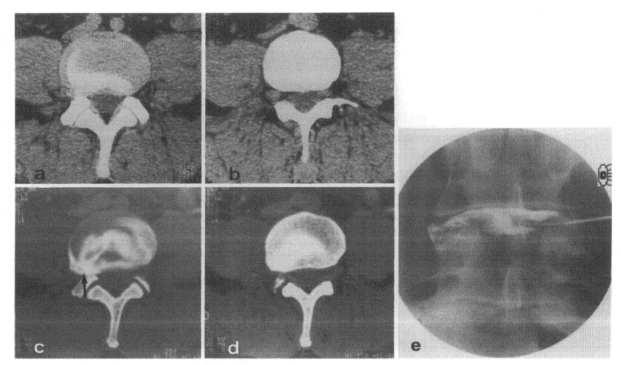

Fig. 136a–e. 51-year-old man. Right femoral pain. *CT:* **a** Right lateral L4–L5 herniation with disappearance of extraspinal fat surrounding L4 ganglion. No abnormalities of posterior margin of disk. **b** L4–L5 foramen. Large right L4 root. Localized inflammation or an associated small contiguous fragment? *Postdiskography CT at L4–L5:* **c** Diskal plane: Right lateral fissure (→) with accumulation of contrast medium in the extraspinal lateral herniation. **d** Overlying foraminal plane: no passage of contrast medium through the foramen, large isolated root. **e** *Diskography:* Confirmation of right lateral passage of contrast medium

CT-Surgery Correlations

Surgery is essentially indicated in pure *foraminal* herniations resulting in maximum nerve root compression within an unyielding bony framework. Severe clinical signs (paralytic sciatica) may even prompt emergency surgery.

On the other hand, *lateral* herniations are seldom candidates for surgery. They constitute a peculiar type of herniation: the nucleus pulposus, which is extruded outside the lumbar spinal canal, compresses the nerve root ganglion extraspinally, and the clinical signs improve in a few weeks despite their often hyperalgesic nature. There is actually a particular type of healing of the herniation and the radiculitis. Their extreme lateral location necessitates a wide surgical approach (laminectomy), often with a facetectomy, which may be a source of residual postoperative lumbar pain and vertebral instability. The diskectomy should be extensive. Exploration at surgery is difficult and may even prove negative [6]. Thus, such patients seem to be rather good candidates for *chemonucleolysis* or *intradiskal corticosteroid injection;* however, this is not universally recommended, since these hernias are classically extruded [94, 142]. In practice, despite the possibility of a transligamentous free fragment, it has long time been known that such herniations can be injected by diskography [2]. Certain authors go as far as to recommend the performance

Fig. 138a–d. 42-year-old man with left femoral pain. *CT:* **a** Large left L4 ganglion associated with an anterior free fragment *(arrowhead).* **b** Small posterolateral L4–L5 herniation. *Postdiskography CT:* **d** Partial opacification of foraminal free fragment. The posteriorly located ganglion can be distinguished. **d** Passage of contrast through a small orifice lateral to the articular pillar (→) which gave exit to the overlying fragment

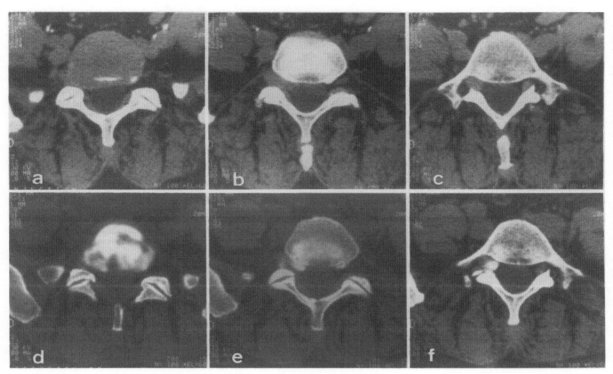

Fig. 137 a–f. 58-year-old woman with left L5 irradiation of sciatic pain resistant to medical treatment. Right L5–S1 lateral herniation. *CT:* **a** Right lateral L5–S1 herniation. **b** Extruded disk fragment in overlying foramen. **c** Large right L5 root below the pedicle: free fragment or inflammatory manifestation? *Postdiskography CT:* **d** Opacification of a degenerated disk with a right lateral extraspinal extension. **e** Overlying foraminal fragment opacified; ligamentous perforation with passage of contrast posterior to the root. **f** Opacified fragment extends upward considerably, reaching the plane of the right L5 pedicle

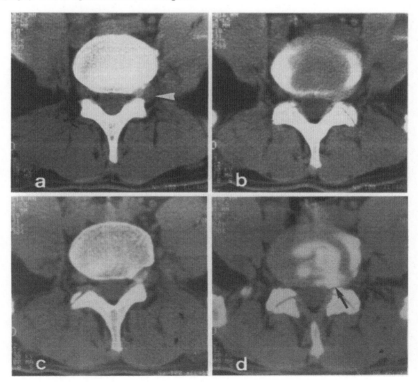

of a *diskoscan* (a postdiskography CT scan) in order to confirm the diagnosis [6] or the spread to the fragment of the injected chymodiactin (Figs. 135–138). The ascending foraminal free fragment is injected via the underlying herniation. The opacification of such herniations guarantees the subsequent diffusion of the enzyme or corticosteroid up to the disk fragment. The use of diskoscans may possibly reveal a small disk fragment in a certain number of cases usually classified as isolated radiculitis.

Postdiskography CT

The value of postdiskography CT in lateral or foramino-lateral herniations lies in its ability to demonstrate the pathophysiologic mechanisms involved, which are identical to those observed in common posterolateral or posteromedian intraspinal herniations. The extrusion orifice is located laterally or within the foramen. Extrusion of the nucleus pulposus occurs towards the foramen (site of maximum nerve root compression), or even furtherout, in the extraspinal space and in contact with the root ganglion.

Postdiskography CT scans confirm what has already been shown by standard CT, i. e., that femoral pain formerly labeled "idiopathic" is in most cases due to nerve root compression by a lateral disk herniation often located at L4–L5 or L3–L4 (see Fig. 138).

Furthermore, in case of isolated radiculitis, postdiskography CT scans are perfectly capable of showing the integrity of the disk and the absence of a small fragment adherent to the edematous nerve root (see Fig. 137).

It should be noted that lateral herniations responsible for typical femoral pain are excellent indications for chemonucleolysis, or, possibly, the intradiskal injection of long-acting corticosteroids.

Double Herniations

The association of two herniations at two different disk segments is a rare finding (6% of our series) which may make it difficult to decide on the segment in need treatment if the clinical picture is unclear. As a general rule, neurosurgeons operate only on the level responsible for the clinical signs. No age group is particularly affected; double herniations may be observed at any time after the age of 20 years. In all cases, the disk herniations were found at L4–L5 and L5–S1.

CT Features [74]

Routine investigation of the last two lumbar disk segments may reveal two associated herniations at L4–L5 and L5–S1 even when the clinical picture is one of typical monoradicular involvement.

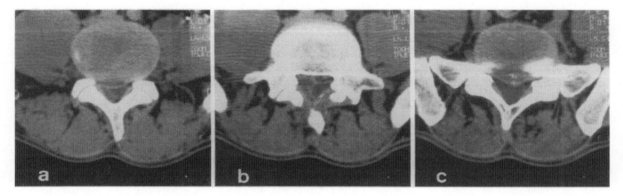

Fig. 139a–c. 31-year-old man with a right L5 sciatica of 4 months' duration, without neuro-deficit. **a** *L4–L5 disk:* posteromedian herniation with a hypodensity (free fragment) having an irregular outline. Unusual posterolateral migration with respect to the thecal sac (ligamentous perforation). **b** Unusual ascending migration is confirmed. **c** *L5–S1 disk:* Fortuitously discovered posteromedian herniation. *Operative findings:* on the clinical evidence, the operation involved only one level. Large L4–L5 free fragment with ligamentous perforation

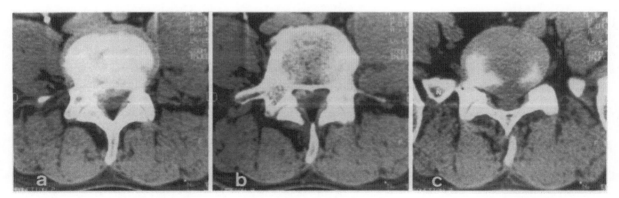

Fig. 140a–c. 40-year-old man. Left lumbosciatic pain of several years' duration. Hyperalgesic right L5 sciatica of 2 months' duration. **a** *L4–L5 Level:* Section through lower portion of disk; bulging associated with a right posterolateral herniation. **b** Section through facet joint plane: large edematous right L5 root which appears hyperdense (radicular lesion). Relatively narrow lumbar canal. **c** *L5–S1 Level:* Major posteromedian herniation. *Operative findings:* In view of the clinical signs (a recent hyperalgesic right sciatica), only the L4–L5 level was operated upon, with ablation of a large free fragment

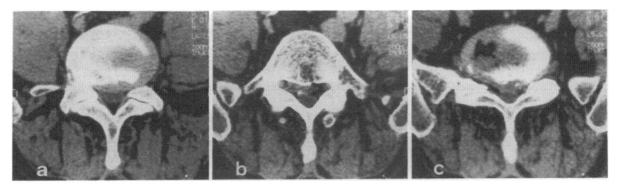

Fig. 141a–c. 53-year-old man: right sciatica with L5 and S1 root suffering of 2 weeks' duration and discrete neuro-deficit. **a** *L4–L5 disk:* posteromedian herniation. **b** Image discontinuity with migratory free fragment descending toward the axilla of the right L5 root, which is partially calcified (old free fragment?). **b–c** *L5–S1 disk:* vacuum disk phenomenon; significant posteromedian herniation. Left paramedian herniation compresses the thecal sac against the posterior arch. *Operative findings:* both levels. – At L4–L5: collapsed disk; little material; soft free fragment which was slightly compressive. – At L5–S1: Disk fragment adherent to right S1 root

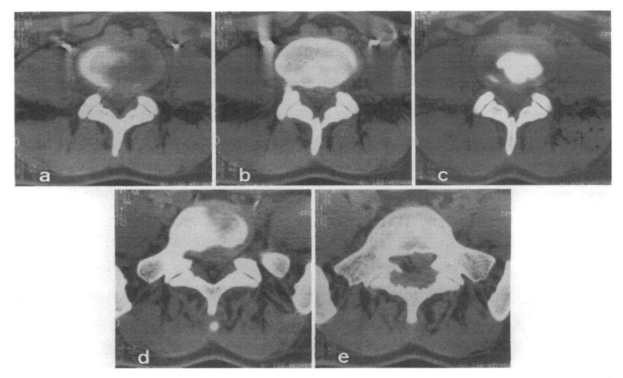

Fig. 142a–e. 27-year-old woman. Incomplete left sciatica of 2 months' duration: suspected double herniation (L4–L5 and L5–S1). *L4–L5 Level:* **a–b** There seems to be a minor descending posteromedian herniation. **c** Postdiskography CT at L4–L5: homogeneous opacification of the nucleus. No fissures of the anulus fibrosus. What previouly resembled a herniation is in fact the anterior epidural veins. *L5–S1 Level:* **d–e** Descending left posterolateral herniation compressing the S1 root in the lateral recess. *Comment:* In view of the negative results of the postdiskography scan at L4–L5, only one chemonucleolysis was performed, at the L5–S1 level

Two different situations may be present:

— In most cases there is monoradicular pain at
L5 or S1 but there is a second herniation at
the adjacent level which is a fortuitous CT
finding. This situation does not present any
problems; the segment responsible for the
clinical signs is the one which will be operated upon. Nevertheless, it is necessary to be
aware of the second herniation site for follow-up purposes, as it may give rise to symptoms following surgery due to the altered mechanical conditions. In fact, the evolution of
clinically "silent" herniations is usually favorable as regards reduction in size and eventual
disappearance (Figs. 139, 140).
— In other cases, the clinical signs are not clear
and there is usually *biradicular* involvement
of L5 and S1. CT should be used to search
for signs of root involvement at both levels
(Fig. 141) and to identify the most pathological segment.

Complementary *myelography* may be performed
to determine the level at which nerve root sheath
compression is greatest. It is particularly useful
in differentiating between a bulging L4–L5 disk
with a locally narrowed spinal canal, and a true
L5–S1 herniation. In difficult cases, this CT-
myelography combination may restrict operation
to one level.

CT investigation of the two segments may also be combined with diskography to confirm the
double involvement in young subjects, who may
be candidates for a double chemonucleolysis.
Such a diskoscan may help to differentiate between a bulging anulus fibrosus, and a true herniation with a torn anulus and extrusion of the
nucleus pulposus (Fig. 142).

Nevertheless, the radiologic work-up may be
unable to guide the neurosurgeon sufficiently to
avoid surgery at both levels with hemilaminectomy. Both herniations may prove to be genuinely
compressive, but in other cases one of the segments proves to be only slightly abnormal, with
little material or soft material which is only
slightly compressive.

Difficult Cases

There are numerous problems in the interpretation of CT scans of disk herniations. Aside from artifacts (due to poor patient cooperation or obesity) and drawbacks in technique (i. e., the exploration is limited to two segments), the evaluation of CT abnormalities may be tricky and result in errors. An image of inferior quality, a poorly visualized posterior disk margin and difficult identification of a nerve root in the superior portion of the lateral recess are all problems often encountered by the radiologist. The most frequent cause of difficulties is the association of a narrow spinal canal and a disk herniation or simple protrusion (bulging) at L4–L5. Myelography remains particularly valuable in all these cases. We first examine the causes of false-negative findings and then of false-positives.

False-negatives

Disk Herniation with Narrowed
Lumbar Spinal Canal

This is the major cause of false-negatives in spinal CT scans.

Lumbar spinal stenosis is of three types [167, 299]:

— *Developmental spinal stenosis* exists at birth as one element of more serious malformations (e. g., lumbar agenesis, dysraphism).
— *Congenital spinal stenosis* forms part of an idiopathic developmental dysmorphism, with shortened pedicles, laminae which are higher and more frontal than normal, and articular facets which are more sagittal (4 cases with a mean age of 31 years in our series). These comprise:
dysplasias, essentially achondroplastic;
dysostoses, which can be divided into: isolated congenital lumbar spinal stenosis [298]; this is the commonest type, moderate and often asymptomatic unless acquired lesions are superadded;

cheirolumbar dysostosis [299], a familial condition with a shortened long axis and lengthened small axis of the long bones of the hands and sometimes the feet;
basal cell nevus syndrome and the Wyers-Thiers oculovertebral syndrome, which are less common forms with vertebral synostosis.
— *Acquired spinal stenosis* is the commonest type; it often precipitates symptoms in a congenital stenosis between the fourth and fifth decades of life by added disk degeneration and facet hypertrophy. It is not always simple to differentiate between acquired and congenital spinal stenosis, especially in older subjects, in whom osteophytic encroachment related to the posterior vertebral body surface, thickened ligamenta flava and an increase in the size of the articular pillars may all contribute to a narrowing of the spinal canal similar to that observed in congenital stenosis.

Spinal stenoses are readily diagnosed and quantified on axial CT. Routine measurements (anteroposterior diameter; interpedicular distance; interfacet distance; pedicular length; Jones-Thompson index) do not necessarily indicate the pathogenic nature of the stenosis. Nevertheless, it is generally accepted that an anteroposterior diameter of less than 10 mm is certainly pathogenic, and that stenosis of between 10 and 12 mm is relative, usually being decompensated by degenerative changes. Measurements of the lateral recess are difficult to obtain because of the obliquity of its posterior aspect; only measurements performed in its superior portion, which has the smallest anteroposterior diameter (over 3 mm) are valid [21, 60, 167, 205, 206]. However, these measurements are not very reliable, being too dependent on the gantry angle.

The structure of the spinal canal and the relationship between the bony canal and its contents are much more important. The spinal canal may have an oval or triangular appearance in cases of congenital spinal stenosis, and usually a cloverleaf or trefoil appearance in cases of acquired stenosis complicating congenital stenoses. In acquired spinal stenosis, hypertrophy of the articular pillars (of degenerative or dysplastic origin) may result in compression of the thecal sac and

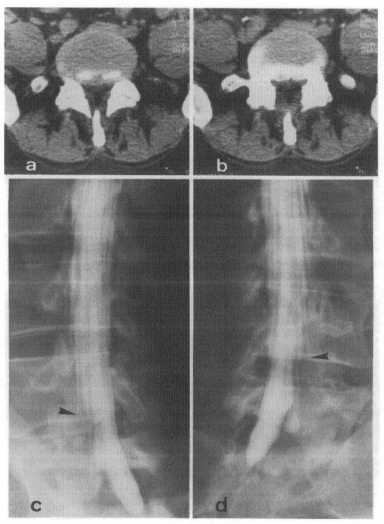

Fig. 143 a-d. 40-year-old woman. Alternating L5 sciatica. Left root involvement: median L4–L5 bulging and spinal stenosis. **a** Posteromedian L4–L5 bulge with diskal protrusion. Posterior margin of disk is poorly visualized. Lateral epidural fat normal. **b** In the upper portion of the lateral recess, the nerve roots appear normal. Previous sections show few signs of compression at the L5 radicular emergences. **c-d** *Lumbar myelograms:* Severe compression of both left and right L5 roots, with amputation of their sheaths *(arrowhead).* *Operative findings:* Significant diskal bulging with compression of L5 roots at their emergence from the thecal sac. Bilateral internal facetectomy

especially of the lateral recess. We have already described this anatomico-surgical entity (cf Radioanatomy). The nerve root which courses in it may be compressed by an isolated posterolateral disk herniation, but also by associated degenerative hypertrophy of an articular pillar or by an isolated lesion of the pillar. Although spinal stenosis is usually multisegmental, it may be confined to one segment, usually L4–L5 (Fig. 143). Pure central spinal stenoses are rare in comparison to the lateral or combined types; degenerative spondylolisthesis gives rise to a central stenosis which may be associated with a lateral stenosis. The lateral recesses should always be carefully investigated for a minimal disk lesion or moderate facet joint arthropathy, either of which may suffice to decompensate a preexisting congenital narrowing of the lateral recess [167, 178, 206, 226, 259, 299].

The identification of a herniation in this context may prove difficult, since both the epidural fat and most of the thecal sac CSF are absent

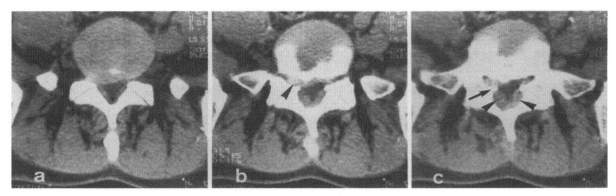

Fig. 144a–c. 33-year-old woman. Right S1 sciatica of 2 months' duration: right L5–S1 herniation and spinal stenosis. **a** L5–S1 disk: common type of right posterolateral herniation in a predisposed subject (spinal stenosis). **b** Disk substance in the upper portion of the right lateral recess and a slightly descending herniation *(arrowhead)*. **c** Right lateral recess stenosis *(→)*. Trefoil appearance of spinal canal and hypertrophied ligamenta flava *(arrowhead)*. Right S1 root differentiated with difficulty. *Operative findings:* Partial perforation of posterior longitudinal ligament; large preligamentous free fragment

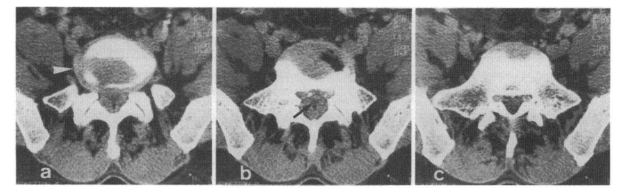

Fig. 145a–c. 53-year-old woman. Alternating S1 lumbosciatic pain of 4 months' duration: L5–S1 bulging and spinal stenosis. **a** L5–S1 disk: posteromedian bulging; spinal stenosis; hypertrophied ligamenta flava. Thecal sac compression by the disk and ligmenta flava. Peripheral enhancement of the disk *(arrowhead)*, which is particularly frequent in cases with disk degeneration. **b** Virtual obliteration of thecal sac *(→)* as a result of the diskal bulging and ligamentous hypertrophy. **c** As is usually the case, the roots below a severe compression appear quite normal. This is observed only within this particular context. *Operative findings:* Large, median preligamentous herniation

and these are normally major aids to CT contrast within the spinal canal. The ligamenta flava are often hypertrophied; the dura mater, nerve roots and the herniation are in close contact with the neighboring densities [206]. There is less CSF bathing the roots of the cauda equina and there is an increase in the densities of the thecal sac contents [299]. In the absence of fat, the posterior disk margin may be poorly visible. The intravenous injection of contrast medium (Iopamiron 300) is essential in defining the posterior limits of the disk. An increased number of sections should be performed, both in the overlying foramen and lower down in the lateral recess. A migratory free fragment has be found in the lateral recess (Fig. 144); its identification may be difficult in case of degenerated or old disk material, which has a lower density than usual. Thecal sac constriction often appears minimized on CT; the diameters above and below the suspected level should be compared (Fig. 145).

All cases of spinal stenosis, especially at L4–L5, should be routinely investigated for disk protrusion or bulging. When bulging is present, the degenerated nucleus pulposus displaces the stretched (but not torn) anulus fibrosus laterally, resulting in extension of the disk margins and a decrease in disk height. CT show a circumferential overlap of the disk in all directions, which extends beyond the vertebral bodies [304, 308]. Contrast uptake may appear as a thin rim at periphery of the disk. Uptake sometimes occurs in normal disks, but is more frequent and intense in disk degeneration (see Fig. 145). The pathogenesis of this contrast uptake is debated; certain authors suggest a renewed vascularization through the cartilaginous plates into the adjacent disk. At a more advanced stage, edema, granulations and scarring may be evident [89, 312]. The presence of gas (nitrogen) within these degenerated disks is not uncommon. Gas bubbles may also be found within the spinal canal, whether close to the disk, straddling a tear in the anulus, or in relation to a remote free fragment [148, 284] (Fig. 146).

The distinction between a disk herniation and a disk protrusion is not merely academic. Protrusion is very common, indeed almost constant after the fourth decade of life, and is usually accompanied by lumbar pain without radiculalgia. Nevertheless, this is not always the case, particularly when there is an associated narrow lumbar spinal canal. In such cases, a protrusion may have the same mechanical consequences as a herniation, resulting in nerve root compression [178, 206]. The degree of such compression often appears minimized by CT; the scan rarely shows signs of nerve root involvement such as deviation or edema, given the chronic nature of the mechanical phenomena (this is comparable to the absence of foraminal vein stasis at the cervical level in case of uncinate process hypertrophy) [160, 162, 310]. This is the only instance in which CT cannot reliably provide indirect radicular signs (see Fig. 143). This is the cause of numerous CT interpretational errors, errors which are more likely if the patient is obese and the image of inferior quality [27].

There should therefore be no hesitation in performing myelography when doubts persist [206]. Myelography will usually show bilateral amputation of the L5 nerve roots. Moreover, CT is unable to investigate dynamic stenosis due to protrusion of the ligamentum flavum or the articular pillars and favored by lumbar lordosis, since scanning is performed on a supine subject with knees flexed, thus reducing the lordosis. Myelography permits a dynamic evaluation (flexion-extension on oblique projections) of both the stenosis in general and of the most pathogenic segment among these often multisegmental stenoses [167, 175].

In such situations, the radiologist should be very cautious, and descriptive rather than dogmatic. It is difficult to evaluate the pathogenic significance of a lesion, given the multiplicity of conditions which may be sources of pain. Simple articular process hypertrophy may result in "pseudosciatic" pain. Similarly, diskal and osteophytic protrusion may be associated. Arranged in

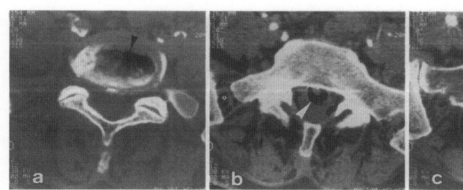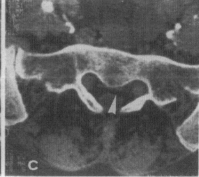

Fig. 146a-c. 62-year-old woman. Intermittent left sciatica of several months' duration. Absent Achilles tendon reflex. **a** Vacuum disk phenomenon at L5-S1 *(black arrowhead)*. Presence of a calcified disk herniation and a calcified ligament. **b-c** Gas bubble below the herniation level around the basisvertebral vein and extending downward to the first left sacral foramen *(white arrowhead)*. *Comments:* The presence of gas is due to degeneration of a descending migratory fragment. This patient had never had epidural injections of antiinflammatory agents

a horizontal perivertebral ring, osteophytes may give rise to axial-section images which are difficult to interpret; because of partial volume effects, they may simulate a calcified disk fragment [71, 206].

One should always keep in mind the clinical aspects during the interpretation of these multiple lesions within the spinal canal. A complete diagnostic work-up is a valuable guide to surgery, which often entails a wider approach than that used in common herniations (laminectomy with or without facetectomy). A narrow lumbar spinal canal associated with a herniation entails a much greater risk of failed chemonucleolysis.

A Large Herniation Merging with the Thecal Sac

This is a commonly encountered and classic source of diagnostic error. Paradoxically, a large posteromedian herniation may be overlooked. It occupies the site of the thecal sac, which it obliterates. Its densities may be close to those of CSF (40 HU). The posterior epidural fat and normal nerve roots may be preserved. It then becomes necessary to explore the posterior disk margin in great detail; the margin shows a defect or a blurred, somewhat irregular aspect. Myelography

will show an almost complete blockage of the contrast column by a herniation which is almost completely extruded [206, 299] (Fig. 147).

Unusual Segments

This is a rather rare possibility, which should be investigated in cases of femoral pain without a lateral disk herniation at L4–L5. If routine CT study of the last two segments is negative in a case of monoradicular sciatica, a search should be made for a possible discopathy at a higher level, especially in elderly subjects. Myelography or a few additional precautionary sections through the L3–L4 segment may be performed, either initially or additionally. It should also be remembered that L1–L2 or L2–L3 herniations are possibilities that cannot be investigated by routine CT scans under any circumstances (Fig. 148).

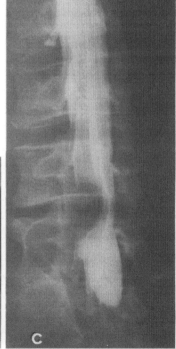

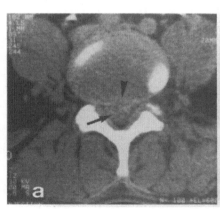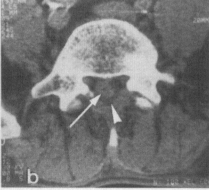

Fig. 147a–c. 51-year-old man. Right L5 sciatica with a discrete neuro-deficit of three months' duration; enormous L4–L5 herniation. **a** L4–L5 disk: posterior margin appears "normal". In fact, there is a median tear *(black arrowhead)*. More posteriorly, the double contour image corresponds to the combination of an enormous herniation (→) and a collapsed thecal sac. **b** L5 roots in the lateral recess are normal.

Herniation (→) has occupied the place of the thecal sac, which has been totally compressed against the ligamenta flava *(white arrowhead)*. **c** These images were initially considered normal; a lumbar myelogram 3 weeks later corrected the diagnostic error. *Operative findings:* Large posteromedian preligamentous herniation

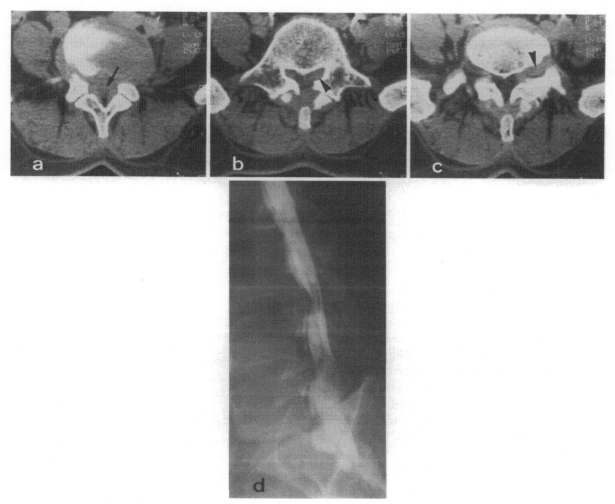

Fig. 148a-d. 48-year-old woman. Alternating L5 and S1 lumbosciatic pain of several months' duration; discrete L5 deficit. **a** L4-L5 disk: bulging associated with posteromedian herniation; spinal stenosis (→). **b** Large L5 root in left lateral recess *(arrowhead)*. **c** Large L5 root associated with a left L5-S1 foraminal herniation *(arrowhead)*. **d** *Lumbar myelography:* performed because of ambiguous clinical signs and a difficult patient. Severe thecal sac compression at L4-L5, as had been shown by CT. Significant overlying L3-L4 herniation. This illustrates the limitations of CT in routine investigations of the last two lumbar levels. *Operative findings:* surgery at levels L3-L4 and L4-L5 was motivated by the myelogram rather than the clinical signs. L4-L5: normal disk material and spinal stenosis. L3-L4: greater bulging of the disk, which was viscous and adherent; spinal stenosis

Pitfalls in CT

It is evident that the examination artifacts dealt with in the chapter on CT technique limit the ability to interpret the images. Patient movement or obesity and insufficient gantry angulation are particular sources of error. To cope with these problems, the patient can be urged to keep still; 5 mm sections are less subject to artifacts in overweight patients; and sagittal reconstructions can be made for an inadequately approached disk. In cases of scoliosis or poor patient positioning, there may well be asymmetry of the thecal sac, nerve root sheaths and epidural fat; bony structure asymmetry and the absence of displaced or compressed nervous structures are valuable findings. Conclusions should not be drawn from a single section of poor quality, but an increased number of sections should be made for fuller investigation of the foramina overlying the disk and the underlying lateral recesses. If a correct interpretation proves to be impossible or if doubts persist, one should not hesitate to resort to myelography [27, 306].

False-positives

Root Emergence Anomalies

These may be nerve roots with conjoined emergences or ectopic origins. Conjoined nerve roots usually involve the L5 and S1 roots. This rare (1%) congenital anomaly is generally unilateral, and was first observed in 1952, during surgery for a disk herniation. The first myelographic observation of conjoined nerve roots was made in 1974 [38, 64, 71, 206, 212, 284, 299, 306].

These anomalies fall into *5 basic types:*

a) a common trunk of two nerve roots which separate after exiting through the same intervertebral foramen: the so-called *"conjoined nerve roots";*
b) a common trunk of two nerve roots which separate, each exiting through its own intervertebral foramen: *"divergent nerve roots";* This is by far the commonest case;
c) two nerve roots exiting through the same intervertebral foramen: *"convergent nerve roots";*
d) nerve root with a horizontal course: *"horizontal nerve root";*
e) anastomosis between 2, or even 3 nerve roots: *"anastomosed nerve roots"* (Fig. 149)

With practice, nerve root emergence anomalies may be identified on CT alone. They appear as a rounded anterolateral opacity with a density equal to or slightly greater than that of the thecal sac (20 to 60 HU). Additional sections can show their progressive junction with the thecal sac. Some may be mistaken for migratory disk herniations. If there is any doubt, myelography provides the diagnosis. It is important that these nerve root anomalies be pointed out to the surgeon. There is debate concerning the painful nature of these isolated radicular anomalies. Nerve root fixity and the considerable volume of the abnormal spinal nerves have been evoked as pathogenic factors, and even a small one associated disk herniation will have aggravated clinical manifestations tending to be multiradicular (Fig. 150).

Radicular Cysts

Radicular cysts include several different anatomic entities which are difficult to differentiate on CT.

Perineural cysts (Tarlov's cysts) should not be confused with a migratory disk herniation in the intervertebral foramen or with a small neurinoma. They have smooth contours and a low density equal to that of the thecal sac. They are found at the spinal ganglion and develop in the perineurium as a result of traumatic or hemorrhagic degenerative changes in the ganglion (Fig. 151).

Extradural arachnoid cysts associated with meningeal diverticula are also possible. In such cases, there may be an expanded spinal canal and scalloping of the adjacent posterolateral surface of the vertebral body, the pedicle and the pedicle-laminar junction. The cortical bone is preserved; there is no osteosclerosis. Lumbar pain may be present. Excessive transmission of CSF pulsation into the subarachnoid space is involved in the pathogenesis of extradural arachnoid cysts; hence, a large thecal sac may be present. The cysts are usually multiple and essentially involve the S1 and S2 nerve roots. There may be associated neurofibromatosis (Fig. 152).

Arachnoid diverticula arise from the evagination of arachnoid through a dural gap; they communicate with the subarachnoid space.

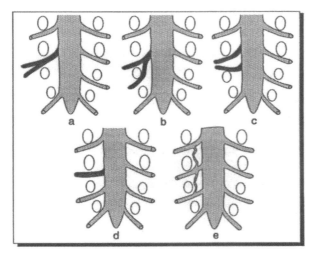

Fig. 149a–e. Difficult cases. Root emergence abnormalities. **a** Conjoined nerve roots. **b** Divergent nerve roots. **c** Convergent nerve roots. **d** Horizontal nerve root. **e** Anastomosed nerve roots

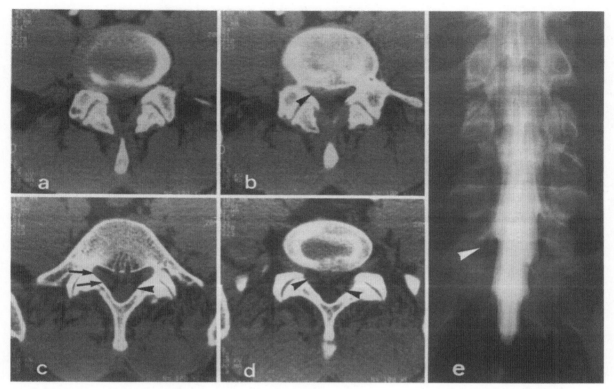

Fig. 150a–e. 32-year-old man. Right lumbosciatic pain: right paramedian L4–L5 herniation associated with an unusually high emergence of the S1 root. **a** Small right paramedian L4–L5 herniation. Asymmetric distribution of lateral epidural fat. **b** Filling-in of right lateral recess; is there downward extension of the hernia *(black arrowhead)?* **c** This is actually an S1 root with a high emergence. Conjoined L5 and S1 right nerve roots are visible in the lateral recess (→). Homologous left S1 root emerges from the thecal sac later *(black arrowhead).* **d** L5 foramen: persistent asymmetry of the S1 roots *(black arrowhead).* **e** *Lumbar myelography:* Plain anteroposterior radiograph confirms the high emergence of the right S1 root *(white arrowhead).* Myelography is unable to show the respective paths a of the right L5 and S1 roots towards the foramen

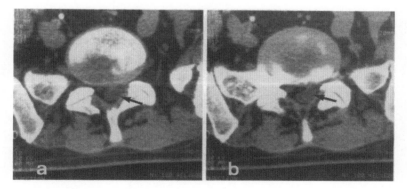

Fig. 151a, b. 40-year-old man. Bilateral S1 sciatica, more pronounced on the left; both Achilles tendon reflexes are absent. At L4–L5 level: very large, descending posteromedian herniation. **a–b** L5–S1 level: posterior margin of disk appears normal: however, there is a questionable hypodensity between the thecal sac and the left S1 root (→). *At Lumbar myelography:* Large radicular cyst originating in the perineurium of the left S1 root. *Operative findings:* Large preligamentous L4–L5 herniation

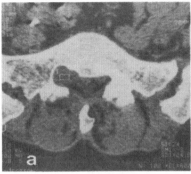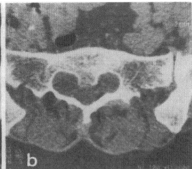

Fig. 152a, b. 58-year-old woman. Lumbosciatic pain: perineurial cysts (Tarlov cysts) of the radicular sheaths. **a** Large structure with a density comparable to that of CSF, which entirely occupies the right lateral recess. **b** Section 9 mm lower-perineural cyst of the left S1 root, also a deformed recess

Epidural Veins

This is a classic, but usually avoidable, diagnostic pitfall. The basivertebral veins are retrocorporeal (but not retrodiskal), opposite the basivertebral foramen and frequently associated with a small bony spur. The only confusion possible is with a migratory disk herniation. However, the veins are more irregular and serpentine in appearance and anastomose with other typical epidural veins. Their densities are comparable to those of a disk fragment. True epidural varices may be found. Once again, careful examination of the posterior disk margin is essential, since it is normal. Furthermore, there are no or few associated partial volume effects [71, 206, 306] (Fig. 153).

Spondylolysis and Spondylolisthesis

Degenerative spondylolisthesis has already been discussed in the context of acquired spinal stenosis [51, 206, 299]. The associated degeneration of facet joints and disks permits the simultaneous sliding of the entire vertebral body and intact neural arch. If there is a preexisting spinal stenosis, subluxation of even a few mm may be enough to result in pronounced clinical symptoms (cauda equina syndrome).

Spondylolysis and nondegenerative spondylolisthesis, which has a different etiology, can be diagnosed on plain radiographs using anteroposterior, lateral and oblique projections. Nevertheless, CT is often needed to determine the etiology of associated lumbosciatic pain.

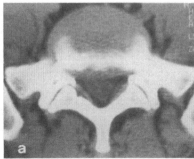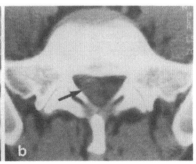
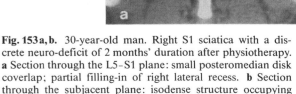

Fig. 153a, b. 30-year-old man. Right S1 sciatica with a discrete neuro-deficit of 2 months' duration after physiotherapy. **a** Section through the L5-S1 plane: small posteromedian disk coverlap; partial filling-in of right lateral recess. **b** Section through the subjacent plane: isodense structure occupying the right paramedian region, which was diagnosed as a descending L5-S1 herniation (→) No injection of contrast medium. *Operative findings:* This was not a large disk fragment but an enlarged varicose epidural vein

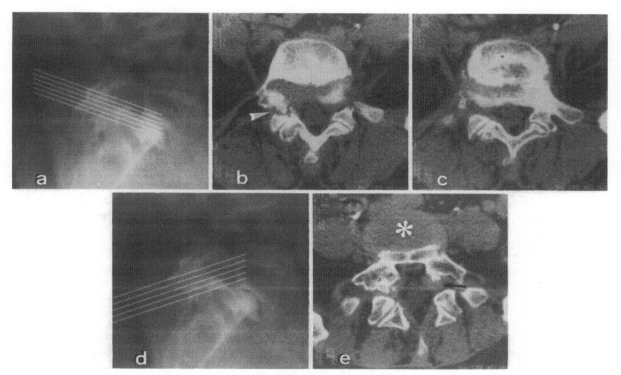

Fig. 154a–e. 61-year-old woman. Right L5 and S1 lumbo-sciatic pain: L5–S1 spondylolysis with severe forward subluxation of L5 on S1. **a** Sagittal scout view: L5–S1 spondylolisthesis. Even maximal gantry angulation is insufficient for correct study of the disk. **b–c** L5–S1 disk: posterior disk margin is normal; intraforaminal portion of the right L5 root is poor-ly visualized. Unilateral right pars interarticularis defect *(white arrowhead)*. **d** Sagittal scout view: sections parallel to posterior arch of L5. **e** This projection shows the bilateral pars interarticularis defect particularly well, as well as the swelling of the joint capsule which predominates on left (→). L4–L5 disk is seen in this section (✱)

Isthmic spondylolisthesis may be the result of a stress fracture. It tends to appear between 5 and 7 years of age, much more seldom between 7 and 18 years. By age 18, 5 to 7% of the general population have a spondylolysis. There is a familial propensity, involving congenital hypoplasia of the pars interarticularis. These pars interarticularis defects are usually bilateral; L5 shows a defect in almost all cases and L4 less frequently. Several levels, as well as pedicles and laminae, may be involved. A simple elongation of the pars interarticularis may correspond to a healed stress fracture.

Within this framework, lumbosciatic pain may have several etiologies, which are best investigated by CT:

— Persistent unilateral sciatica should prompt a search for osteofibrous callus and which develops anterointernally at the fracture site, compressing the nerve root posteriorly in the lower portion of the lateral recess. CT sections through the axial plane of the neural arch are best for exploring such a callus or possible ossification centers. Osteosclerosis of the contralateral neural arch (vertebral anisocoria) should not be confused with an osteosclerotic tumoral lesion (Fig. 154).

— Unilateral sciatica of rapid onset should suggest a disk herniation at the overlying level. A herniation is very seldom found at the same level as the pars defect (Fig. 155). Pseudobulging of the disk, due to significant diskal tilt and an insufficiently angled CT section plane, should not be confused with a herniation (Fig. 156). Reconstructed sagittal views may be especially helpful [107, 249].

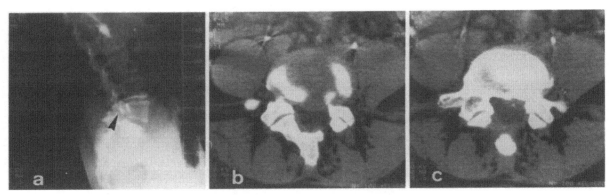

Fig. 155a–c. 28-year-old woman. Left L5 sciatica of 6 months' duration; L5–S1 spondylolysis and left posterolateral L4–L5 herniation. **a** Sagittal scout view: spondylolysis is clearly visible *(arrowhead)*, with no associated forward subluxation. **a–c** Discrete descending L4–L5 herniation is clearly visible in the left lateral recess. *Operative findings:* Considerable preligamentous L4–L5 herniation. The herniation associated with spondylolysis usually occurs at the level above

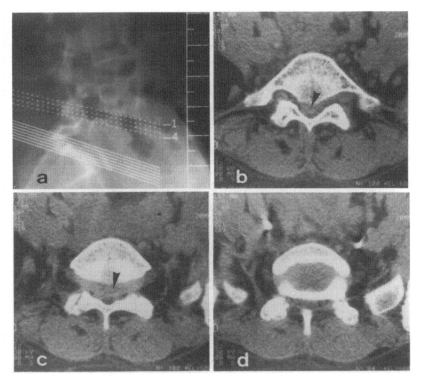

Fig. 156a–d. 33-year-old woman. Right S1 lumbosciatic pain of 2 months' duration with a discrete neuro-deficit, onset after physical exertion: right L5–S1 spondylolysis with forward subluxation. **a** Sagittal scout view: L5–S1 disk cannot be properly investigated (gantry angle greater than 20°). **b** Section through midportion of the body of L5: hyperdense appearance of the lumbar canal *(arrowhead)* (ascending free fragment? considerable venous stasis?). **c–d** Sections show that the apparent herniation is in fact due to a technical limitation (the gantry cannot be angled parallel to the disk). The abnormal apparent size of the lumbar canal (a small anteroposterior diameter) is due to a beam angulation artifact. These sections had suggested an ascending disk herniation. *(arrowhead) Operative findings:* L5 root was highly compressed between the S1 vertebra and the L5 lamina. Substantial impression of S1 root; stepped appearance due to spondylolithesis. No disk herniation. Spinal stenosis

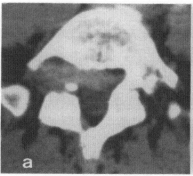 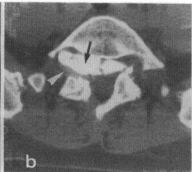

Fig. 157a, b. 53-year-old woman. Right L5 sciatica; bilateral spondylolysis with forward subluxation of L5 on S1. **a** CT at L5-S1: Foraminal asymmetry due to lumbar scoliosis; on the right side it is difficult to differentiate between a foraminal herniation and an isolated L5 radiculitis. **b** Postdiskography CT at L5-S1: substantial opacification of the entire disk, which appears degenerated (→). There is no foraminal free fragment; the disk is rendered more visible by the forward subluxation and scoliosis. The slightly displaced L5 ganglion is clearly seen *(white arrowhead)*. *Comments:* Absence of a typical foraminal herniation on postdiskography CT is a contraindication to chemonucleolysis

— Bilateral atypical (truncated) sciatica should prompt a search for nerve root compression due to spinal stenosis or for root elongation due to significant slip. Physical therapy may destabilize this condition. CT may reveal an isolated radiculitis, without a directly compressive lesion.

In over two-thirds of the cases, nerve root compression is multifactorial.

Postdiskography CT
This examination demonstrates that standard CT yields pseudoimages, since the sections performed are not parallel to the diskal plane, which is very oblique, especially in case of spondylolisthesis, whereas gantry angling is limited to 20°.

In these very specific cases, postdiskography CT may help in confirming a common diskal bulging in a predisposed subject, in contact with an inflamed or merely elongated nerve root (Fig. 157).

Other Diagnostic Pitfalls

Discovery of Asymptomatic Lesions

This is a most difficult problem, and one to which we have already alluded in discussing double herniations. It is tempting to assign a clinical repercussion to every abnormality detected on CT, yet 35% of CT examinations in asymptomatic subjects reveal disk or facet joint abnormalities. It is very important to rely on the clinical examination, which should be as thorough as possible concerning the segmental nerve roots.

Intraspinal Infectious and Tumoral Lesions

Diskitis with vertebral osteomyelitis can be easily diagnosed using plain radiographs, when the typical clinical syndrome is present [71, 127, 206, 306]. Suggestive findings on CT are: a heterogeneous disk which takes up contrast and sometimes exhibits an intradiskal air-fluid level; bone erosion and lytic defects; and spread to paraspinal soft tissues. Nevertheless, the differential diagnosis of disk herniation may arise in certain cases of isolated diskitis with an epidural abscess but no bone involvement. In such cases, one should look for evidence of infection (e.g., brucellosis), disk hypodensity, and for epidural soft-tissue spread generally extending over more than one intervertebral space (Fig. 158).

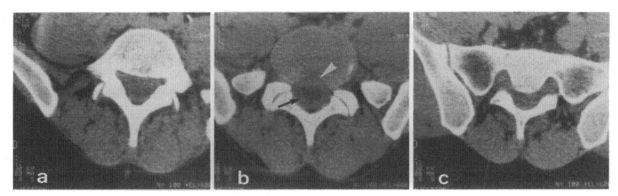

Fig. 158a–c. 22-year-old man. Acute lumbar pain followed by bilateral lumbosciatic pain of 3 weeks' duration. Development of cauda equina syndrome. **a** Section through midportion of body of L4: no epidural fat visible between the roots and the thecal sac. **b** L5–S1 disk: no fat present between the ligamenta flava and the thecal sac, which seems to be surrounded by a thin hyperdense rim (→). Hypodensity within the posterior portion of the disk *(white arrowhead);* this is not an artefact **c** Subjacent section. Fat is also absent in all planes of section studied. Disk fragments would be incapable of obliterating the fat simultaneously at several levels. The disk hypodensity should suggest an infectious process. Patient had contracted brucellosis 3 weeks earlier. *Operative findings:* Cheesy pus anterior to thecal sac and at the level of the right S1 axilla. Sclerosed epidural tissue at the L5 axilla. Partially necrotic disk. Brucellar diskitis

We have never had any diagnostic problems with tumoral lesions; all atypical painful syndromes have led us to perform either myelography or Iopamidol-enhanced CT scans or, more recently, MRI.

Benign tumors (*neurinoma* of the cauda equina) are very rare. They take up contrast medium; however, their density may be close to that of the thecal sac, so that they pass unnoticed on routine CT scans. If there is the slightest doubt (nocturnally exacerbated pain), myelography or MRI should be performed to study the entire cauda equina and medullary cone [57].

We have already seen that a neurinoma in the intervertebral foramen may simulate a far lateral foraminal disk herniation. Classically, the foramen is enlarged with osteosclerotic contours. Nevertheless, large herniations of more than a year's standing may lead to cortical erosion of the vertebral body, and to enlargement and sclerosis of the foraminal walls [196].

An *intradural disk herniation* [189] may simulate an intradural tumor. The incidence of such herniations is very small (0.13%). They are frequently accompanied by lingering lumbosciatic pain with acute episodes and severe neurologic deficits involving several nerve roots. Myelography or a myeloscan can provide the diagnosis by showing an irregular or lobular intradural mass. Disk fragments may migrate within a nerve root sheath or be associated with a gas bubble [148]. A firm fixation of the ventral dural mater to the posterior longitudinal ligament favors such migrations. Among the factors favoring intradural herniations are: degenerative and inflammatory disk lesions; microtraumas; and previous surgery [110, 148].

Invasive epidural tumors (e.g., lymphoma, metastatic epiduritis) are usually more diffuse and poorly defined. They have lower densities and are associated with bone lesions.

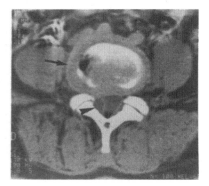

Fig. 159. 51-year-old man. Right L5 sciatica resistant to treatment; right L4–L5 synovial cyst. L4–L5 disk: bulging associated with intradiscal gas; peripheral enhancement after IV injection of contrast medium (→). Small, hypodense fluid-filled sac originating in the upper part of the right lateral recess immediately median to the L4–L5 pars interarticularis *(arrowhead).* There is a faint peripheral enhancement

Finally, an *intraspinal synovial cyst* may simulate a disk fragment. Classically, this is a cystic formation with parietal calcifications; which is adjacent to a degenerated facet joint (usually L4–L5). Lumbar pain may be present, and is more indicative of degenerative lesions of the underlying facet joints than of compression of the thecal sac or a nerve root [36, 127] (Fig. 159).

Postoperative Follow-up

In case of recurrent pain, it may be difficult to distinguish between postoperative *fibrosis* and *recurrent herniation*. The following chapter is devoted to such cases.

Although CT is established as a primary investigation before surgery or chemonucleolysis of a disk herniation, the findings should always be treated cautiously and any anatomic abnormality should not be too readily regarded as the cause of the pain. The radiologist should always keep the clinical findings in mind, and not hesitate to perform a myelography if there is doubt or poor CT-clinical concordance. Myelography is especially indicated in the following cases: a degenerative narrow lumbar spinal canal, in order to identify the most pathogenic segment; congenital spinal stenosis, in order to define the extent of the laminectomy atypical sciatica or low back pain (though this is debatable in young subjects; cf chapter dealing with lumbago); and, finally, suspicion of tumoral pathology, although MRI is now capable of replacing myelography to good advantage.

The Postintervention Lumbar Spine

The Postoperative Lumbar Spine

When therapy has failed, a follow-up CT examination is performed. This may be postoperative long considered as difficult to interpret, or postchemonucleolysis, which the popularity of this procedure has made increasingly common.

The recurrence of lumbosciatic pain following diskectomy for a lumbar disk herniation presents difficult clinical and radiologic problems in terms of both diagnosis and management. There are two main causes of symptoms: recurrent herniation and epidural fibrosis. It is often impossible to differentiate between the two on the basis of the clinical or myelographic findings. Determination of the etiology is nevertheless necessary, since recurrent herniation may improve after a second operation, whereas postoperative epidural fibrosis is often not amenable to treatment. The term "postoperative fibrosis" is a poorly chosen one, since some scar formation is more or less inevitable. In our experience of postoperative CT examinations, active epidural fibrosis with nerve root entrapment has proved extremely rare (Fig. 160).

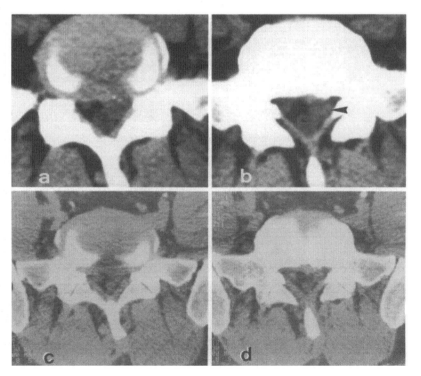

Fig. 160a–d. 50-year-old man. Left S1 lumbosciatic pain of 4 weeks' duration, no neuro-deficit: left L5–S1 disk herniation. *Initial CT:* **a** L5–S1 disk: left posterolateral herniation. Left S1 root is no longer distinguishable. **b** Migratory fragment between thecal sac and left S1 root *(arrowhead). CT 9 months later:* Favorable clinical course under medical treatment. **c–d** Rectilinear appearance of posterior margin of disk. There remains only a small asymmetry of the left S1 radicular sheath, in comparison to its fellow. Disk fragment between the thecal sac and nerve root has almost completely disappeared

Clinical Considerations

It may be difficult to differentiate between a recurrent disk herniation and epidural fibrosis on the basis of the clinical findings. Nevertheless, it is generally accepted that a progressive aggravation of symptoms one or more years after diskectomy is in favor of epidural fibrosis, whereas a sudden onset of symptoms after a variable period is in favor of a recurrent herniation [37, 281, 312].

The great majority of patients are seen late, over a year after surgery.

CT Features

Most authors recommend performing CT scans before and after the intravenous injection of large quantities of contrast medium [30, 89, 195, 227, 282, 299, 301, 302, 312], and even performing myeloscans [263, 264, 281]. Our own routine employs a single injection of contrast medium over one to two minutes.

The images obtained on postoperative CT vary with the type of surgery performed. This may range from (a) bilateral multisegmental laminectomies and facetectomy (leading to articular facet instability) in which retraction of the thecal sac may lead to hemorrhage and arachnoiditis, completed by a total diskectomy, to (b) the present more conservative trend to a minilaminectomy, with a small fenestration, partial removal of the ligamentum flavum, an approach to the particular nerve root involved, and resection of the disk fragment [152]. The subsequent scarring is a normal physiologic healing process, which will be less extensive if the bony and ligamentous elements have been spared.

The following figures describe a classic interlaminar approach with surgical fenestration:

Surgical approach to the laminae and interlaminar space (the dotted line indicates the extent of ligamentum flavum removed) (Fig. 161).

Excision of the ligamentum flavum (Note that incision of the ligamentum flavum begins medially; a swab protects the dura mater) (Fig. 162).

Enlargement of the interlaminar approach (by resection of a small portion of the superior and inferior laminae) (Fig. 163).

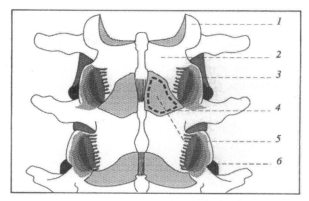

Fig. 161. Postintervention. Approach to the laminae and interlaminar space. The *dotted line* indicates the extent of ligamentum flavum excision: *1,* superior articular process; *2,* lamina; *3,* joint capsule; *4,* ligamentum flavum incision; *5,* ligamentum flavum; *6,* intervertebral disk

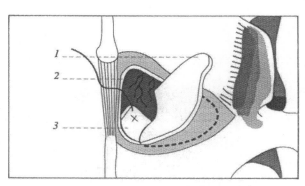

Fig. 162. Postintervention. Excision of the ligamentum flavum. Incision of the ligamentum flavum begins medially; a swab protects the dura mater: *1,* excision of the ligamentum flavum; *2,* dura mater; *3,* swab

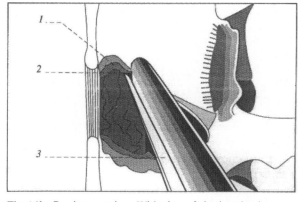

Fig. 163. Postintervention. Widening of the interlaminar approach. This is done through the ablation of a small portion of both the superior and inferior laminae. *1,* epidural fat; *2,* ligamentum flavum; *3,* ablation of the lamina and ligamentum flavum

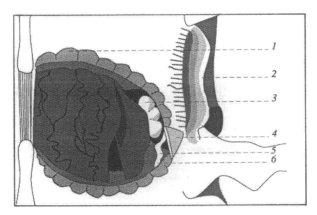

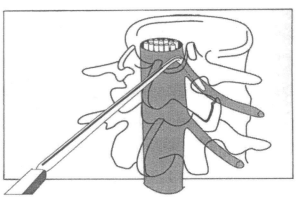

Fig. 164. Postintervention. Approach after ablation of bone and the ligamentum flavum. The ligamentum flavum proximal to the joint capsule is left undisturbed: *1,* sectioned border of the superior lamina; *2,* joint capsule; *3,* extruded nucleus pulposus; *4,* ligamentum flavum; *5,* epidural vein; *6,* nerve root

Fig. 166. Postintervention. Exploration of the intervertebral foramen after disk ablation. The probe is guided anteriorly through the intervertebral foramen and towards the nerve root: exploration of the intervertebral foramen

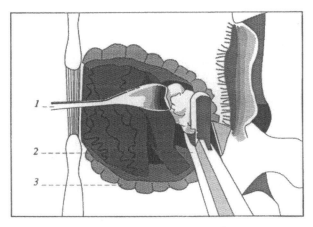

Fig. 165. Postintervention. Ablation of the disk fragment with forceps. The nerve root emergence is displaced medially: *1,* medial retraction of nerve root; *2,* extraction of the ruptured nucleus pulposus; *3,* sectioned border of inferior lamina

Surgical approach after resection of bone and ligamentum flavum (Note that the ligamentum flavum adjacent to the joint capsule is left intact) (Fig. 164).

Extraction of the disk fragment with forceps (*Note* that the nerve root is retracted medially at its emergence) (Fig. 165).

Exploration of the intervertebral foramen following disk extraction (*Note* that the probe is guided forward through the intervertebral foramen and toward the nerve root) (Fig. 166).

Epidural Fibrosis

Fibroblast proliferation and scar formation frequently occur at the site of the surgical procedure. There are changes in the blood-vessels, the fluid and formed elements of the blood, and the neighboring connective tissue. The region is invaded by highly vascularized connective tissue. Blood-flow at this neovascularized site increases and chemotactic factors modify the endothelial layer, thereby increasing vascular permeability [301].

Epidural fibrosis appears in CT as soft tissue classically taking up contrast media and having a density close to or slightly greater than that of the disk. It faces the fenestration site posteriorly, and may extend toward the surgical approach, along the lateral aspect of the thecal sac, and anteriorly to reach the posterior disk margin. The lateral recess is often filled in by fibrosis, which impairs visualization of the corresponding nerve root, though this is not displaced. The fibrosis may extend cephalad and caudad over more than one intervertebral space. It gives rise to either a slight or no partial volume effect; the homolateral nerve root and thecal sac are retracted toward the epidural fibrosis and the fenestration site, particularly if the ligamentum flavum has been removed [89, 263, 264, 281, 282, 312].

Uptake of the circulating contrast medium depends only on its blood concentration, where-

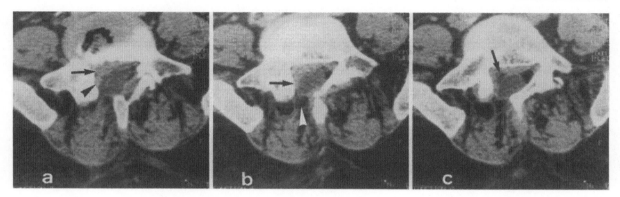

Fig. 167a–c. 48-year-old woman who had been operated on for a right L4–L5 disk herniation 2 years earlier. At present, right L5 lumbosciatic pain. **a** L4–L5 disk: vacuum disk phenomenon. Clearly visible recurrent herniation, oriented to right (→), with displacement of the corresponding root *(arrowhead)*. Absence of scar tissue at the laminectomy site; thecal sac is drawn toward the surgical approach (pseudomeningocele, no ligamente flava). **b** Filled-in right lateral recess. Nerve root cannot be distinguished. Scar tissue running along the right anterolateral aspect of the thecal sac (→). Fat and soft tissues at laminectomy site undisturbed *(white arrowhead)*. **c** L5 root is once again visible in the lateral recess as a hypodense nodule surrounded by scar tissue (→) (15%). Small meningocele at the laminectomy site (50%). *Operative findings:* Residual lateral disk bulging

as *epidural fibrosis enhancement* also depends on the local blood-flow, the vascular perfusion and the interstitial distribution of the contrast medium. This last factor is certainly the most important [301, 302]. Contrast medium uptake by the epidural fibrosis is usually homogeneous, with limits which are even, well-defined and linear, though uptake may be slightly greater at the borders of the fibrosis [89] (Fig. 167).

It is important to recognize three variations:

— The fibrous tissue may consist of several layers, or enclose fatty tissue or a nerve root, all of which result in a heterogeneous uptake of contrast medium. With practice, this is easily distinguished from a recurrent herniation, given the lack of *partial volume effects* and the perfectly round appearance of a hypodense nerve root within the contrast-enhanced fibrosis in the lateral recess or close to the intervertebral foramen [282] (Fig. 168).
— Opacification of the adjacent epidural venous plexus may take the epidural fibrosis appear larger [215].
— Recent studies have shown that uptake of contrast medium by the fibrosis is inconstant, being absent in approximately 35% of cases [89, 282, 299].

There is disagreement concerning the degree of contrast uptake as a function of the duration of the epidural fibrosis. Some authors find no correlation [282], whereas others assert that contrast enhancement decreases with increasing duration (over one year) [230, 301]. We observed no fibrosis (whether on CT or at surgery) in one patient 6 months after surgery, whereas a second patient showed significant enhancement 13 years after surgery. Contrast uptake seems to vary greatly from one individual to the next and to have no particular significance.

Epidural fibrosis is the most frequently observed phenomenon in patients with a recurrence of lumbosciatic pain. Its incidence varies from 54% to 100% in different series [30, 73, 227, 264, 282, 301, 312]. The earlier CT is performed after surgery, the more visible the epidural fibrosis appears (Fig. 169). Localized fibrosis may lead to a mistaken diagnosis of a herniation. Very firm hypertrophic tissue with small calcifications and an altogether unusual *mass effect* on the thecal sac is a classic source of diagnostic error [89, 282, 299] (Fig. 170).

The essential problem in determining the *pathogenic nature* or not of isolated epidural fibrosis is in a patient whose symptoms persist postoperatively, who may experience severe socioprofessional repercussions, and who may claim invalidity benefit. The psychological con-

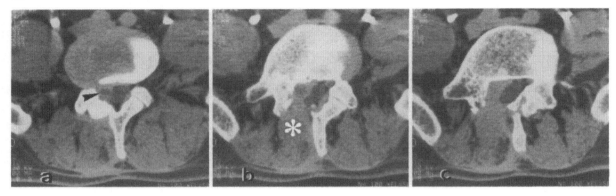

Fig. 168 a-c. 46-year-old man operated for a right L5 sciatica 2 months earlier. Sudden appearance of a right L5 sciatica of 3 weeks' duration. **a** L4–L5 disk, hypodensity due to recurrent right L4–L5 herniation *(arrowhead).* **b** Free fragment is difficult to differentiate from the intra- und extraspinal fibrosis (✳). **c** Fibrous tissue formation in the soft tissues affected by the neurosurgical approach, and extending into lateral recess. Fibrous tissue formation may be significant in the early postoperative period, leading to difficulties in interpretation. IV injection of contrast delineates the fibrosis and distinguishes any residual or recurrent free fragment (hypodensity)

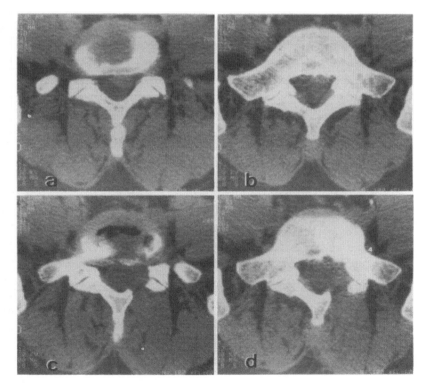

Fig. 169 a-d. 37-year-old woman. Left S1 sciatica resistant to medical treatment. Left L5–S1 herniation. *Preoperative CT:* **a–b** Large left posterolateral L5–S1 herniation descending into axilla of S1. *Postoperative CT* (at 3 months): performed for recurrence of pain and paresthesia in the same territory. **c** Intradiskal gas (vacuum disk phenomenon). Posterior margin of disk appears normal. **d** Filling-in of left lateral recess. *Comment:* Scar tissue is usually found during the early postoperative period, especially in the lateral recess. The clinical signs are not always consistent with the postoperative CT

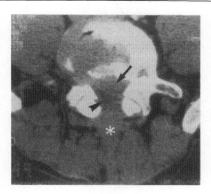

Fig. 170. 70-year-old man operated for an L4–L5 herniation associated with spinal stenosis, one month earlier. Hyperalgesic left L5 sciatica of two weeks' duration (discitis?). L4–L5 disk: posterior margin poorly visualized. There seems to be a posteromedian herniation with leftsided extension. Dense material anterior to thecal sac and filled-in epidural fat (→). Identical findings posterior to the thecal sac, which appears constructed *(arrowhead)*. Filling-in of subcutaneous tissue opposite the bilateral laminectomy (✱). Recent operation renders interpretation difficult: considerable fibrosis due to hemorrhage or infection? *Operative findings (emergency):* Very dense fibrous tissue; fibrous tissue anterior to thecal sac; no free fragment

text is unfavorable and there is lumbar pain without evidence of a disk lesion in approximately 20% of cases [286]. Although epidural fibrosis and secondary nerve root retraction have been implicated as causes of recurrent pain, these CT signs have been observed postoperatively in asymptomatic subjects. It is rash to speak of CT differences between symptomatic and asymptomatic epidural fibrosis, although certain authors report marked contrast uptake by a hypertrophic and abnormally active scar, and absent or very slight uptake by a stabilized scar [299]. CT-clinical correlations are therefore essential.

Recurrent Herniations

A recurrent herniation may be diagnosed on the basis of:

— *direct signs* of herniation, as already discussed in the chapter on common herniations (Figs. 171, 172);
— *indirect signs* of mass effect on the homolateral nerve root and thecal sac.

In this difficult postoperative context, it is especially important that a positive diagnosis of disk herniation be either made or excluded. Detailed

CT investigation is tricky and it is risky to be too assertive about the integrity or otherwise of the posterior longitudinal ligament. In cases without epidural fibrosis, the diagnosis of a recurrent herniation is no different from that of unoperated herniations. Only those cases in which the disk herniation is associated with epidural fibrosis are difficult to interpret.

The injection of contrast medium plays a very important part in efforts to differentiate between them. As we have seen, the basic principle is enhancement of the neovascularized fibrosis, which surrounds the avascular and therefore hypodense disk fragment with a dense rim [30, 89, 299]. Earlier studies noted the constant appearance of a fibrous band following diskectomy, which emphasized the posterior margin of the new herniation [152, 263, 264, 281, 282] (see Fig. 168; Fig. 173). We have observed this in only 20% of cases.

Several reasons may explain this:

— the relatively low frequency of fibrosis associated with the herniation, which is probably due to the interval (over 1 year) between surgery and CT evaluation being longer than in other series;
— the type of surgery, which was probably more conservative and less conducive of fibrosis than in Anglo-American series;
— the contrast injection procedures, which differed from ours in using greater quantities (up to 300 ml) in some series and, even more often, in maintaining an IV line during the investigation ration in other series. Moreover the epidural fibrosis enhancement is described as being short-lived;
— the high frequency of transligamentous migratory disk herniations which are remote from possible sites of fibrosis formation.

Recent studies have pointed out the possibility of a *homogeneous uptake of contrast* by the disk fragments, without providing a satisfactory explanation [69, 89, 282]. We have not been able to observe this phenomenon, since our patients had been initially injected with contrast medium. Nevertheless, two-thirds of the herniations had a homogeneous appearance on medium-enhanced sections. It is difficult to determine whether this relates to residual fragments overlooked during the initial surgery or to true recurrence.

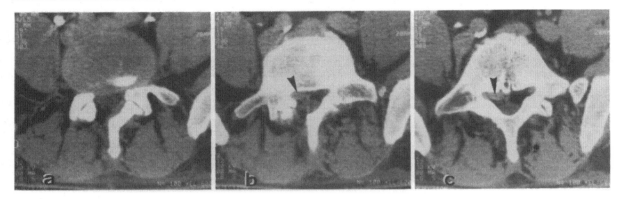

Fig. 171a–c. 48-year-old man, operated for a right L4–L5 herniation 5 years earlier. Several episodes of right lumbosciated pain. Right L5 sciatica with a neuro-deficit of 10 days' duration. **a** L4–L5 disk: small right posterolateral herniation. Presence of epidural fat at site of previous laminectomy, no fibrosis. **a–b** A large root (associated fragment is visualized?) Below the disk in the right lateral recess *(arrowhead)*. **c** Migratory fragment is readily visualized between the thecal sac and the root *(arrowhead)*. *Operative findings:* Perforated ligament; moderate bulging of disk beneath the L5 axilla; free fragment entering lateral recess

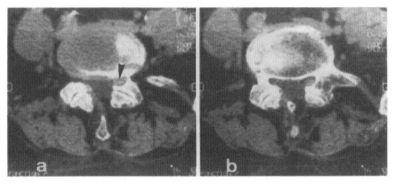

Fig. 172a,b. 61-year-old woman, operated for a left L4–L5 herniation four years earlier. Left L5 sciatica of two months' duration, no neuro-deficit. **a** L4–L5 disk: small, very lateral, left herniation (buttonhole type) *(arrowhead)*, with filling-in of the osteoarthritic lateral recess. **b** Large dense root (associated free fragment?). *Operative findings:* Torn ligament, large free fragment, narrow lateral recess

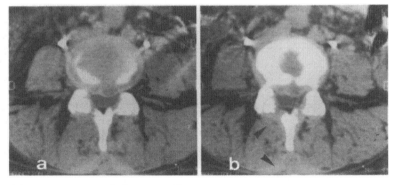

Fig. 173a,b. 39-year-old woman operated for a median L4–L5 herniation 3 months earlier. Alternating L5 sciatica of 2 months' duration. **a** Diskal plane at L4–L5: recurrent herniation with two clearly visible hypodensities (free fragments), with enhancement of peripheral fibrous tissue. **b** Poor differentiation of the roots, especially in right lateral recess. Fibrous tissue surrounding the thecal sac and defining the previous surgical approach; it can be enhanced by contrast medium in the early postoperative period (50% of all cases) *(arrowhead)*. *Operative findings:* Free fragments; recurrent herniation

Postoperative increase of an extradural mass has been advanced as an argument in favor of a recurrent herniation, in contrast with epidural fibrosis which does not have a spontaneous tendency to increase in size [281].

Postdiskography CT

In these difficult situations in which a residual or recurrent herniation and scar tissue are associated, postdiskography CT performed several weeks after surgery may be of great help. In one case intradiskal injection opacified a small posterolateral herniation near the orifice of a previous diskectomy; it also showed a small free fragment in the underlying lateral recess and adherent to the nerve root (Fig. 174).

Other Complications

Other, more infrequent complications should be routinely looked for in cases of persistent postoperative pain [227].

Spondylitis with Diskitis. This very rare condition may present diagnostic problems, especially since cartilaginous plate erosion and disk collapse may be secondary to the curettage. There is a heterogeneous uptake of contrast by the interverbral disk (due to inflammation and neovascularization); exceptionally, there may be a soft-tissue abscess or fragmentation of the vertebral body with infraction of the cortical bone. An epidural abscess may simulate a recurrent disk herniation [89, 282, 312].

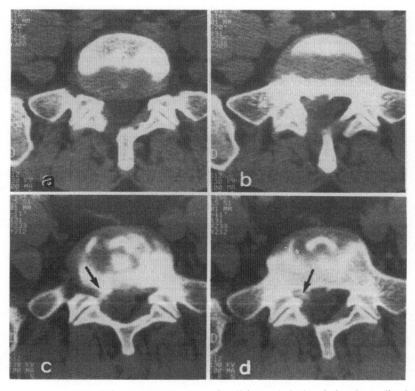

Fig. 174a–d. 38-year-old man operated for a right L5–S1 sciatica 3 years earlier. Recurrence of right S1 sciatic pain. *CT at L5–S1:* **a** Filling-in of right lateral epidural fat on the diskal plane. Hemilaminectomy. **b** Increased filling-in of right lateral recess: free fragment probably in contact with right S1 root. *Postdiskography CT at L5–S1:* **c** Heterogeneous diffusion of contrast medium within the entire operated disk. Small buttonhole herniation immediately anterior to the S1 root emergence (→) – Epidural leakage of contrast medium: torn ligament or opacified free fragment? **d** Opacified free fragment in lateral recess (→). *Operative findings:* Confirmation of recurrent right L5–S1 herniation. Subjacent free fragment found in the lateral recess, using the operating microscope

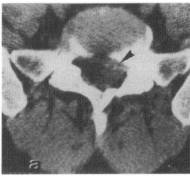 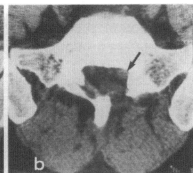

Fig. 175 a, b. 42-year-old man operated for a left L5–S1 herniation 10 years earlier. Left S1 sciatica of 3 months' duration. **a** L5–S1 disk: defect of left posterolateral margin of disk: left S1 root is obscured; upper part of the lateral recess is occupied by material of disk density *(arrowhead)*. **b** Section through midportion of vertebral body once again shows the root, which is enlarged (→). *Operative findings:* Unusually enlarged S1 root; torn radicular sheath; torn posterior longitudinal ligament. Several remote free fragments are visible within the S1 radicular sheath

Pseudomeningocele. This is a cystic formation containing CSF, resulting from a dural tear at surgery.

A Large Nerve Root. A large inflamed nerve root may persist (sometimes becoming calcified), especially if there is a narrow spinal canal. It is important to exclude any associated disk fragments (Fig. 175).

Arachnoiditis. A hyperdense thecal sac may be mistaken for a herniation. Localized arachnoiditis may appear as a segmental thickening of the thecal sac walls with a variable and irregular uptake of contrast. It may be difficult to differentiate between extradural fibrous tissue extending to the thecal sac wall, and thickening restricted to the dura mater. The diagnosis always rests on myelography (especially in moderate forms), even though its repetition under these conditions may be difficult. Iopamidol-enhanced CT shows clumped intradural nerve roots and, at a more advanced stage, a small stenotic thecal sac with the nerve roots no longer visible. A single homolateral nerve root may take up contrast, indicating the existence of fibrosis within or around the nerve root sheath [89, 282, 299] (Fig. 176).

Facet Joint Instability. Typical findings are subluxation and residual apophyseal joint arthropathy.

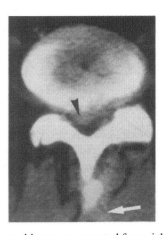

Fig. 176. 32-year-old woman, operated for a right L5–S1 herniation two months earlier; persistence of a left S1 sciatica. L5–S1 disk: presence of posteromedian high-density tissue *(white arrowhead)*. Contrast enhancement of soft tissues lining the surgical fibrosis (granulation tissue) (→). *Operative findings:* No disk herniation; isolated arachnoiditis. Iopamidol myelography may sometimes be useful in investigating postoperative arachnoiditis

Other postoperative findings are not true complications, since they may all be observed in asymptomatic patients:

– disk-space collapse, which is virtually constant;
– vacuum disk phenomenon, due to release of gas (usually nitrogen), from fissures in the degenerated disk. It is usually a sequel to recent surgery, though it may be visible 6 to 7 months after diskectomy (see Fig. 169);

— thecal sac retraction towards the fenestration or laminectomy site, and a possible pseudomeningocele; this is a rather frequently observed phenomenon (see Fig. 167);

— marked hypertrophic changes.

CT thus appear to be the most reliable diagnostic tool; it is slightly invasive, requiring only one intravenous injection, and should be the primary investigation for painful postoperative recurrence of a lumbar disk herniation. In a significant number of cases, even when in contradiction with the clinical picture, CT may indicate the need for reoperation. Some authorities currently favor postoperative chemonucleolysis. Recent studies have shown that CT scans without contrast were capable of providing the correct diagnosis in 50% to 60% of cases. The injection of contrast yielded additional information in 23% of cases [89, 312]. We have found comparable or even somewhat greater reliability with a primary injection of contrast medium. This is the more noteworthy, now that the accepted notion of a constant enhancement of the fibrosis following injection of contrast medium is being questioned and in view of the fact that the enhancement may be heterogeneous and that disk fragments may also take up the contrast. Thus, more information can be derived from structural considerations and from indirect signs in enhanced sections (eg. mass effect) than from density variations.

Although the diagnosis of recurrent herniation presents few problems by a year after therapy, it is much more difficult in the immediate postoperative period, which favors errors (i. e., false-positives). In this last instance, MRI, possibly complemented by the IV injection of gadolinium, may be very helpful [95].

Postchemonucleolysis

Surgery on an intervertebral disk requires exposure of the spinal canal. This implies resection of muscle and ligaments, and sometimes resection of the articular facets and handling of the nerve roots. There is a risk of extra- and intradural fibrosis due to the postoperative hematoma, which is also a source of stubborn lumbar and radicular pain. In order to avoid these problems, certain authors (Smith 1964 and others subsequently) have advocated chemical diskectomy by *chemonucleolysis using chymopapain,* a procedure that has gained popularity in France over the past five years. However, a failure rate of 20% to 40% and a far from negligible complication rate (although rarely severe) account for chemonucleolysis not yet being a significant alternative to surgery. A *follow-up operation* is necessary in 10% to 20% of cases [64, 68], but since the reduction in pain, may be slow surgery is not usually indicated before a minimum delay of four to six weeks.

CT Features

In order to understand the appearance of an intervertebral disk following chemonucleolysis, it is important to be acquainted with its mechanism of action.

Mechanism of Action

Chymopapain is a proteolytic enzyme of plant origin, extracted from the latex of Carica papaya [16, 17, 18, 19, 25, 32, 181, 215, 230, 290]. Its enzymatic activity is not highly specific. Like all other proteolytic enzymes, it has immunogenic potential; therefore, the patient may only be injected once during his lifetime. Since its intradiskal injection may provoke an anaphylactic reaction, some degree of patient selection is necessary.

In the doses usually administered, chymopapain acts only upon proteoglycans. It affects the *carrier proteins* of the glycosaminoglycans (GAGS). The large proteoglycan molecules are depolymerized, liberating polysaccharides and losing their hydrophilic properties (Fig. 177).

The macroscopic effects on the disk quickly become evident; in 10 to 30 minutes the normal structure of the nucleus pulposus becomes profoundly altered. The nucleus becomes globally condensed, with contraction of the more peripheral layers close to the anulus fibrosus. After four hours, the chondromucoid substance making up the nucleus becomes fragmented. After 24 hours it is replaced by more or less heterogeneous clusters separated by large fissures reaching the deeper layers of the anulus.

Chymopapain itself is rapidly inactivated by a circulating enzyme inhibitor (plasma - 2-mac-

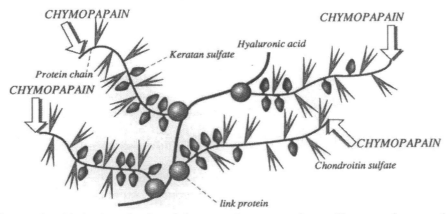

Fig. 177. Postintervention. Mechanism of action of chymopapain on proteoglycans. Chymopapain acts at the level of the proteins bearing the glucosaminoglycans (GAGS)

roglobulin) and destroyed by the reticuloendothelial system. It has a less spectacular action on degenerated disks, where aging has brought about spontaneous proteoglycan decomposition and nuclear dehydration.

The reasons for sciatic pain reduction following chemonucleolysis are poorly understood. Certain authors suggest that a *volume reduction* of the disk and its herniated fragment decrease nerve root compression by disk material. Yet it is well-known that there may be clinical improvement following chemonucleolysis without any change in the size of the herniation on follow-up CT [100, 101]. Furthermore, it is possible that the activity of chymopapain is more than just mechanical. Certain authors have postulated an antiflammatory activity. Others believe that the decrease in disk height usually observed one month after chemonucleolysis may decrease nerve root tension and compression by its *ligamentous attachments,* without any decrease in the size of the herniation.

Following chemonucleolysis, most patients experience lumbar pain which may be very unpleasant but which differs from the original symptoms.

CT Modifications Following Chemonucleolysis

Although CT follow-up is not justified if there is good clinical resolution following chemonucleolysis, numerous authors have nevertheless studied the usual disk modifications on CT and the possibility of CT-clinical correlations.

Disk Collapse
Disk collapse is evaluated on sagittal sections (scout view), and is an index of the enzymatic activity [32, 53, 186, 250]. It is observed early, from the third day. After three months, almost all contrast-enhanced disks are collapsed, then remain stable for a year. After one year, reexpansion may be found in 20% of patients; young subjects retain the ability to synthesize new proteoglycan molecules.

The Vacuum Disk Phenomenon
As may be the case following diskectomy (20%), intradiskal gas may be observed in approximately 25% of cases following chemonucleolysis [186, 250] (Fig. 178).

Decrease in Size of Disk Herniation
Reduction in the size of herniation is difficult to evaluate, given the difficulty in obtaining completely superimposable CT sections from different examinations. It is tempting to establish a parallelism between the decrease in the size of the disk fragment and the clinical improvement;

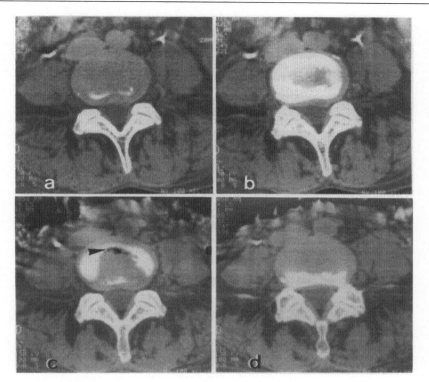

Fig. 178a–d. 54-year-old woman with left S1 sciatica without neuro-deficit. Left L4–L5 herniation. **a–b** Preoperative CT. Small left posterolateral L4–L5 herniation with a hypodensity: preligamentous free fragment. Treatment: chemonucleoly- sis (chymodiactin) **c–d** Follow-up CT at 3 months: vacuum disk phenomenon *(arrowhead)*. Peripheral bulging exhibited by the collapsed disk. Complete disappearance of the left posterolateral herniation

but such a correlation is debatable and influenced by the interval between the chemonucleolysis and follow-up CT examination [186]. Moreover, one the natural history of a herniation usually entails a reduction in size.

Follow-up CT one month after chemonucleolysis is too early; in 47% of cases the size of the herniation is unchanged, even when the clinical course is favorable [250]. On the other hand, evaluation at twelve months is too late, given the poor correlation between the persisting disk abnormalities and the clinical results [156, 157]. An interval of three months appear to be the most appropriate, with a rather good CT-clinical correlation. In about 75% of cases the herniation has either disappeared or decreased in size [156, 157, 250] (see Fig. 178). In the remaining 25% there are no changes in the size of the disk fragment but the clinical course is quite often satisfactory (Fig. 179).

Bulging

It is equally important to note that in most cases (33% to 80% in various series), a decrease in nerve root compression by the herniation occurs in parallel with the appearance or increase of a diffuse bulging of the anulus fibrosus [32, 156, 157, 250]. This bulging is explained by a decrease in disk height, together with preservation of the integrity of the collagen fibers in the anulus (see Fig. 180). Thus, chemonucleolysis is not indicated when compression of a nerve root or the thecal sac is due solely to a bulging anulus, since it can only accentuate the condition [156, 157].

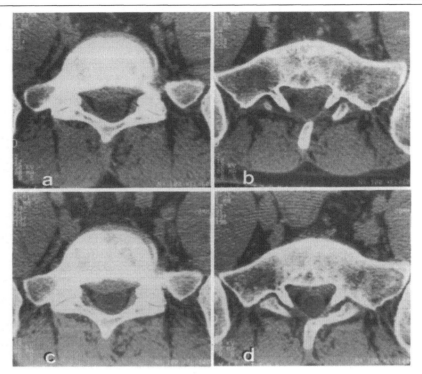

Fig. 179a-d. 28-year-old man with left S1 sciatica resistant to medical treatment. Left L5-S1 herniation. **a-b** Preoperative CT: posteromedian L5-S1 herniation with small leftward extension in lateral recess. Treatment: chemonucleolysis of L5-S1 (chemodiactin). **c-d** Follow-up CT at 2 months: persistent median bulging. Partial disappearance of herniation in left lateral recess. *Comment:* Despite a good clinical outcome, there is no correlation between the radiographic and clinical findings, since CT scans show only partial regression of the herniation

Disk Density Modifications

This is also difficult to evaluate from one CT examination to the next, given the minor density variations, but there may be a moderate increase (of approximately 10 HU) in overall disk density due to dehydration. MRI appears to be more sensitive in detecting such modifications, which give rise to a loss of the disk signal in T 2-weighted sequences and a decreased anulus-nucleus differentiation [132].

Negative Signs

No changes were detected in the inferior articular processes or lateral recesses one year after chemonucleolysis. The lumbar spinal canal appeared unchanged on CT sections.

No epidural fibrosis has ever been observed following chemonucleolysis [156, 250]. Nevertheless, there may be adhesions at the nerve root level, with inflammatory and hypervascularized scar tissue.

Failed Chemonucleolysis

Although follow-up CT scans are of little importance when there is good clinical progress, they are essential in cases with persistent or recurrent pain. The two principle causes to be considered are:

- a recurrent herniation (usually at the same level)
- foraminal stenosis (essentially lateral recess stenosis)

CT is the examination best suited to distinguish between these.

Recurrent herniation

In our experience, this is usually a free disk fragment which is either detached from the nucleus pulposus or still has a thin pedicle; it accounts for 25% of failures [41, 45, 63, 64, 135, 136]. Its location may be:

— Transligamentous, with a perforation of the posterior longitudinal ligament. The fragment may remain close to or in partial contact with the intervertebral space; it may also easily migrate. CT is the best examination for making the diagnosis (cf chapter "migratory herniations") (Figs. 180, 181). The herniation may be contemporary with the chemonucleolysis, or may appear secondarily after a clinical remission. Epidural leakage of contrast medium during diskography is not a definitive argument in favor of an extruded herniation; it only calls for a slow injection of the chymopapain [286, 292, 293].

— Subligamentous. This is much more rare; it detaches the posterior longitudinal ligament (which nevertheless remains intact), and usually migrates below the intervertebral space. Classically, a migratory herniation is the prime cause of failure, since the enzyme cannot reach the free fragment. Despite the possibility of opacifying migratory free fragments on discoscans, failure is often noted between 4 and 6 months after chemonucleolysis and after a temporary remission. Chymopapain produces only partial dissolution of the fragment. The increasingly simple detection of migratory free fragments by CT prior to chemonucleolysis tends to reduce the failure rate through a strict selection of patients.

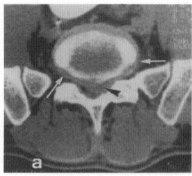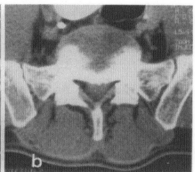

Fig. 180a, b. 25-year-old man. Left L5–S1 chemonucleolysis one month earlier. Recurrence of left S1 sciatica. **a** L5–S1 disk: large herniation with a hypodensity (free fragment) (black arrowhead) occupying two-thirds of the lumbar spinal canal. Peripheral bulging of the disk (—►). **b** Poorly visualized left S1 root in lateral recess. Spinal stenosis. Thecal sac is pressed against ligamentum flavum. *Operative findings:* Perforated ligament; free fragment (25% of all causes of chemonucleolysis failure). *Comment:* In general, large disk herniations are not good indications for chemonucleolysis, especially when there is a free fragment associated with spinal stenosis

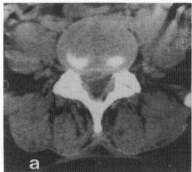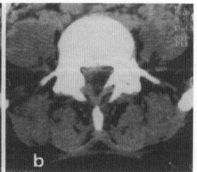

Fig. 181a, b. 45-year-old woman. L4–L5 chemonucleolysis for right herniation three years earlier. Several episodes of L5 sciatica since, with a diminished right Achilles tendon reflex. **a** L4–L5 disk: right posterolateral herniation with a hypodensity (free fragment). **b** Herniation into right lateral recess (6 mm below diskal plane). *Operative findings:* Transligamentous buttonhole disk herniation. *Comment:* Occurring after a symptom-free period of several years, the cause is a recurrent herniation rather than a residual fragment

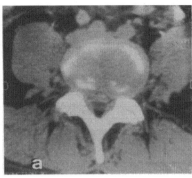 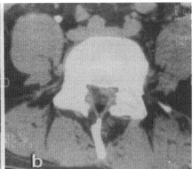

Fig. 182a, b. 36-year-old man. L4–L5 chemonucleolysis 2 months earlier; persistent left L5 sciatica without neurodeficit. **a** L4–L5 disk: bulging associated with a posteromedian herniation which appears significant in a narrowed canal. **b** Herniation in left lateral recess. CT is unable to show if this is really compressive. *Operative findings:* Very discrete bulging of soft tissues; no disk fragment; empty disk; lateral recess stenosis. Foraminotomy and facetectomy. *Comment:* Follow-up CT at two months after chemonucleolysis did not show regression of the herniation

Subligamentous Disk Herniation and Protrusions

A subligamentous herniation is a less frequent finding. It is then difficult to explain the recurrence. The inefficacy of the enzyme may be due to *improper positioning of the needle* during the injection. Certain authors have suggested an *interaction with the contrast medium* injected during the diskography, prior to injection of the enzyme. Nevertheless, absence of enzyme activity inhibition by the contrast medium has been shown in vitro.

A degenerate disk with a high collagen content, but poor in water and proteoglycans and insensitive to chymopapain, is only slightly affected by enzyme. In such cases, the amount of disk material removed by the neurosurgeon varies; it may be very abundant or almost nil. Its consistency may also vary widely, from a very firm fragment to soft tissue adherent to the cartilaginous endplates) (Fig. 182). Genuine hard free fragments are sometimes extracted from within soft disk substances, testifying to the "biochemical failure" of chymopapain at this level.

Lateral Recess Stenosis

Lateral recess stenosis may be associated with a subligamentous disk herniation or be an isolated finding. In either case, there is a narrow lateral recess which may or may not be associated with a narrow lumbar spinal canal.

In there is a preexisting *isolated lateral recess stenosis,* its possible aggravation by chemonucleolysis must be borne in mind. A moderate lateral recess stenosis does not represent an absolute contraindication to chemonucleolysis. Nevertheless, one should recognize the increased failure-rate, warn the patient; and make a collaborative choice between surgery and chemonucleolysis (Fig. 183).

Disk collapse is often associated with an even bulging of the anulus fibrosus (55%). Certain authors have suggested the possibility of nerve root compression by an "isolated disk resorption syndrome". Following disk collapse, the pedicle descends and the superior articular process of the next lower vertebra subluxates upwards. Nerve root compression may occur in the intervertebral foramen, as well as in the lateral recess, between the disk margin and the ligamentum flavum protruding into the foramen. In fact, this phenomenon appears to be very rare; the immobilization produced at this level by the disk collapse is actually beneficial for the nerve root, offsetting the relative decrease in the size of the lateral recess [63, 64] (see Fig. 182).

Such a lateral stenosis, which can be easily diagnosed on CT, is an indication for a more or less extensive resection of the superior articular process (i. e., facetectomy) or even a foraminotomy.

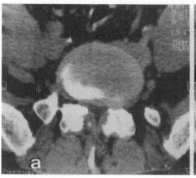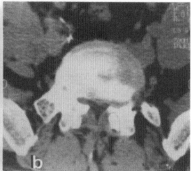

Fig. 183a, b. 43-year-old man. L5–S1 chemonucleolysis for a left herniation two months earlier. Persistence of left S1 sciatica. **a** L5–S1 disk: asymmetric left portion of disk. Very narrow lumbar spinal canal. **b** Bilateral facet joint arthropathy associated with stenosis of lateral recess. Trefoil appearance of spinal canal; hypertrophy of ligamenta flava; total absence of lateral epidural fat. *Operative findings:* Isolated lateral recess stenosis; no disk herniation found. *Comments:* Lateral recess stenosis and spinal stenosis are frequent causes of failure of chemonucleolysis

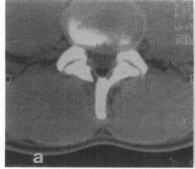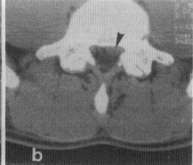

Fig. 184a, b. 26-year-old man. Left L4–L5 chemonucleolysis 1 months earlier. Persistent left L5 sciatica without neuro-deficit. **a** L4–L5 disk: Asymmetric left disk prolapse with thecal sac impression. **b** Hyperdense material in contact with the nerve root (migratory free fragment?) *(arrowhead)*. *Operative findings:* Adherent root surrounded by a very vascular gelatinous substance (inflamed adherent roots account for 15% of chemonucleolysis failures). Discrete bulging; little disk material. Foraminectomy. *Comment:* CT cannot accurately evaluate the consistency of diskal material following chemonucleolysis

Localized Nerve Root Inflammation

A large isolated inflamed nerve root may be found on CT, the differential diagnosis being from a residual free fragment. The surgeon finds a red swollen nerve root adherent to the disk. There is no relationship between the degree of inflammation and the significance of the disk herniation, it such is actually present. Sometimes the nerve root is covered with fibrosis, making dissection almost impossible ("fixed root") (Fig. 184).

CT is not routinely repeated for early failure of chemonucleolysis (3 to 4 weeks); ordinary radiographs are sufficient for investigating a decrease in disk height possibly evoking diskitis and thus contraindicating surgery. On the other hand, CT examination becomes essential when failures occur at a later stage (between 3 and 8 months).

The conditions of surgery following chemonucleolysis are identical to those of the initial operation. No adhesions or epidural fibrosis can be attributed to the chemonucleolysis. At most, one finds a few nerve root adhesions; however, such an appearance is not exceptional in disk surgery, especially if the sciatica is of long duration and the herniation is transligamentous. The surgical approach may be unilateral, but should be relatively wide in new of the frequency of lateral recess stenosis; microsurgery is not suitable for this type of operation. Certain authors go as far as advising against touching the disk itself, so as not to destabilize the fibrous tissue formed after chemonucleolysis, and content themselves with extracting the disk fragment or freeing the nerve root from bony compression.

The best means of reducing the failure-rate in chemonucleolysis is to be mindful of the contraindications to this procedure:

Absolute contraindications:
— paralytic sciatica and/or cauda equina syndrome;
— previous chemonucleolysis;
— allergy to chymopapain; allergic background;
— pregnancy.

Relative contraindications:
— poorly conducted conservative medical treatment;
— narrow spinal canal and/or lateral recess stenosis;
— migratory disk herniation;
— very large herniation (more than 75% of the spinal canal);
— calcified herniated disk;
— previous disk surgery.

Strict patient selection is also fundamental; preliminary CT plays a major part in specifying the nature of the herniation and of the surrounding bony structures. Nevertheless, CT alone cannot provide the indication for chemonucleolysis; it is a criterion of great value, but one which should always be considered together with the clinical findings. The best indications are small- and medium-sized disk herniations in young subjects, without a ligamentous tear and occurring in a lumbar spinal canal of normal size. The role of intradiskal injection of corticosteroids (hexatrione) remains to be settled; one good indication seems to be extraspinal lateral herniations; but small herniations and relative spinal stenoses may also qualify [16, 18, 19, 197, 286].

Lumbago

Introduction

Lumbar pain is a very widespread condition which is presently one of the major reasons for patients to consult physicians. Does it represent a disease caused by Western civilization? Affluence? Is the lack of regular participation in sports in "modern" society one of the reasons for its emergence?

One should differentiate acute lumbago from the general clinical picture of lumbar pain; the former is a paroxysmal, painful event characterized by lumbar pain of rapid onset and a feeling of spinal blockage. This is classically (and mistakenly) referred to as "kidney pain" (French: "Tour de rein") by patients. It represents one of the most characteristic clinical manifestations of disk degeneration.

Clinical Aspects

At the onset of lumbago, the patient sometimes experiences a click or displacement concomitant with a sharp lumbar pain and the sensation of vertebral blockage. This lumbar pain usually affects young men or women (i. e., usually in their forties). It occurs suddenly and is incapacitating, taking place in the morning upon waking or sometimes in the evening after a full day of activity. Blockage phenomena due to reflex splinting are frequent and render daily activity difficult or even impossible; relaxation therapy is essential. Everyday activities such as driving an automobile may become much more difficult.

Episodes of lumbago may be recurrent and disabling over the long term (i. e., a period of several months). The relief afforded by anti-flammatory agents and exercise programs for the shoulder and pelvic girdles is of limited value, since their effects are transient.

Physical examination reveals a pain-avoidance posture comprising spinal curvature and a flattening of the normal lumbar arch. The absence of signs of nerve root suffering and of sphincter lesions should also be confirmed.

In general, the patients concerned are motivated; their impaired capacity to work and clinical condition justify work stoppage. One sometimes finds in the past medical history of these patients episodes of less severe lumbar pain.

In the vast majority of cases, acute lumbago regresses spontaneously in 3–8 days. In other cases, it may cause lasting disability, persistent discomfort indicative of a recurrence in the near future (i. e., recurrent acute lumbago), radicular sciatica, or chronic lumbar pain. When confronted with the very peculiar clinical picture of recurrent disabling lumbago, often affecting young subjects, the physician may be led to resort to radiodiagnostic procedures.

Radiological Investigations

It is commonly accepted that lumbago results from a partial posterior rupture of the L4–L5 or L5–S1 anulus fibrosus, causing the nucleus pulposus to compress the more posterior disk fibers (which are the only ones innervated) and the posterior longitudinal ligament (which is richly innervated).

Routine X-Rays

The three most common views of the lumbar spine (i. e., in the anteroposterior, lateral, and oblique planes) are taken with the patient standing and are centered on the L4–L5 and L5–S1 disks. Roentgenograms may confirm a pain-avoidance stance, demonstrate a posterior or lateral bulging of one of the last two intervertebral spaces, and sometimes show a disk lesion indicative of a preexisting disk degeneration.

CT Scans

We are especially concerned here with the classical CT investigation performed as a work-up examination of choice in cases of typical sciatica not responding to proper therapy.

During an episode of disabling (and we stress the fact) lumbago, the radiologist understandably focuses his attention on the last three lumbar segments to detect a possibly curable condition, particularly a disk abnormality. He also examines the bony lumbar spinal canal (using appropriate window settings) in order to study in an almost ideal fashion the facet joints at the level of the lumbosacral joint.

What contributions can CT scans make in these very specific clinical cases of acute or sometimes chronically evolving lumbago? It has been known for a long time that disk herniations may be cause lumbar pain, by simply tensing the posterior longitudinal ligament. However, our experience has been that the value of radiological procedures does not lie in showing a more-or-less significant number of posteromedian herniations on CT scans, responsible for major lumbar pain in young subjects.

In fact, the disk abnormalities one should look for are often minor ones, such as a banal bulging at the L4-L5 or L5-S1 levels along with a minimal image of a small posteromedian overlap hardly evoking a median disk herniation, wich in any case on axial sections do not appear to involve the emerging roots.

MRI

Sagittal and parasagittal sections of the lumbosacral spine have recently attracted great interest. They clearly show the canal's dimensions and the size of the intervertebral spaces (and, thus, that of the disks). In particular, a possible posteromedian bulging can be properly and immediately evaluated by comparing it with the overlying or underlying levels.

T2-weighted images show a nucleus with a normal hyperintense signal. One may sometimes observe a simple signal extinction at either one or both of the last two levels without there being a very significant posterior abnormalitiy (i.e., a relatively frequent appearance of disk lesion). These images may very often be considered to be insignificant in a given population; the severe clinical picture observed does not prompt one to favor a particular feature of the MRI sections obtained (i.e., loss of T2 signal or bulging), prior to deciding upon appropriate treatment.

Postdiskography CT Scans

Given the minimal images of focalized bulging or posteromedian overlap without other associated abnormalities, such as a narrowing of the intervertebral space in question or possible signs of a narrowed spinal canal at the same level, the idea of a complementary exploration has progressively gained ground; it should be emphasized that the clinical picture and gravity of the cases underlined this need. Given the possibility that a disk lesion is responsible for the lumbago but is unsatisfactorily demonstrated on CT scans and MRI sections, postdiskography CT scans have gradually attained a place of their own. They are CT sections performed 0.5–1 h after the intradiscal injection of contrast medium.

Postdiskography CT scans are obtained by a recently developed technique involving diskography followed by computed tomography; they usually permit a direct visualization of disk herniations, both at the lumbar and cervical levels. In the group of patients with disabling lumbago and in whom standard CT scans only showed a focalized bulging at the L4-L5 or L5-S1 levels, diskography was performed under local anesthesia or neuroleptanesthesia. The *technique* calls for fluoroscopy-controlled puncture localization of the offending intervertebral space, with the patient in the right lateral decubitus position. A trocar and a thin needle with a curved tip is placed in the center of the intervertebral space. Finally, 1 or 1.5 ml Iopamiron 300 are injected, and routine anteroposterior (i.e., aligned disk) and lateral views are taken in order to verify the correct location of the contrast medium at the center of the intervertebral space.

Second, 45–60 min after the intradiscal injection, a CT examination is performed at the diskography level (i.e., postdiskography CT scans). Investigation of the injected segment then reveals a certain number of abnormalities; a normally opacified nucleus is seldom found following the median opacification of the nucleus pulposus. One sometimes finds a classic herniation which had been diagnosed on routine CT scans and which may or may not be associated with signs of disk degeneration. In the latter case, the portion of the disk involved is of course the posteromedian section; the opacification touches not only the herniation but also the entire posteromedian section.

In half of a series of 35 patients investigated, in the most interesting cases – because of their

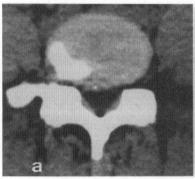 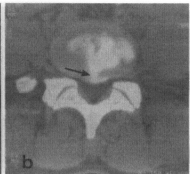

Fig. 185 a, b. *Lumbago:* Recurrent lumbago within a context of posttraumatic low back pain, causing episodes of disability in a 32-year-old woman. **a** CT: isolated posteromedian bulging at L4–L5. **b** Postdiskography CT ½ h after L5–S1 diskography. Clear signs of posterior leakage (very localized peripheral rupture of anulus fibrosus) (→). *Comment:* In view of these findings secondary chemonucleolysis was performed, resulting in decreased low back pain within 2 months after the injection of chymodiactin

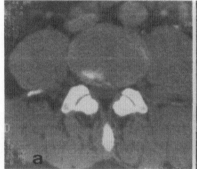 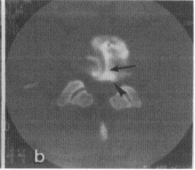

Fig. 186 a, b. *Lumbago:* Chronic lumago in a 54-year-old man, resistant to long-term treatment (6 months) with antiinflammatory agents. Frequent episodes of lumbar rigidity. **a** CT: isolated L3–L4 bulging (the L4–L5 and L5–S1 levels are normal). **b** Postdiskography CT ½ h after diskography (1 ml of Iopamiron 300). Demonstration of posterior leakage through anulus fibrosus (→), with passage of nuclear substance *(arrowhead). Comment:* Fissuring of the peripheral anulus fibrosus is always posteromedian. Secondary lumbar chemonucleolysis results in a reduction of lumbar pain

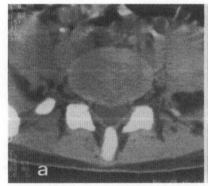 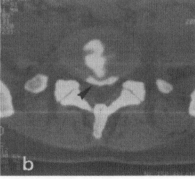 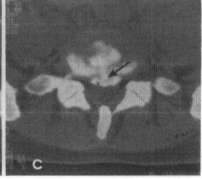

Fig. 187 a–c. *Lumbago:* Disabling lumbago recurring over a period of 6 months in a 23-year-old woman. **a** CT shows an ordinary posteromedian bulge at L5–S1; **b–c** Postdiskography CT ½ h after L5–S1 diskography (injection of 1 ml of Iopamiron 300). There is a central distribution of the contrast medium within the nucleus pulposus. There is an image of a thin median channel traversing through the anulus fibrosus (→) which leads towards a small posteromedian accumulation of contrast *(arrowhead). Comment:* These postdiskography images are indicative of a fissuring of the anulus fibrosus at a very early stage of a disk herniation; the passage of nuclear substance through the fissure in the anulus is evident. Secondary chemonucleolysis (chymodiactin) at the L5–S1 level. Slow improvement of the limited back motion and of the lumbago over a period of 8 to 10 weeks

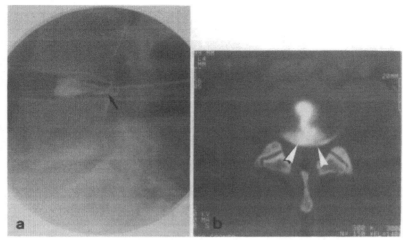

Fig. 188 a, b. Acute lumbago in a 39-year-old man with several recurrences over the preceding nine months. CT scans were normal at L4–L5 and L5–S1, but showed bulging at L3–L4. **a** Diskography at L3–L4 (1 ml of Iopamiron 300). Sagittal view: minor posteromedian leakage (→). **b** CT ½ h after diskography: contrast medium can be seen in the nucleus pulposus. There is a fissure in the posterior portion of the anulus fibrosus. In this instance, the accumulation of contrast medium in the posteromedian portion of the disk appears different, corresponding more to disk degeneration associated with the fissure in the anulus *(white arrowhead). Comment:* In view of the posteromedian leakage, L3–L4 chemonucleolysis was performed 4 weeks after the postdiskography CT. After a follow-up of 6 months, good results with respect to the recurrence of lumbago

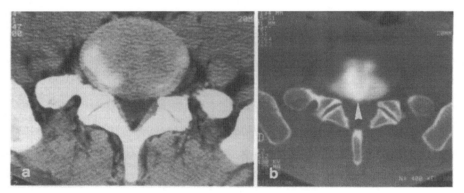

Fig. 189 a, b. Recurrent lumbago with various episodes of back rigidity. **a** CT: isolated L5–S1 bulging. **b** CT ½ h after L5–S1 diskography (1 ml of Iopamiron 300). Opacification of the nucleus; no images of posterior leakage through an orifice in the anulus. On the other hand, there is an opacification of the posteromedian portion of the disk, with no anulus-nucleus differentiation *(white arrowhead). Comment:* In this particular case, no therapy was envisaged (i.e. no chemonucleolysis), since there was posteromedian degeneration of the L5–S1 disk rather than a rupture of the anulus fibrosus

novelty and unexpected nature – there was a small accumulation of contrast medium at the level of the bulging thanks to a rigorously posteromedian channel. This channel is evidence of a very thin and very focalized rupture of the peripheral annulus fibrosus, resulting in the posteromedian migration of an admittedly very small quantity of nucleus pulposus substance, against the posterior longitudinal ligament. The sections performed are among the most detailed obtainable within the framework of disk abnormalities; they probably correspond to very incipient herniations, which are only visible on postdiskography CT sections at 1-mm intervals (Figs. 185–189).

Therapeutic Approach

In patients with minimal disk abnormalities actually consisting of a median (i. e., or almost always median) radiate fissure of the anulus fibrosus, it is very tempting to propose a more interventionist therapeutic approach than a plastered lumbosacral support or an exercise program for the pelvic girdle. Chemonucleolysis was proposed to 20 young and motivated patients whose mean age was less than 40 years. We found the results to be less spectacular than in cases of classic sciatica due to disk herniation. The lumbar pain receded slowly over 3–4 months, and all the patients in our series were able to resume normal work activity 4–6 months after the injection of chymopapain and found that their lumbar pain decreased in intensity, becoming less disabling. Blockage phenomena in particular disappeared after a few weeks. Percutaneous nucleotomy may also be of great therapeutic value in these very specific cases of median rupture of the peripheral anulus fibrosus shown on postdiskography CT scans.

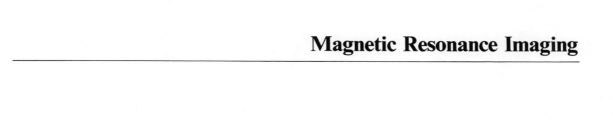

Magnetic Resonance Imaging

Magnetic resonance imaging (MRI) is a rapidly growing method of diagnosis. Although it is acknowledge to be the technique of choice for the study of the brain and spinal cord, it is still little used for the investigation of disk herniations because of the scarcity of machines and the duration of the examination. However, it has many advantages compared with other examinations such as myelography and CT. In addition to the harmless and simple acquisition of a multidimensional image (sagittal, transverse frontal and oblique) not requiring patient immobilization, the use of appropriate surface coils provides excellent anatomic detail, especially since its contrast resolution of soft tissues is vastly superior to that of CT. MRI avoids the artifacts due to beam hardening, which limit CT scans. It also readily permits the identification of nuclear degeneration [23, 38].

This new technique may appear to be more complex than other methods of radiologic investigation since three physiochemical factors are directly involved in the creation of the image, whereas ordinarily there is only one. During an MRI examination, the patient is not subjected to ionizing radiation but to the harmless effects of:

— *A constant magnetic field,* which is both uniform and intense and produces magnetization of the atomic nuclei in the various tissues of the body;
— *A radiofrequency pulse* which enables one to obtain the "resonance" phenomenon by disrupting the equilibrium state of the magnetization;
— *Variable magnetic fields,* which are nonuniform and of low intensity, and enable one to obtain a tomographic image of the organ studied.

The image so obtained is no longer a simple description of the anatomic structures. For each magnetized microvolume of the organ studies, the image depends on three parameters characteristic of this magnetization:

— the density of hydrogen nuclei
— the T 1 relaxation time
— the T 2 relaxation time, which describes the variation in the local magnetization over time [53]

MRI of Degenerative Joint and Disk Lesions at the Cervical Level

Anatomy

The vertebral bodies and intervertebral disks at the cervical level do not differ essentially from those at the lumbar level.

T1-weighted sequences enable one to demonstrate the spinal cord surrounded by the hyposignal of the subarachnoid spaces (Fig. 190). At the cervical level, it is important to know the relationship between the spinal cord, the subarach-

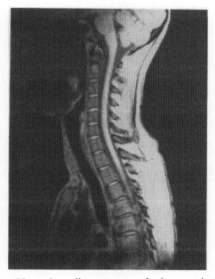

Fig. 190. Normal radioanatomy of the cervical spine. T1-weighted median sagittal section (TR = 500 msec; TR = 16 msec; 4 excitations). – The cervical spinal cord appears slightly hyperintense in this gradient echo sequence. – The cervical disks are also hyperintense in this rapid sequence. – Hyposignal appearance of the cortical bone of the cervical vertebrae and especially of the posterior aspect of the vertebral body. – Hyposignal appearance of the subarachnoid spaces. *Comment:* The true anteroposterior diameter of the cervical spinal canal cannot be correctly evaluated using sagittal echo-gradient sequences, because of lack of proper differentiation between the subarachnoid space and the cortical bone

noid spaces and the spinal canal; this can be achieved by means of T2-weighted sequences which provide a myelographic effect (Fig. 191). In these sequences the CSF has high signal intensity. Artifacts due to blood circulation and CSF pulsation sometimes appear as high-signal lines parallel to the spinal cord; they are reduced by cardiac gating, though this prolongs the examination time [52, 55, 59, 81].

Regardless of the sequence used, the cortical bone of the vertebral bodies, as well as the ligaments, the dura mater, the anulus fibrosus, degenerated disks and osteophytes do not give rise to a signal. Their visualization is therefore indirect, by means of neighboring structures.

The spinal nerves may be distinguished within the intervertebral foramina; they appear as structures with a low intensity signal which are visible on axial sections (Fig. 192), but especially on oblique sections through the long axis of the root or perpendicular to it [28, 29] (Fig. 193). The nerve roots are surrounded by epidural fat with high signal intensity, but found in only limited quantities at the cervical level. The anterior epidural veins and intervertebral veins are particularly note worthy. Although these veins usually have low signal intensity, they may take up contrast medium after the injection of Gadolinium, thus becoming hyperintense [40] (Fig. 194). According to certain authors [26], these veins appear hyperintense on rapid (gradient-echo) sequences because their blood-flow is slow, stagnant and sinusoidal; on sagittal sections, these veins are identifiable behind the vertebral bodies as linear segmented bands having high signals. There is also a naturally-occurring enhancement at the anterolateral angle of the spinal canal on axial sections, which is identical to the enhancement

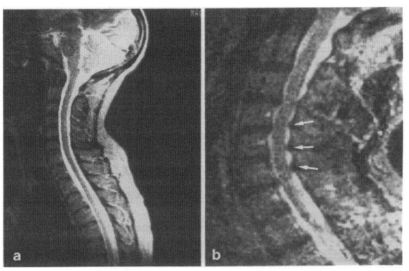

Fig. 191 a, b. Median sagittal section through the cervical spine. T2 - weighted sequence (TR=2000 msec; TE=40; 4 echoes). **a** Myelography effect is obtained with the last echo (TE=160 msec). Hyperintense appearance of the subarachnoid spaces; the cervical spinal cord is well defined (hypointense), as is the true anteroposterior diameter of the cervical spinal canal. *Note* the signal loss at the level of the lower cervical and upper dorsal disks (hypointense appearance).

b T2-weighted median sagittal sequence (TR=1800 msec; TE=40 msec; 4 echoes). Myelographic effect is perfectly obtained with the last echoes (4 th echo=160 msec). Cervical spinal cord is hyposignal in comparison to the hyperintense subarachnoid spaces. *Note* the tiered disko-osteophytic protrusion in this 54-year-old patient, associated with hypertrophy of the ligamenta flava (→)

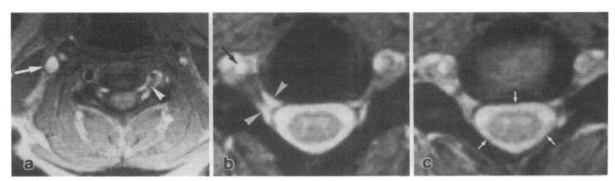

Fig. 192 a-c. Axial sections (C5–C6) through the foraminal plane. Gradient echo, T1 - weighted sequence, TR=300 msec, TE=14 msec, 4 excitations. **a** The spinal cord is clearly visualized; intermediate signal. Peripheral CSF gives a hypointense signal. Nerve roots are well seen in the two intervertebral foramina (hyposignal) *(white arrowhead)* enhanced by the hypersignal of the foraminal veins (slow flow, entry sequence). The disk is poorly identified on axial sections. *Note* the hypersignal of the low flow of both internal jugular veins (→). **b-c** T2 - weighted sequence, axial sections, TR=1800 msec, TE=40 msec, 3rd echo=120. In this sequence, the hypersignal from the foraminal veins *(white arrowhead)* highlights the nerve roots in the two foramina. Rapid flow (vertebral artery) also gives a hypersignal (→). Subarachnoid spaces are hypersignal (→) (T2 - weighted sequence=myelographic effect) surrounding the meningeal membranes. Intrathecal roots are identified; good differentiation between the gray and white matter of the spinal cord

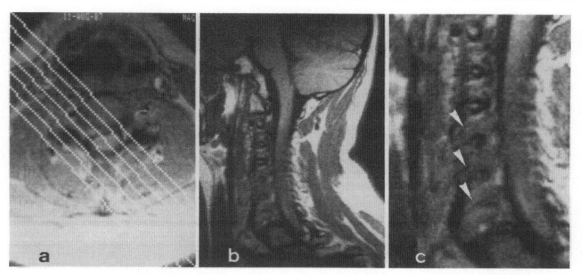

Fig. 193a-c. Oblique sections: sagittal oblique section derived from a transverse scout view. **a** Transverse scout view. Section plane passing through the major axis of the foramen, and therefore of the root studied. **b-c** Oblique sections (spin echo, T1 - weighted sequence, TR = 500 msec, TE 28 msec): projections are comparable to the oblique views in cervical myelography. *Note* the foraminal passage of rootlets on two levels *(white arrowhead)*, below the corresponding pedicles

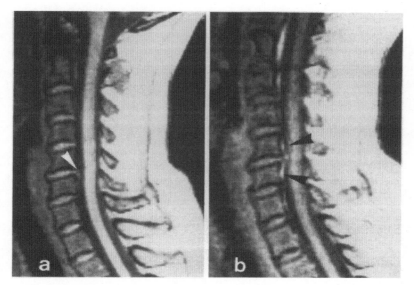

Fig. 194a, b. Left C5-C6 cervicobrachial neuralgia. C5-C6 disk herniation. MRI: T1-weighted left paramedian section; TR = 500 msec; TE = 16 msec; 4 excitations. **a** Small image evoking an isointense C5-C6 disk herniation with partial amputation of the anterior subarachnoid space *(white arrowhead).* **b** Same section after IV injection of Gadolinium-DTPA. Observe the enhancement of the retrovertebral veins above and below the herniation at C5 and C6 *(black arrowhead). Comment:* This illustrates the venous stasis found above and below the disk herniation

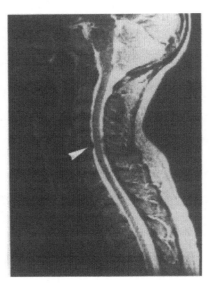

Fig. 195. 50-year-old patient. Spastic paralysis of both lower limbs. Sagittal T2 – weighted section, TR = 1800 msec, TE = 40 msec, 4th echo = 160. Myelographic effect of good quality. At C5–C6, existence of a hyposignal due to a disko-osteophytic lesion *(white arrowhead)*. A solely osteophytic origin cannot be postulated in this case

provided on CT sections by the IV injection of contrast medium; this enhancement is due to the foraminal veins [26].

Degenerative Joint and Disk Lesions

Since they are composed of compact bone, osteophytes do not give rise to MRI signals. Their visualization is therefore indirect, either by an impression on the spinal cord or subarachnoid spaces or by the filling-in of an intervertebral foramen (Fig. 195). Just as in the lumbar spine, degenerative joint lesions result in a remodeling of the spongy bone of the vertebral body, giving a high signal intensity on T1-weighted images.

A recent disk herniation has high signal intensity and is readily distinguished from degenerative joint lesions [3] (Figs. 196, 197). The herniation may displace the spinal cord or the subarachnoid space, or fill in the intervertebral foramen; displacement of venous structures has been described [3] which is identical to that detected on CT (see Fig. 194). Just as at the lumbar level, a degenerated disk has a loss of signal, especially on T2-weighted sequences; thus, a soft

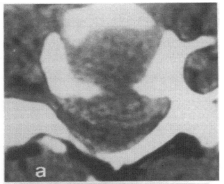

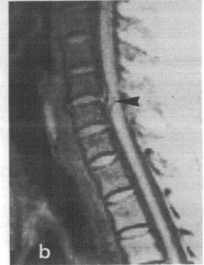

Fig. 196a, b. Posteromedian C5–C6 herniation: tetraparesis developing progressively over several days in 36-year-old patient. **a** CT: large soft disk herniation markedly displacing the spinal cord against the posterior arch. **b** MRI: sagittal T1-weighted section. Herniation gives a signal identical to that of the disk opposite *(black arrowhead)*: recent soft disk herniation. Significant spinal cord compression associated with the herniation

disk herniation of long standing and one which has occurred in a degenerated disk will have the same signal as an osteophyte [10], and there is no way to differentiate between them. Nevertheless, certain authors have improved the discrimination between a soft and a hard disk herniation through the use of adequate sequences [5] (Fig. 198).

Degenerative lesions at the cervical level express themselves as two very different clinical syndromes: degenerative compression myelopathy and radiculopathy.

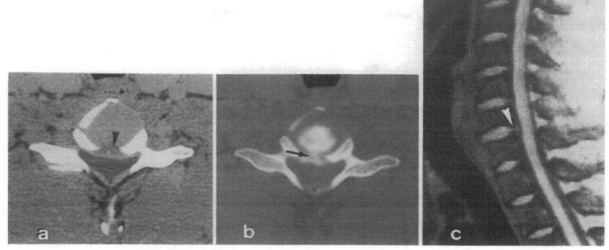

Fig. 197a–c. Left C6–C7 cervicobrachial neuralgia in a 36-year-old patient. **a** Left posterolateral C6–C7 herniation with a small posteromedian hypodensity *(black arrowhead).* **b** Postdiskography CT following cervical chemonucleolysis: selective nucleography with filling-in of a small posteromedian herniation through a small orifice (→). **c** MRI, sagittal T1 - weighted section, TR = 450 msec, TE = 17 msec, 4 excitations. Observe the perfect condordance with postdiskography CT: posterior rupture of the anulus with passage of nuclear material through a small orifice *(white arrowhead)* and a posteromedian herniation

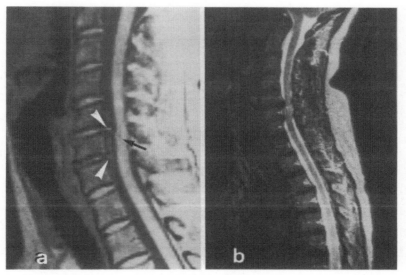

Fig. 198a, b. Cervical arthritic myelopathy in a 54-year-old man. Plain films show the existence of retrovertebral osteophytes at C5–C6 and C6–C7. **a** Median sagittal T1 - weighted section, TR = 450 msec, TE = 14 msec, 4 excitations. Presence of isosignal material in contact with the retrovertebral space at C5–C6 and C6–C7 *(white arrowhead).* Deformation of the facing spinal cord and existence of a small cavity (→). **b** Median sagittal T2 - weighted section, TR = 1800 msec, TE = 40 msec, 4th echo = 160 msec. Disko-osteophytic material is better analyzed than on T1 - weighted sections: better visualization of the subarrachnoid space. Better visualization of spinal canal narrowing and of spinal cord compression, evidence of intramedullary damage. Postmyelography CT scans are more effective than MRI for specific the hard or soft nature of the diskopathy prior to surgery

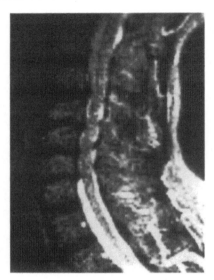

Fig. 199. 74-year-old man with cervical arthrotic myelopathy. Median sagittal T2 - weighted sections (TR = 1800 msec, TE = 40 msec, 4th echo) show multisegmental amputation of the anterior subarachnoid spaces from C3-C4 to C6-C7

Degenerative Compression Myelopathy

Sagittal sections show the spinal cord displacement and compression on T1-weighted sequences and the repercussions on the subarachnoid spaces on T2-weighted sequences, provided there is no scoliosis (Fig. 199). Spinal cord compression may be anterior and of diskal or osteophytic origin, or posterior and due to hypertrophy of the ligamenta flava. It is possible to evaluate the degree of spinal cord atrophy (which implies an unfavorable prognosis), and to demonstrate spinal cord involvement (edema or defect opposite the obstacle) [3, 11] (Figs. 200-202). These sections are capable of exploring the entire cervical spinal cord and determining the most pathogenic segment, information that was formerly provided by cervical myelography [64].

Spinal stenosis, ligamentous calcifications and lateral recess stenosis can also be evaluated using axial sections, which certain authors believe show axial rotation and compression of the spinal cord better than sagittal sections [12].

MRI is the most efficient method for investigating cervical myelopathies, whether their origin is degenerative, tumoral or other [13].

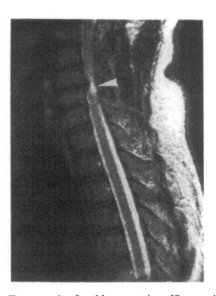

Fig. 200. Tetraparesis of sudden onset in a 57-year-old woman. Sagittal T2 - weighted section, TR = 1800 msec, TE = 40 msec, 4th echo = 160 msec. Major hyposignal lesion at C6-C7 which markedly displaces the spinal cord against the posterior arch. *Note* the concomitant spinal cord edema (hypersignal) *(white arrowhead)*. *Comment*: There was a soft disk herniation, which is difficult to differentiate from an associated osteophyte

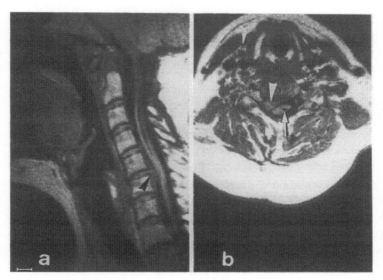

Fig. 201a, b. 41-year-old woman: Chiari malformation associated with syringomyelia operated 7 years previously by trephination and laminectomy. Recent paraparesis associated with right C6 cervicobrachial neuralgia. **a** Sagittal T1-weighted section, TR = 550 msec, TE = 26 msec, 4 excitations. Syringomyelia is clearly seen from C1 to C4. C5–C6 soft disk herniation compressing the spinal cord against the posterior arch *(black arrowhead)*. **b** Axial section through C5–C6. Right posterolateral herniation is clearly visible *(white arrowhead)*, as well as the intramedullary cavity (→)

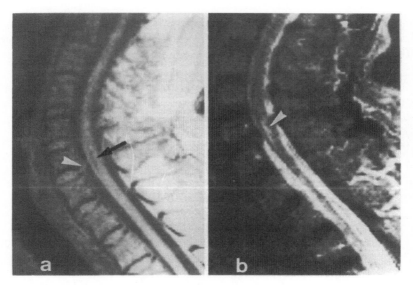

Fig. 202a, b. 55-year-old woman with right C7 cervicobrachial neuralgia and suddenly increased reflexes. **a** MRI median sagittal sections, T1 – weighted sequence, TR = 450 msec, TE = 14 msec, 4 excitations. Hyposignal herniation which deforms and compresses the anterior subarachnoid space *(white arrowhead)*. Observe the intramedullary hyposignal indicative of edematous lesion (→). **b** Same section, but with a T2 – weighted sequence, TR = 1800 msec, TE = 40 msec (4th echo = 160 msec). Hyposignal herniation: the exact limits of the spinal cord are better evaluated, and especially the edema opposite the recent obstacle *(white arrowhead)*

Radiculopathy

Because of the orientation of the intervertebral foramina, the usual techniques using sagittal sections are not adequate for the study of radiculopathies [4]. It is necessary to perform axial and especially oblique sections, either through the long axis of the nerve root or perpendicular to the axis [19, 20]. The relationships between the nerve roots, uncinate processes and the disk are clearly shown.

We favor oblique sections through the axis of the nerve root, which permit one to explore its entire course (Fig. 203). Other authors prefer the axis perpendicular to the nerve root, visualizing the latter in the lower portion of the foramen [1].

Oblique sections thus improve the sensitivity of MRI, which approaches that of Iopamidol CT scans [41, 42, 43]. It is possible to diagnose a herniation only in the absence of degenerative joint lesions, though lateral recess stenosis may mask a small herniated fragment [69]. No comparative studies have yet been performed between CT after the IV injection of contrast medium and MRI, but we believe that a small herniation associated with degenerative joint disease or a migratory fragment within an intervertebral space will be better detected either by CT scans with intravenous contrast, or by postdiskography CT.

To sum up, MRI appears to be the most sensitive examination for investigating degenerative compression myelopathy, since it enables one to identify the most pathogenic segment, to evaluate the condition of the spinal cord, and to eliminate other possible etiologies (Fig. 204). Routinely cer-

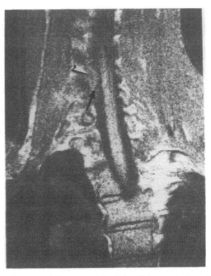

Fig. 203. 38-year-old man with right C6 cervicobrachial neuralgia. Sagittal oblique section derived from a transverse scout view. This oblique section reveals the next lower nerve root, C7 (→). At the overlying level, the herniation amputates the subarachnoid space laterally and is in contact with the C6 nerve root *(black arrowhead)*

vical degenerative myelopathy are first investigated by sagittal MR sections. When it is possible to perform good-quality oblique sections, MRI also exhibits great sensitivity in detecting the level of nerve root compression. Nevertheless, CT scans appear to be more specific in differentiating between a soft disk herniation and a hard one; like other authors [69], we therefore perform Iopamidol CT scans as part of the preoperative work-up of patients with degenerative compression myelopathies or radiculopathies.

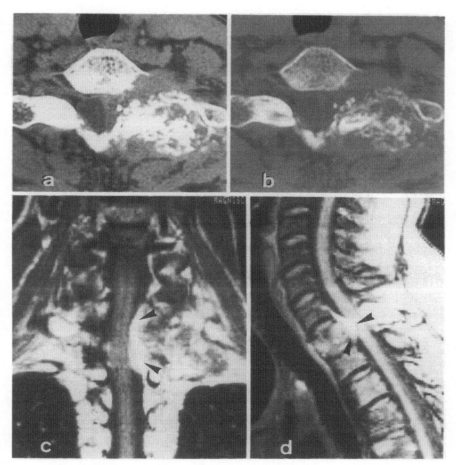

Fig. 204 a–d. A 48-year-old woman with left C8 cervicobrachial neuralgia: spastic paralysis of both lower extremities. **a–b** CT Filling-in of left C7–T1 foramen associated with a large bony out growth originating in the posterior arch of the C7 vertebra. **c–d** Frontal and sagittal MRI sections after IV injection of DTPA Gadolinium, T1 - weighted, TR = 500 msec, TE = 18 msec. The anterior and posterior aspects of the tumor are perfectly seen on sagittal sections; tumor spread is to the left, immediately above the lung apex. The component within the spinal cord (epidural tumor mass) is clearly visible *(black arrowhead)*. Operative findings: a chondrosarcoma originating in the posterior arches of C7 and T1 vertebrae

MRI of Lumbar Disk Herniations

Examination Technique

Our experience with MRI in the diagnosis of lumbar disk herniation is recent. The apparatus used was a 0.5-Tesla MAGNISCAN CGR. The limited access to such equipment prevents the rapid acquisition of a large series of examinations; approximately 300 patients suffering from a disk herniation have been examined so far [5, 6, 8, 17, 18, 22, 57, 58, 59, 78, 79, 88, 89, 90, 93, 97].

Oblique sections have seemed especially useful in visualization of the nerve roots, starting at their emergence from the thecal sac and continuing throughout their entire foraminal and even extraspinal course. Most disk herniations are posterolateral and directly affect the subjacent nerve root at the involved level. CT permits a good diagnosis of nerve root compression of disk origin in most cases. However, oblique MRI sections furnish a better direct anatomic image of the disk, the herniated nucleus, and the nerve root involvement in particular, of a quality superior to any three-dimensional CT reconstruction. All patients initially underwent a CT examination (CGR CE 10000), and the MRI examination was performed and oriented according to the CT images. Only significant herniations were considered.

Patient positioning is more comfortable than for CT scans. A cushion is placed beneath the knees, although reduction of the lumbar lordosis is not essential since the incidence angles of the sections are not restricted by the mechanical limitations of the gantry. The arms remain beside the body, since they do not produce artifacts as in CT. The patient is asked to remain totally motionless, and to breathe calmly and regularly. No injection of paramagnetic contrast medium is performed, since it is of no diagnostic help in disk pathology except in postoperative follow-up. Similarly, cardiac gating is of little aid in this type of pathology.

The technique relies exclusively on surface coils in order to approach the spinal segment involved as closely as possible. Positioning of the coil should be perfect, and centered on the pathologic segment. If necessary, a correction can be made at the beginning of the procedure, after a rapid sagittal scout view using an gradient-echo technique.

The examination starts with sagittal views (gradient-echo), in order to identify the pathologic segment. A 250 mm field is used, which visualizes the entire lumbar spine, lumbosacral junction and medullary cone with a satisfactory spatial resolution (i. e., a pixel of approximately 1 mm^2). This reveals two different situations according to the level involved:

- *L 4–L 5 disk herniation:* axial (transverse) gradient-echo sequences are then performed in order to define two oblique section planes:
  FOT: frontal oblique views in the long axis of the intervertebral foramen (i. e., frontal oblique section derived from a transverse scout view); *SOT:* sagittal oblique views perpendicular to the intervertebral foramen (i. e., sagittal oblique section derived from a transverse scout view).
- *L 5–S 1 disk herniation;* strictly frontal sections are performed, followed by oblique sections derived from the preceding ones:
  SOF: sagittal oblique views of the S 1 nerve root throughout the length of its intrasacral course (i. e., sagittal oblique section derived from a frontal scout view).

Axial (transverse) spin-echo sequences are sometimes performed, permitting a comparison with CT sections which is especially valuable postoperatively. The smallest field is used (200 mm), thus giving a better spatial resolution and limiting the number of motion artifacts due to abdominal and pelvic structures.

The thickness of the image obtained should be small, given the small size of the structures to be examined and in order to reduce partial volume effects as much as possible. We perform 5-mm thick MR scans (axial and oblique) in order to study the nerve roots. When necessary, these slices were used in the sagittal plane, in T 2-weighted sequences, so as to obtain late echoes which still have a satisfactory signal, but only for study of the disk signal and the posterior longitudinal ligament.

We always use a 192×256 matrix, except for scout views, which may be performed with a low resolution (128×128). The choice of sequences should take into consideration the total length of the examination, which should not exceed half an hour, this being the patient's tolerance limit. Localization images are obtained using an gradient-echo sequences. Other MR section planes are obtained with T 1-weighted spin-echo sequences with only one echo (TR 500–600 msec; TE 26–28 msec), and 4 excitations in order to preserve a satisfactory signal-to-noise ratio. We prefer the use of a TR of 600 msec, which provides sufficient images during multislice sequences (10 contiguous 5-mm-thick sections). When the length of the examination permits it, we perform sagittal T 2-weighted spin-echo imaging (TR 1800 msec; TE 40 msec; 3 echoes) with 2 excitations, passing through the herniation.

The duration of MR imaging remains much greater than that of CT. Nevertheless, improvements in the design of surface coils (i.e., much smaller coils placed at the exact level of the nerve-root compression) and in the gradient strength should yield a definite improvement in the signal-to-noise ratio. This should reduce the acquisition time by 75% or reduce the slice thickness, while improved resolution would diminish the partial volume effect. Although 5-mm slices are satisfactory, a slice of 3 mm or less would be preferable.

Limitations and Artifacts

Absolute Contraindications

— cardiac pacemakers (and spinal cord stimulators)
— intracerebral ferromagnetic surgical clips (heart valve prostheses, even metallic ones, are not contraindications)
— other prostheses or ferromagnetic objects (i. e., intraocular fragment)

Artifacts

There are various types of artifacts [10, 21, 56, 60, 100]:

— *Artifacts due to metallic objects* (eg. osteosynthesis material). Only ferromagnetic prostheses result in significant deterioration of the image. In practice, metallic artifacts are often smaller with MRI than with CT. They may appear as loss of signal, peripheral hypersignal, or deformation of the adjacent image.
— *Motion artifacts* may be significant, given the prolonged acquisition times. CSF pulsations in themselves may create artifacts. A pulsatile and turbulent flow of CSF results in dephasing and localized signal loss. A typical example is the situation at the cerebral aqueduct, but this also applies at the thoracolumbar junction. There is an increased CSF signal at the level of the dural cul-de-sac; this is due to a relative decrease in the mobility of the CSF at this level and to the elimination of dephasing phenomena.
— *Technical artifacts* are numerous and have various origins: nonuniform main field or radiofrequency pulse; faulty gradients (involving linearity and calibration); chemical shift (eg. the cortical bone of the superior endplates of the vertebral bodies is thicker than that of the inferior ones); image reconstruction (i. e., truncation artifacts with images of alternating intensity: the Gibb phenomenon).
— Finally, claustrophobia, may prevent completion of the examination in a few patients.

Normal Anatomy

The physical principles determining magnetic resonance images are altogether different from those involved in CT images obtained with X-rays; similarly, the appearance of the image is entirely different. The contrasts of the lumbar spine canal and its contents vary from T 1-weighted to T 2-weighted sequences.

T 1-weighted Sequences
(TR 600 msec; TE 26 msec)

These provide the best anatomic details [2, 23, 47, 48, 54, 62, 75, 76, 80, 99, 101].

Sagittal and Parasagittal Sections

Cortical bone appears as a line devoid of signal which frames the vertebral body; this is due to the lack of mobility of the hydrogen protons in compact bone. The cortical layer, which appears white and dense on CT, appears black on MR images. It is an important factor in image contrast; however, absence of this signal may render the localization of calcifications within the vertebral canal more difficult than on CT (Fig. 205).

The spongy bone of the vertebral bodies gives a signal isointense with that of muscle. This relative intensity may increase with age and after irradiation of the spinal column, because of the replacement of bone marrow by fat.

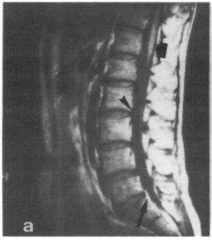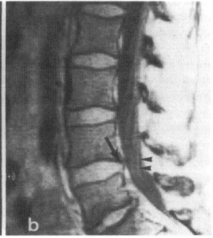

Fig. 205 a, b. *Sagittal T1 - weighted section* (spin echo, TR = 600 msec, TE = 30 msec, 4 excitations). **a** Cortical bone of the vertebral bodies is devoid of signal. Inferior vertebral end-plates appear thicker than the superior ones, because of the chemical shift in the direction of the frequency-encoding axis. The posterior half of the vertebral spongy bone gives a higher signal (spinal cord fat). Basivertebral veins not visible in this sequence. Intervertebral disks give a signal which is less than that of spongy bone. The anulus fibrosus gives no signal and is indistinguishable from the vertebral end-plate *(black arrowhead)*. CSF appears dark because of its long T1. This sequence is inadequate for studying the relationship between the disk and the thecal sac posterior to the disk. It is impossible to differentiate between the anulus fibrosus, the posterior longitudinal ligament, the dura mater and the CSF (all of which give similar weak signals). The anterior epidural fat posterior to the vertebral bodies gives a high signal, greatest at L5–S1, where it clearly defines the anulus (→). The

medullary cone can be studied on the same section if a sufficiently large field is used (at least 25 cm). It gives a signal similar to that of spongy bone (➡). The uppermost portions of the cauda equina roots are distinguishable in the posterior half of the spinal canal (supine patient) and often have poorly defined limits (root mobility). **b** *Sagittal gradient-echo section* (T1 - weighted, TR = 450 msec, TE = 16 msec, 4 excitations). Gradient-echo sequences are very useful for anatomic studies, since they are more rapidly performed and provide remarkable detail. They are essentially T1 - weighted. However, the nucleus gives a higher signal with shorter TRs; the signal is greater than that of spongy bone, permitting good definition of its posterior margin with respect to the weak signal of the thecal sac CSF (→). The cauda equina roots are very well defined by the use of a fast sequence *(arrowhead)*. Even the posterior longitudinal ligament is sometimes visible, posterior to the vertebral bodies and surrounded by the anterior epidural fat

Pedicles, articular facets and laminae also appear as structures with a signal equal to that of spongy bone, framed by a thin black rim of cortical bone.

Ligaments (particularly the posterior longitudinal ligament and the ligamenta flava) also have a very weak signal, their highly organized structure making them only slightly mobile. Whereas with CT two different windows are necessary for a good analysis of bony structures and soft tissues, one window is sufficient in MRI.

In the posterior half of the vertebral body the basivertebral veins of the anterior epidural plexuses may give either a low or high signal, depending on the degree of blood-flow and the type of sequence used. Their structural appearance is characteristic.

Intervertebral disks have a signal slightly less than that of spongy bone; they are framed by the cortical layer of the vertebral end-plates. The inferior end-plate may appear thicker than the superior because of a chemical shift, an artifact usually observed with high-field devices (i. e., T5 Tesla and greater). This phenomenon is due to differences in the resonance frequencies of the protons in water and in fat; it is usually observed along the axis of the frequency-encoded gradient (usually the inferior end-plate). With age and/or degeneration, there is a progressive loss of signal intensity due to disk dehydration. The anulus fibrosus gives a signal identical to that of cortical bone and appears as a slightly convex band with loss of signal, limited posteriorly by CSF with an identical or intermediate signal on sagittal sections. It may be difficult to distinguish between the CSF and the anulus, since they sometimes have similar signals. On parasagittal images, the foraminal fat defines the contours of the anulus much more satisfactorily. In fact, just as in CT scans, in which it has negative densities, the fat makes a very important contribution to image contrast. It is the tissue with the most intense (i. e. white) signal, given its relatively short T1.

The dorsal root ganglion is clearly visible in the upper third of the fat-filled intervertebral foramen, just below the pedicle. The spinal nerve is very well highlighted in the midst of the fat, since it has a low intermediate signal similar to that of the CSF in the thecal sac.

The CSF of the thecal sac, given its relatively long T1, has a low signal and therefore a dark-gray appearance on images. The image is influenced by CSF mobility within the thecal sac. At the level of the dural cul-de-sac, the CSF may exhibit a higher-intensity signal than at the thoracolumbar junction, because of the stagnation and lack of flow-related phase shifts.

It is not usually possible to differentiate between the posterior cortical bony layer, the anulus fibrosus, ligaments, dura mater and thecal sac CSF, since all these structures give signals which are quite low and similar on sagittal sections. Nevertheless, if there is abundant anterior epidural fat and anterior detachment of the thecal sac, it is sometimes possible to distinguish the detached posterior longitudinal ligament posterior to the vertebral bodies; it appears as a black band highlighted on both sides by the brightness of the epidural fat and the anterior venous plexuses.

The signal intensity of the *medullary cone* is high and similar to that of spongy bone. It is easily recognizable within the thecal sac and usually ends at the level of T12–L1.

The cauda equina nerve roots are often visible below, forming a column with a signal lower than that of the medullary cone but higher than that of the CSF. The contours of the cauda equina may appear blurred because of the mobility of the nerve roots. It is posteriorly located in a supine subject.

Axial (Transverse) Images

These may be strictly axial views or oblique axial views (TOS) through the intervertebral disk. These images are easier to interpret, because of their analogy with CT section planes (Fig. 206).

The thecal sac appears as a rounded structure with a low signal intensity, surrounded by the bright hypersignal of the epidural fat.

Nerve roots can often be identified in the thecal sac as tubular structures isointense with muscle. Because they have some mobility, their contours may appear blurred on sagittal sections. Only CT myelography with the intrathecal injection of contrast medium permits an equivalent examination. Beyond the dura mater, the emerg-

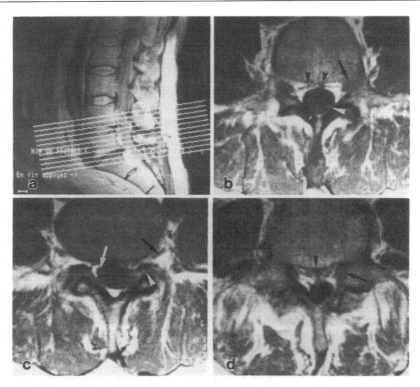

Fig. 206 a–d. Transverse oblique sections derived from a sagittal scout view. Spin echo, T1 - weighted sequence, TR = 500 msec, TE = 26 msec, 4 excitations. **a** *Oblique scout view section:* the transverse oblique sections derived from a sagittal scout view are identical to CT scans parallel to the intervertebral disk (gantry angle of 9°). Image contrast obtained with MRI differs from that of CT scans. **b** *Section through L4–L5 intervertebral foramen:* the thecal sac is dark (long T1) and the cauda equina roots are visible within it (as in postmyelography CT) as posteriorly located rounded structures with a higher signal than that of CSF *(white arrowhead).* L4 ganglia are clearly visible within the high-signal foraminal fat; their signal is comparable to that of CSF (—►). Anterior epidural veins are silhouetted against the lighter surrounding fat, posterior to the vertebral body *(black arrowhead).* **c** *Section through the L4–L5 disk:* the disk is poorly distinguishable from the adjacent end-plates (similar signals in 6-mm-thick sections). Extraspinal L4 roots run along the lateral part of the intervertebral disk (—►). Intrathecal portion of the right L5 root is already visible just before its emergence *(white arrow).* Cortical bone of the laminae and the articular processes gives no signal. Ligamenta flava give intermediate signals; their lateral extension towards the joint capsule of the articular processes is clearly seen *(white arrowhead).* **d** *Section through the L5 facet joint:* L5 roots are easily seen in lateral recesses (—►). Basivertebral vein posterior to the vertebral body has a dark irregular appearance *(black arrowhead)*

ing roots are very clearly identified and highlighted by the epidural fat, often in a more distinct fashion than by CT. The nerve roots may be followed laterally into the intervertebral foramina and over their extraspinal course.

The epidural veins are particularly well seen on axial views, appearing as sinuous structures devoid of signal and immediately posterior to the posterior cortical layer of the vertebral bodies.

It should be noted that it is difficult to distinguish a normal disk on axial sections, since its signal is similar to that of the vertebral body and there is a partial volume effect which is significant on 5-mm slices. A degenerated disk is easier to spot, since it has a much lower signal intensity and thus gives better contrast.

Oblique Views

One of the difficulties with surface coil MRI lies in obtaining a detailed analysis of the lateral recess and the intervertebral foramen on sagittal and axial views [24, 58, 71, 94]. Recent studies have shown the value of oblique views in the investigation of these regions at the cervical level [20, 71]. At the lumbar level, oblique views permit a better study of the nerve roots by exposing and aligning them after their emergence from the thecal sac. The roots are well highlighted, whether in the vertebral canal and intervertebral foramen or outside the spinal cord, thanks to the significant brightness of the fat.

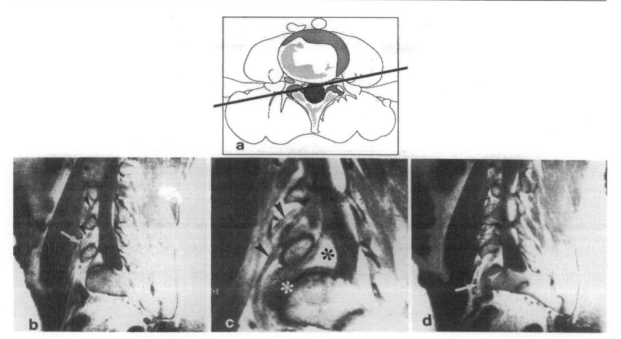

Fig. 207 a–d. Frontal oblique section derived from a transverse scout view. (T1 – weighted images, TR 500 msec, TE 28 msec). **a** Oblique sequence derived from a transverse (axial) section and following the major axis of the neural foramen of the root to be investigated. Gantry angle is less than 45°. **b** The similarity to oblique projections using plain films (lumbar myelograms) is evident. Nevertheless, all the roots cannot be captured on one section; they appear successively on several adjacent sections. The L3, L4 and L5 roots are clearly visible over a longer distance than on lumbar myelograms: the portion below the pedicle is also seen (ganglion *(arrowhead)* and fasciculus of nerve (→)). **c** L4 root helps constitute the lumbosacral plexus and its pelvic branches *(arrowhead)* L5 axilla and its epidural fat are clearly visible (✻) and are in close contact with the underlying L5-S1 disk *(white star).* **d** Presacral course of L5 is shown (→), as well as emergence of the S1 root *(white arrowhead)*

The *FOT* are identical to the oblique antero-posterior projections performed in myelography. Their intepretation is also familiar, with a good exploration of the roots at their emergence and particularly at their axillae. The L3, L4 and L5 roots are particularly well investigated with this obliquity. The slices are parallel to the long axis of the foramen and align the nerve root over a long distance, below the pedicle and also over several centimeters outside the spinal column. One can readily identify the early division of the extraspinal nerve roots, particularly of the anterior branches of L3 and L4 to form the femoral nerve of the lumbar plexus. The L5 root is well highlighted, before its sudden directional change to adopt a vertical presacral course. In contrast to myelography, in which all the nerve roots are visible on the same oblique projection, MRI shows the nerve roots progressively on serial sections (Fig. 207).

The *SOT* are perpendicular to the long axis of the intervertebral foramen. The foramen is clearly seen, with its bilobed aspect, on strictly "transverse" views. The nerve root surrounded by its sheath of foraminal veins is well shown in the upper third of the foramen, as are the bony contours (pedicle, articular processes, and adjacent vertebral bodies) and the posterolateral disk margin. Parasagittal views may provide comparable information; however, their inclination is not optimal, and there is foraminal deformation as well as frequent partial volume artifacts (Fig. 208).

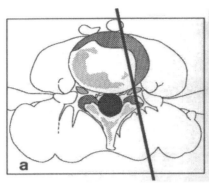 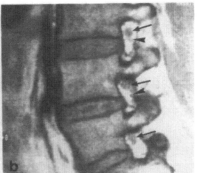

Fig. 208a, b. Sagittal oblique sections derived from a transverse scout view (T1 – weighted images; TR 500 msec, TE 28 msec, 4 excitations). **a** Oblique sequence: starting with a transverse plane, sections are made perpendicular to the axis of the foramen of the root to be studied. **b** Intervertebral foramina at several levels are well studied on the same section.

Epidural fat underlines the root particularly well in the upper part of the foramen (→), as well as the accompanying foraminal veins *(arrowhead)*. Posterolateral margin of the disk is well defined by the fat. This projection is particularly useful for studying strictly foraminal herniations

The *SOF* are less often used. They provide excellent demonstration of the S1 nerve roots. The S1 roots descend vertically within the sacral canal towards the first sacral foramen, and are well aligned by strictly frontal images. SOF views permit good demonstration not only of their emergence from the thecal sac, but also of their entire intrasacral course and of the nerve root ganglion in particular (which is poorly shown on CT). Distal to the ganglion, the nerve rami may be distinguished as thin parallel branches (two groups of rami are usually visible) (Fig. 209).

The *TOF* may be grouped with the SOF projections. They align the L5 or L4 roots, based on frontal scout views; they are particularly useful for exposing the uppermost portion of the corresponding lateral recess (Fig. 210).

Finally, we have already considered the TOS, which are simply variants of rigorously axial views and align the intervertebral disk in the same manner as CT scans (see Fig. 206).

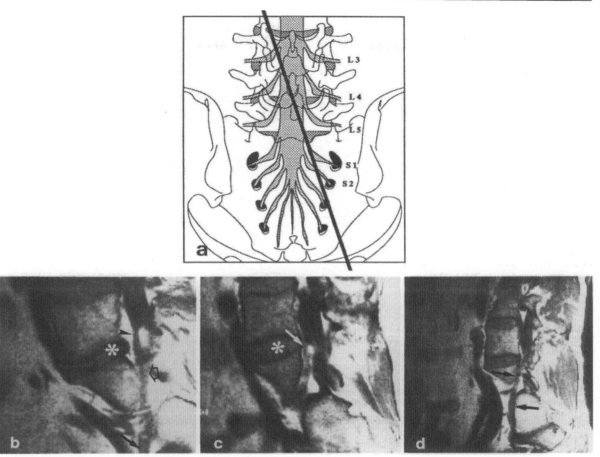

Fig. 209 a–d. Sagittal oblique section derived from a frontal scout view, T1 – weighted sequence, TR = 650 msec, TE = 28 msec, 4 excitations. **a** *Oblique scout view sections:* the strictly vertical orientation of the S1 roots enables them to be seen on a simple frontal view. Sagittal oblique sections derived from a frontal scout view are oriented according to the major axis of the S1 root within the sacral foramen. **b** S1 root can be traced particularly well, starting at its thecal sac emergence *(arrowhead)* contiguous with the L5-S1 disk (✻), and anteriorly as far as the intrasacral ganglion *(empty arrow)*. The underlying nerve fasciculi can often be seen (usually two bundles) (→). **c** L5 root is more difficult to trace on this oblique view; two adjacent sections are necessary. L5 root emergence (→) is traced posterior to and below the L4-L5 disk (✻). Axillary fat of the L5 root is seldom seen. **d** An adjacent section shows the very short course below the pedicle as well as the directional change of the L5 root, which becomes vertical in its extraspinal presacral segment (→). Usually, this segment is the only one clearly seen

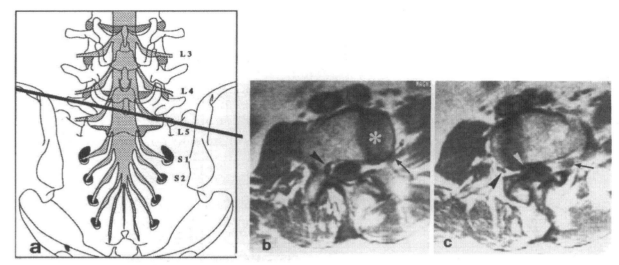

Fig. 210a–c. *MRI:* Transverse oblique section derived from a frontal scout view. (SE; T1 - weighted images; TR 500 msec, TE 28 msec). **a** *Oblique sequence:* this is comparable to that of sagittal oblique sections derived from a frontal scout view, although with a smaller gantry angle (less than 45°). These sections are parallel to the root course below the pedicle. The sections differ from axial ones in that the left and right sides are asymmetric. **b** On the right, the L3 root is still within the lateral recess *(arrowhead),* against the internal aspect of the pedicle. On the left, the extraforaminal L3 root is visible in the prevertebral fat (—►) in contact with the psoas muscle and the intervertebral disk ✻. **c** *Subjacent section:* The left

L3–L4 foramen investigated appears enlarged in this section: the deformed L4 ganglion, which is enlarged by the oblique projection is more easily identified against its bony background (—►). Right L4 root is not yet visible, since it is still within the thecal sac *(white arrowhead).* Right L3 ganglion *(black arrowhead)* is investigated anterior to the posterolateral margin of the L3–L4 disk. *Comment:* We seldom use this method; it is especially useful for showing the L4 and L5 roots as they pass through the lateral recess and neural foramen (i. e., in isolated radiculitis or a large root associated with a spondylolisthesis)

T2-weighted Sequences [18, 40, 80, 120]

T2-weighted sequences of sagittal views were made only to better define the posterior margin of the intervertebral disk and its relations with the posterior longitudinal ligament and the thecal sac [2, 15, 23, 25, 61, 72, 76] (Figs. 211, 212).

The signal of the spongy bone of the vertebral bodies decreases with the late echoes, hampering the distinction between the cortical layer and the spongy bone.

The *cortical layer* continues to be devoid of signal.

The *facet joint space* appears as a hyperintense line, because of the presence of synovial fluid.

The *basivertebral veins* now contrast strongly, appearing as hypersignal areas on median views.

On sagittal MRI views, normal lumbar disks may be differentiated into nucleus and anulus by using sequence settings favoring T2-weighted images and proton densities, both of which are

sensitive to hydration changes. There is a significant difference in water content between the healthy anulus and nucleus. A normal nucleus has a signal whose intensity increases when T2 increases (i. e., 120 msec). A longer TR seems to offer an optimal combination of a high signal-to-noise ratio and a maximum nucleus-anulus contrast (we use a TR of 1800 msec; certain authors recommend much longer TRs of about 3000 msec, but the acquisition time then becomes so long as to prevent its routine use).

Most normal disks (over 90%) exhibit a central intranuclear cleft with a low intensity signal, which gives a notched or biconcave appearance to the nucleus, identical to the appearance at diskography [1]. This cleft communicates posteriorly in 81% of cases. The percentage of disks with this central intranuclear defect increases appreciably with age. In patients over 30 years of age, all normal and abnormal disks with a residual high-intensity signal have such a cleft. MRI of disks removed at autopsy shows this intranuclear defect,

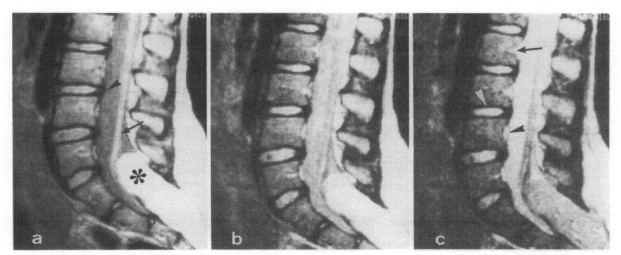

Fig. 211 a–c. Sagittal section, spin echo, T2 – weighted sequence, TR = 1800 msec, TE = 40–120 msec. Tethered cord in a 10-year-old child, associated with an intrasacral lipoma. **a** *1st echo (40 msec):* Signal of the vertebral spongy bone is still high, but tends to decrease with subsequent echoes **(b–c)**. The cortical bone never gives any signals. The nucleus is easily seen and gives a high signal which increases with subsequent echoes **(b–c)**. Nuclear signals in children are intense and homogeneous (richly hydrated). Low-signal anulus already has a signal weaker than that of CSF *(black arrowhead)*. Fat gives an intense signal (intrasacral lipoma) (✻). The tethered cord and thickened filum terminale give a stronger signal than CSF (→). **b** *2nd echo (80 msec):* reinforced nuclear and CSF signals. Tethered cord is no longer visible (crossover point of the T2 decay curves of the spinal cord and CSF). Lipoma signal tends to decrease. **c** *3rd echo (120 msec, strongly T2 – Weighted):* CSF gives a very intense signal (long T2) and appears white ("myelographic effect"). Reversal of contrast with respect to the tethered cord. Fat signal of the lipoma decreases rapidly. Nucleus gives a very intense signal and remains homogeneous *(white arrowhead)*. The more internal anular fibers are indistinguishable from the nucleus. Anterior limits of the thecal sac are more accurately seen. Posteriorly, the posterior epidural fat hampers accurate definition. Posterior disk margins are well defined. Posterior longitudinal ligament is still visible behind the vertebrae *(black arrowhead),* adherent to the posterior surface of the disks. Basivertebral veins give an intense signal (→)

with a signal indistinguishable from that of the peripheral anulus. This transaxial extension of lamellar substance dividing the nucleus into superior and inferior fragments is also found on histologic sections, especially in the posterior portion of the disk, thanks to staining properties similar to those of the anulus. Diskography in adults also typically shows a filling-in of the nucleus as two parallel plates which communicate posteriorly, whereas in children and young adults the contrast opacifies the entire nucleus. The invagination of the anular lamellae into the nucleus becomes evident during the second and third decades of life.

The *CSF* acquires a much more intense signal because of its prolonged T2 relaxation time. It appears white on late echoes (i.e., 120 msec); both the cauda equina roots and the medullary cone appear as hyposignal structures surrounded by the bright CSF. This high intensity CSF signal highlights disks and/or osteophytes which may project into the vertebral canal. It is only by us-

ing these sequences that the precise contours of the thecal sac may be determined. Heavily-T2-weighted sequences are particularly useful for increasing the contrast between the intervertebral disk and the thecal sac when there is little epidural fat, resulting in what is almost a myelographic effect.

The posterior longitudinal ligament was visualized in our series by means of such sequences; it is shown on median sections, posterior to the vertebral bodies, where it is normally detached. Its close attachment to the posterior margin of the intervertebral disk make it distinguishable from the anulus fibrosus, which has a low-intensity signal close to that of the ligament.

Because of flow effects, the CSF signal may be nonuniform and reticular in appearance, thus preventing good analysis of the image. These artifacts, are particularly sensitive at the cervical level and may necessitate the use of cardiac gating here.

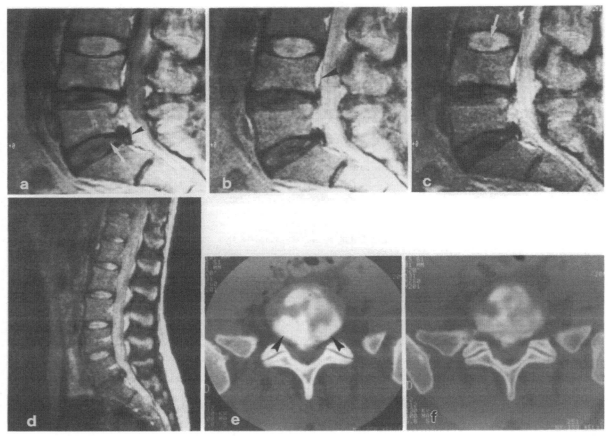

Fig. 212a–f. MRI: Disk degeneration. **a–c** Sagittal section (SE; T2 weighted images; TR 1800 msec, TE 40, 80 and 120 msec). Nuclear portion of a normal L3–L4 disk gives a high signal, which is reinforced by late echos **(c)**. Presence of an intranuclear cleft, which is better seen on the third echo (→). This cleft is present in all patients over 30 years old and is an expression of transaxial extension of lamellar material. There is partial concordance with the images furnished by postdiskography CT. T2 - weighted images increase the size of the nucleus, with the more internal fibers of the anulus contributing to the central hypersignal. A high nuclear signal cannot be found if a herniation is present. Posterior longitudinal ligament is clearly seen, bounded anteriorly by the epidural fat and veins and posteriorly by the high signal of the CSF (2rd echo) **(b)** *(black arrowhead)*. *Note* the disk degeneration present at the last two levels. Nuclear dehydration results in collapse, signal loss and loss of the nucleus - anulus differentiation. Intranuclear cleft is barely visible **(a)**. Although a disk herniation is always accompagned by an altered signal, the converse is not always true. The anulus, which no longer gives a signal, bulges into the spinal canal but is not fissured **(a)** *(black arrowhead)* Nuclear material remains at a distance **(a)** (→). **d–f.** Right S1 sciatica in a 31-year-old woman. **d** Median sagittal. T2-weighted MRI section (2nd echo; TR = 1800 msec; TE = 40 msec). Incomplete myelographic effect; Hyposignal L5–S1 herniation is clearly visible, elevating the posterior longitudinal ligament. Note the hyposignal appearance of the L5–S1 disk, indicating its degeneration. **e,f** Postdiskography CT one hour after L5–S1 chemonucleolysis: this confirms the good accessibility of the herniation to the contrast and therefore to the enzyme. *Note* the significant signs of L5–S1 disk degeneration *(black arrowhead)*; there is no nucleus-anulus differentiation. *Comment:* The disk degeneration associated with herniations in young subjects is not a contraindication to chemonucleolysis

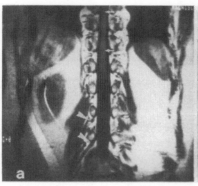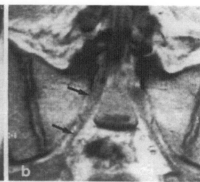

Fig. 213a, b. T1 – weighted frontal view. **a** Spin echo, TR = 600 msec, TE = 28 msec, 4 excitations. Medullary cone has an intermediate signal greater than that of CSF. Central canal of the spinal cord appears as a thin median line giving a hyposignal (→). Root emergences can be easily studied at each level, as well as their course beneath the pedicle to the root ganglion *(white arrowhead)* which is not visible on a comparable frontal myelogram. **b** Gradient echo, TR = 600 msec, TE = 14 msec, 4 excitations. On a single section, the S1 roots are visible within the two sacral foramina as well as in the pelvis (→). The roots give a higher intermediate signal in this sequence than in the preceding one

Gradient-Echo Sequences

These sequences are very often used for performing scout views; however, in order to shorten the examination, it is possible to use them for one or two projections. Satisfactory anatomic details can be obtained with sufficiently long TRs (i.e., of about 300 to 500 msec) and at least 4 excitations. The images are compositely weighted, being T1-weighted for the bony structures, fat and nervous structures (thecal sac and nerve roots). The cauda equina nerve roots are often individualized better by such sequences, with a much more rapid acquisition time of about 5 mn. Intervertebral disks give a hyperintense and homogeneous signal; it is not possible to distinguish the anulus from the nucleus. Large disk fragments also have an identical signal which is quite high, and stronger than that of the spongy bone of the vertebral bodies. These sequences are also much more sensitive to venous blood-flow; thus, the basivertebral veins are hyperintense and well highlighted by the surrounding bone (Fig. 213).

Lumbar Disk Pathology

Disk Degeneration

Changes in the degree of disk hydration become more apparent on T2-weighted images (TR 1800 msec; TE 2 e echo 80 msec; 3 e echo 120 msec). The normal nucleus of young adults, consisting of 85% to 90% water, gives a higher intensity signal than that of the anulus [2, 15, 32, 35, 36, 37, 44, 45, 61, 70, 72, 73, 75, 83, 95, 102] (see Fig. 212). With disk degeneration, increasing age, or both, the degree of hydration decreases to 70%. The water content of the anulus, normally 78%, also decreases to 70%. This proportionately greater water loss by the nucleus reduces the distinction between the nucleus and the anulus. The intranuclear cleft may also be less easily identifiable. The appearance of the disk and the cleft range from a simple relative decrease of the nuclear signal, compared with healthy disks in the same patients, to a total loss of contrast between the nucleus and anulus.

The biochemical constitution of the affected disk is also modified, with an increase in the collagen concentration of the nucleus and a decrease in mucopolysaccharides and chodroitin sulfates. The effects of these chemical changes on signal amplitude of each component are not well known; the degree of nuclear hydration seems to be the determining factor in signal generation.

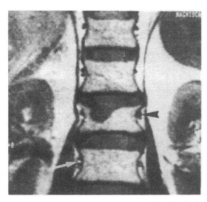

Fig. 214. Right paramedian T12–L1 Schmorl's node. Frontal section (SE; T1 - weighted images, TR 600 msec, TE 28 msec). Disk has not degenerated and still gives a normal signal. *Note* the presence of lateral intervertebral veins *(arrowhead)*. Flows are variable, with paradoxical enhancement of slow flows (→)

T1-weighted sequences may not be sensitive enough to detect a decreased signal intensity. Sagittal views are the most appropriate for evaluating the disk signal, since they minimize partial volume effects (contrary to axial sections) and permit a comparison with all the other lumbar disks on one image.

Disk degeneration is such a frequent finding as to considered nonspecific, whether the subject is symptomatic or not. In asymptomatic patients 8% to 30% of all disk present clear signs of degeneration, and around the age of 50 years 85% to 95% of autopsied subjects have lumbar disk involvement. A decreased T2 relaxation value may be observed in several disks, without there being any disk bulging or herniation. In the case of *Schmorl's node*, although there is a disk herniation through the vertebral end-plate, the disk does not exhibit an abnormal decrease in signal intensity such as that found in all posterior disk herniations. Furthermore, the existence of a herniation within the spongy bone does not appear to be linked to disk degeneration [82] (Fig. 214).

Disk Herniation

MRI appears to be the most sensitive means for the identification of disk degeneration, though this is not necessarily accompanied by disk her-

niation [2, 9, 15, 16, 23, 39, 44, 61, 67, 68, 74, 76, 77, 85, 90, 102]. On the other hand, all herniations are accompanied by signs of degeneration. In a patient with lumbar pain, if the lumbar disk has a normal signal on MRI, a herniation can be excluded (except at a very early stage, since water loss can be confirmed only after 48 hours). The biochemical changes are identical, with a decrease in water content and fibrocartilaginous transformation of the disk, leaving no clear distinction between nucleus and anulus.

Disk herniations should be studied with successive T1-weighted and T2-weighted sequences. Although the *T1-contrast* does not appear useful in the study of a degenerated disk, it is of great value in the structural evaluation of a herniation and a compressed nerve root. T1-weighted sequences furnish subtle anatomic details, due to highlighting by the fat hypersignal and the speed of acquisition. We continue to prefer these sequences, especially with the use of oblique views.

Herniated disk material has a signal intensity similar to or slightly lower than that of the nucleus. Occasionally, it may have a higher signal intensity. The disk herniation has a very characteristic appearance, with nuclear extension towards the epidural fat, the thecal sac, or the intervertebral foramen. It may be difficult to distinguish between a herniation and a disk bulging, especially as both may give rise to symptoms. Structural differences seem to be the most helpful. The herniation is evident when there is anulus rupture (particularly visible on sagittal images) and localized extension of nuclear material through an obvious defect in the posterior hyposignal rim of the anulus (Fig. 215). Concentric disk expansion with an intact but often thin anulus is considered indicative of bulging (see Fig. 212).

Axial (transverse) images or axial oblique images (TOS) identical to those in CT are sometimes obtained. Although it may be difficult to differentiate between the disk and the vertebral body (because of similar signals and partial volume effects with 5 mm slices), a large herniation extending toward the vertebral canal, the filling-in of the epidural fat and the nerve root displacement are all evident, as would be any associated

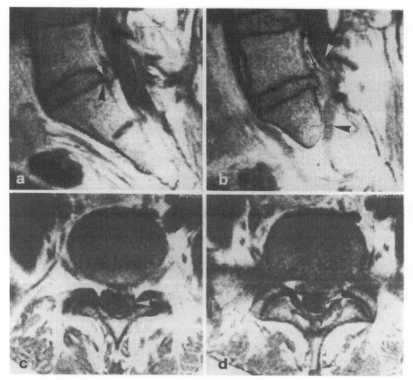

Fig. 215a-d. Left S1 sciatica in a 40-year-old man. Sagittal oblique section derived from a frontal scout view (SE; T1 - weighted images: TR 600 msec, TE 26 msec). **a** Disk hernia-tion can be confirmed; rupture of outermost anulus fibers *(black arrowhead)*. Fissuring of the anulus; nuclear material passes through a small orifice posterior to the anular fibers (→). This appearance is comparable to that obtained by plain film diskography. **b** Adjacent section past the orifice shows nuclear material (→) (intermediate signal) posterior to the anulus fibrosus (hyposignal rim). Root compression by the herniation is particularly evident, being visible throughout its height; displacement of thecal sac and cauda equina *(white arrowhead); displacement and deformation of left S1 root (black arrowhead).* **c** Transverse oblique section derived from a sagittal scout view (SE; T1 - weighted images; TR 600 sec, TE 26 msec). L5-S1 foramen. Left S1 root within the thecal sac is displaced posteriorly, above the herniation *(white arrowhead).* Under no conditions would this be visible on CT. **d** Section through the facet joints: left L5-S1 postero-lateral herniation which is slightly descending. Left S1 root evidently compressed *(white arrowhead)*

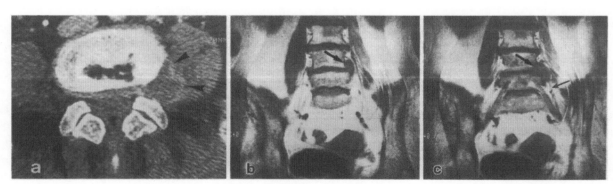

Fig. 216a-c. Left femoral pain resistant to medical treatment in a 78-year-old woman. **a** CT: large left lateral L3-L4 herni-ation outside the spinal canal. *Note* the unusual peripheral enhancement around the disk material *(black arrowhead).* Root is not visible. **b-c** MRI: Frontal sections (SE; T1 - weighted sections; TR 450 msec, TE 28 msec). Confirmation of an ascending and descending herniation outside the spinal canal. Signal is identical to that of the L3-L4 disk; herniation is contiguous with the intervertebral space *(large arrow).* L3 root is visible immediately below the herniation *(small arrow)*

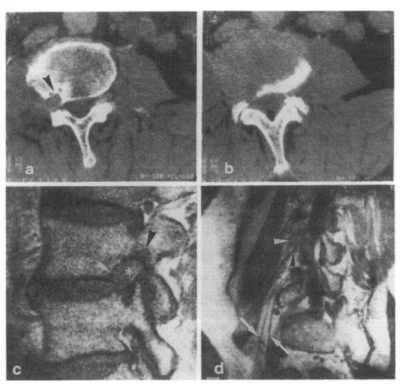

Fig. 217 a–d. Right femoral pain of 3 months' duration. *CT:* **a** L3–L4 intervertebral foramen: Foraminal herniation and filling-in of the fat. Impossible to differentiate between the disk fragment and the nerve root ganglion. End-plate erosion at this level, with a small degree of secondary osteosclerosis; this is usually seen in cases of large old herniations *(black arrowhead).* **b** L3–L4 disk: normal appearance of lateral disk margin; the posterior disk margin is not clearly defined. *MRI:* **c** Sagittal oblique section derived from a transverse scout view; TR 500 msec, TE 28 msec, 4 excitations. Obliteration of the foraminal epidural fat by a disk fragment adjacent to the intervertebral disk, and having an identical signal (✽).

The limits of the anulus are ill defined. Erosion of the adjacent vertebral end-plate *(white arrowhead).* L3 root is displaced posteriorly and compressed against the pedicle *(black arrowhead).* **d** Frontal oblique section derived from a transverse scout view; TR 600 msec, TE 28 msec, 4 excitations. Disk fragment is clearly visible below the L3 pedicle *(white arrowhead)* resulting in compression and displacement of the L3 root just below its emergence from the thecal sac *(black arrowhead).* On this section, one cannot see both the intervertebral disk and the herniation. *Note* the L4 branches contributing to the lumbar plexus (→)

spinal stenosis. Herniations with a transverse location are especially well seen (see Fig. 215). Nevertheless, we consider comparable thin CT sections with a thickness of 1 mm to be just as informative or even more so. The lateral extension of the herniation toward the lateral recess and intervertebral foramen, or even extraspinally in the case of lateral herniations, are well seen of frontal views (Fig. 216) and even better on oblique images.

Though a herniation may be quite easily located on the CT scans or axial MRI images, exact location of the nerve root and its displacement the very site of root compression by the disk are often difficult; this is especially true in

foramino-lateral herniations. In cases where it is difficult to determine on CT scans if the lateral recess stenosis is secondary to a vertebral body osteophyte or a calcified herniation, SOT images may show the intervertebral disk and the herniation to be continuous and to have identical signals. The nerve root may be located with respect to the herniation, being displaced cephalad by an ascending herniation, or caudad and posterior by a lateral herniation; this is essentially done using FOT images. With these oblique projections, it is not possible to visualize both the herniation and the disk on the same image. The two projections are therefore complementary (Figs. 217, 218). They may also provide interesting information in

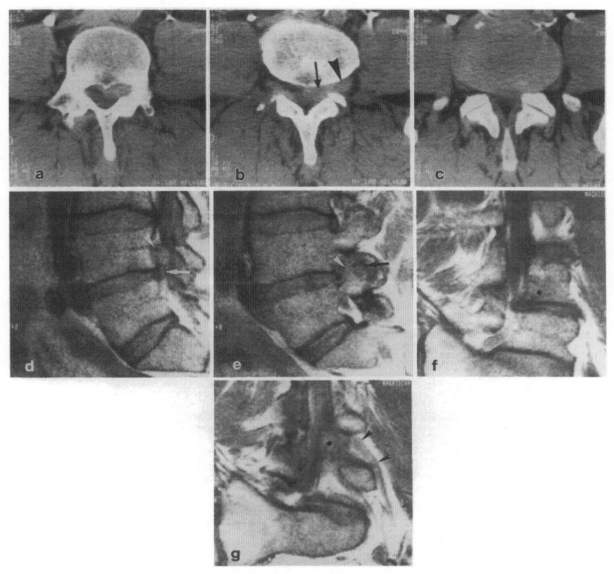

Fig. 218a–g. Left femoral pain; ascending L4–L5 herniation. *CT:* **a** Plane through the midportion of L4 vertebral body: left paramedian disk fragment anterior to the thecal sac. **b** L4–L5 foramen: herniation at the foraminal entrance (→); its external boundaries are ill-defined. L4 ganglion is large and partially obliterates the foraminal fat *(black arrowhead).* **c** L4–L5 disk: moderate asymmetry of the left posterior diskal margin. Extraforaminal L4 root has once again a normal appearance. *MRI:* **d–e** Sagittal oblique sections derived from a transverse scout view (SE; T1 - weighted images; TR 500 msec, TE 28 msec). **d** Disk fragment visible in left lateral recess *(white arrowhead);* it ascends past the anulus (→) to the midportion of L4 vertebral body. **e** Outermost section shows lateral extension of the herniation within the L4–L5 foramen, with partial obliteration of the foraminal fat *(white arrowhead).* L4 root is better visualized than in CT scans; it is clearly deviated posteriorly (→) **f–g** Frontal oblique section derived from a transverse scout view (SE; T1 - weighted images; TR 600 msec, TE 28 msec). **f** Section through the L4–L5 disk; ascending herniation is barely visible (✱) since it has a more internal extension. **g** Disk fragment (✱) is clearly visible in the L4 root axilla, which is elevated and deformed *(black arrowhead)*

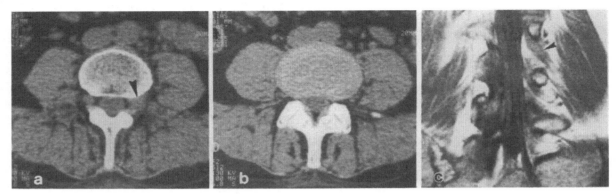

Fig. 219a–c. Left L3 femoral pain in a 52-year-old woman. **a** L3–L4 foramen: partial filling-in on left: isolated inflammatory ganglion?, small associated free fragment *(black arrowhead)?* **b** CT normal L3–L4 disk. No extraspinal abnormalities. **c** Frontal oblique section derived from a transverse scout view (SE; T1 – weighted images; TR 500 msec, TE 28 msec). Left L3 root is clearly identifiable against a bony background; it appears large and isolated *(black arrowhead).* Axillary fat is preserved. *Conclusion:* Isolated left L3 radiculitis. Treatment by intradiscal injection of corticosteroids (hexatrione). Complete recovery

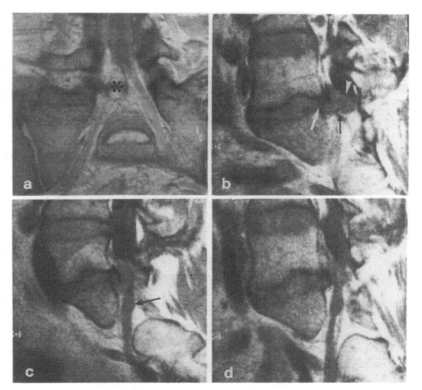

Fig. 220a–d. Right S1 sciatica of one month's duration in a 38-year-old patient. **a** Frontal scout view (gradient-echo; T1 – weighted images, TR 500 msec, TR 16 msec). Full extent of the free fragment is visible (✳); it is in contact with the right S1 emergence. **b** Sagittal oblique section derived from a frontal scout view. (SE, T1 – weighted images; TR 500 msec, TE 28 msec). Nuclear material is extruded into the spinal canal through a large tear in the anulus *(white arrow).* Constricted herniation at site of ligamentous perforation (→). Posterior compression of thecal sac *(white arrowhead).* **c** Right S1 emergence in contact with disk material (nucleus). S1 ganglion is adjacent to compression site and perfectly recognizable (→). **d** Right S1 sciatica in a 35-year-old woman. In certain cases the compression and deformation of the S1 emergence is particularly evident

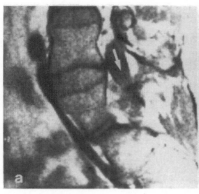 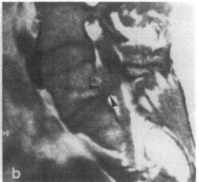

Fig. 221a, b. Right S1 sciatica in a 41-year-old patient. **a** Sagittal oblique section derived from a frontal scout view. (SE; T1 – weighted images; TR 600 msec, TE 28 msec). Considerable deviation of the thecal sac and cauda equina above the herniation (→). **b** Detailed analysis of the root compression by herniation: right S1 emergence is compressed by the disk material. *Note* the rupture of the anular fibers *(arrowheads)*

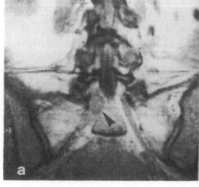 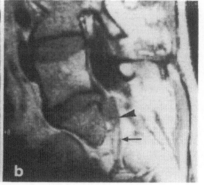

Fig. 222a, b. Right S1 sciatica in a 43-year-old woman. **a** Frontal scout view (gradient echo; T1 – weighted images; TR 450 msec, TE 14 msec). Herniation is identified below the disk, descending toward the first sacral foramen *(arrowhead)*. **b** Sagittal oblique section derived from a frontal scout view (SE; T1 – weighted images; TR 500 msec, TE 28 msec). A migratory herniation compresses the S1 root at the level of its ganglion *(arrowhead)*. *Note* the nerve root fasciculi more remotely (→). Operative findings: confirmation of migratory free fragment and ligamentous perforation

case of isolated radiculitis accompanied by a large nerve root ganglion, in order to rule out an associated foramino-lateral disk fragment (Fig. 219). Although more difficult, post-diskography CT obviously constitutes an even more detailed approach.

Nerve root compression of disk origin may be directly visualized by *SOF* projections over a significant height, and very easily for L5–S1 herniations. The S1 roots descend vertically over a considerable distance toward the first sacral foramen, permitting their alignment over several centimeters on a single oblique view. The posterior displacement of the S1 nerve root, its deformation and compression at the level of the hernia-

tion, and the significant radicular edema distal to the site of root compression by the disk are all clearly visualized. The subjacent nerve root ganglion is easily distinguished form the disk fragment (see Fig. 215; Figs. 220–222). CT can also demonstrate signs of nerve root involvement (i.e., a large, deformed and hyperdense root), but the approach is segmental and much less anatomic (Fig. 223).

There should be close spacing of the *TOF* projections, which on frontal views align the L4 and L5 roots at the lateral recess and their course beneath the pedicle. They give a proper exposure of the uppermost portion of the lateral recess and identify the nerve root at this level.

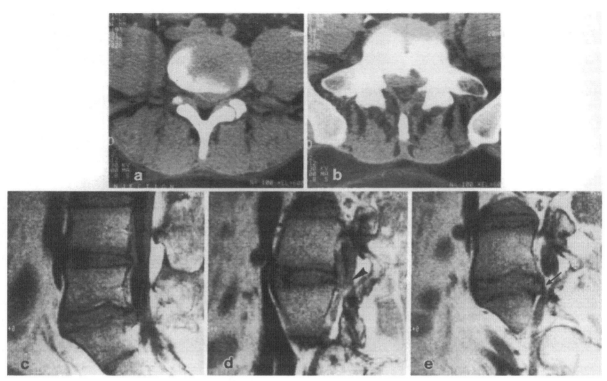

Fig. 223 a–e. Right S1 sciatica of 4 weeks' duration in a 30-year-old man with a history of left L5 sciatica 7 months previously. *CT:* **a** L4–L5 level: left posterolateral herniation with thecal sac indentation. **b** L5–S1 level: right posterolateral herniation descending toward the lateral recess and compressing the right S1 nerve root. *MRI:* **c** Sagittal section; spin echo; T1 - weighted sequence; TR 500 msec, TE 26 msec, 4 excitations. Double L4–L5 and L5–S1 herniations are clearly visible. L5–S1 herniation appears larger on this median section. **d** Sagittal oblique section derived from a frontal scout view; T1 - weighted sequence, TR 500 msec, TE 26 msec, 4 excitations. Moderate displacement of left L5 root at its emergence by the herniation *(arrowhead)* **e** Sagittal oblique section derived from a frontal scout view; T1 - weighted; TR 500, TE 26. Significant compression and deformation of the right S1 root at its emergence (→). *Comments:* In view of the CT signs of double disk herniation a double chemonucleolysis using chymodiactin was performed (although there was only right S1 symptomatology)

Nevertheless, we seldom use these projections, and only when the nerve roots have a rather horizontal course in the lateral recess (Fig. 224), particularly in cases of spondylolisthesis (Fig. 225).

T2-weighted sagittal views are useful (as we have seen) in determining the degree of disk degeneration, but they also provide valuable information concerning the type of herniation. A relative increase in signal intensity of the CSF (i. e., a long T2) together with a long TR and TE in comparison to those of the degenerated disk, results in an inversion and increased contrast between the CSF and the disk. This *"myelographic effect"* permits the herniated disk fragment to be identified as a defect at the level of the subarachnoid space (Fig. 226). On late echoes, signal of the defect may sometimes increase compared to that of the intervertebral space (Fig. 227). This sequence is all the more valuable, since the anterior epidural fat is sparse or almost absent in 10% of patients. Good evaluation of the size, configuration and contents of the thecal sac is possible. It is interesting to observe that the CSF in the ventricles becomes brighter at a shorter TR than that in the thecal sac. The hyposignal of the ligaments and the cortical bone is highlighted by the whiteness of the CSF. In lumbar spinal stenosis, a single sagittal gradient-echo section enables one to evaluate the stenotic segments for the entire lumbar spine (Fig. 228). A T2-weighted sagittal view may be more efficient but takes longer to acquire.

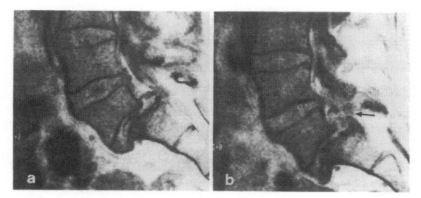

Fig. 224a, b. Spondylolisthesis in a 35-year-old woman. Sagittal section: gradient echo; TR 450 msec, TE 14 msec, 4 excitations. **a** Median section: note the anterior displacement of L5 in relation to S1; the disk remains in place. Posterior margin of L5-S1 disk is in alignment with S1; on axial CT scans, this gives a false image of a posteromedian herniation. **b** Parasagittal section. *Note* the osteocartilaginous canal and the supernumerary ossicles in contact with the lateral recess (→)

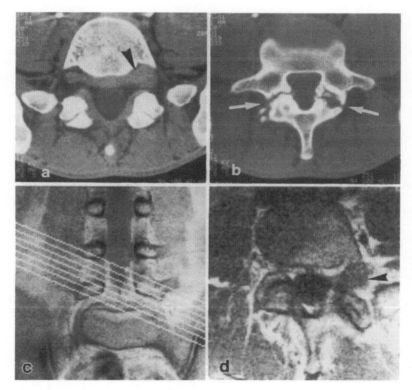

Fig. 225a-d. Left L5 sciatica in a 36-year-old patient. Bilateral isthmic spondylolisthesis at L5-S1. *CT:* Plane parallel to neural arch (gantry angle of 20°). **a-b** The medially located posterior disk margin is clearly seen; there remains a doubt as to a small left latero-foraminal herniation *(black arrowhead)*. *Note* the associated isthmic lysis (→). Supernumerary ossicles. Frontal scout view. **c** Because the spondylolisthesis, the L5 roots are unusually horizontal. **d** Transverse oblique section derived from a frontal scout view; TR 500 msec, TE 28 msec; T1 - weighted section, 4 excitations. Only one large (left) L5 ganglion is found *(black arrowhead)*. This projection artificially improves visualization of the bony foraminal region. *Conclusion:* Left L5 radiculitis without an associated disk herniation

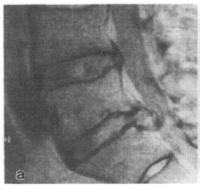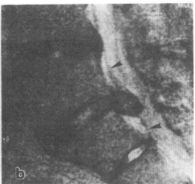

Fig. 226a, b. Sagittal section; T2 – weighted sequence; TR 1800, TE 40, 80, 120 msec. Descending L5–S1 disk herniation with anulus rupture. **a** Disk degeneration at L4–L5 and L5–S1, with a diminished signal especially evident on the third echo **b** Elevation of posterior longitudinal ligament, which is better seen on the third echo **(b)** *(arrowheads);* however, it does not seem to be torn. Evident anterior indentation of the thecal sac. Operative findings: Subligamentous disk herniation

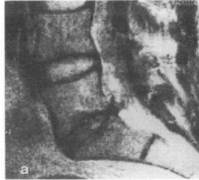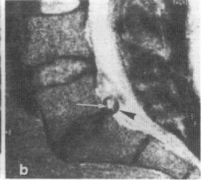

Fig. 227a, b. It is always easy to locate the posterior longitudinal ligament on sagittal T2 – weighted sections. In this case, the herniation has an unusual shape and is composed of two parts: **a** a hypersignal corresponding to the extruded nucleus *(→)* **b** a peripheral component corresponding to the ruptured lamellae of the anulus fibrosus *(arrowhead)*

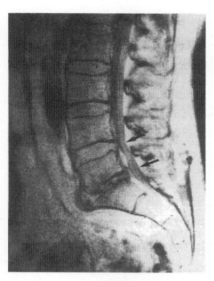

Fig. 228. 36-year-old patient with lumbar pain. Congenital spinal stenosis. MRI: T1-weighted median sagittal section (TR = 450 msec; TE = 14 msec; 4 excitations). Sequence shows very well the anteroposterior narrowing of the spinal canal at L4–L5 and at L5–S1 (—►). Concomitant degenerative disko-osteophytic lesions at the L5–S1 level, especially anteriorly and outside the spinal canal

— The posterior longitudinal ligament, which is directly visible as a thin black rim, is detached and raised by the herniated fragment, which passes through the ligament posteriorly in case of rupture. MRI is the only examination permitting direct visualization of this passage (Fig. 229);

— Finally, certain authors have reported the direct visualization of detached migratory disk herniations located at a distance from the intervertebral space. These migratory free fragments always seem to retain at least a thin pedicle linking them to the disk of origin, even when the migration has been considerable (i. e., over 10 mm). For a descending herniation, the distance measured between the inferior pole of the disk fragment and the intervertebral space seems slightly less than that estimated from CT scans. MRI studies are undoubtedly more precise, as the measurements are directly performed on sagittal views. The obliquity of CT sections is undoubtedly the prime source of error.

In contrast to CT scans, the diagnosis of a free fragment relies only slightly on the structural criteria furnished by axial images (i. e., vertical migration greater than 10 mm, an abrupt shape, a loss of continuity) [65]. Thus, the essential value of a T2-weighted sequence lies in the direct analysis of the *posterior longitudinal ligament* on sagittal views:

— The defect lies posterior to the anterior epidural fat, suggesting a rupture of the posterior longitudinal ligament and thus the existence of a free fragment;

The value of MRI for the diagnosis of subligamentous free fragments remains to be determined.

CT retains a clear advantage in cases of *calcified disk herniation* or *osteophytic* compression. The existence of calcifications may be suspected if hyposignal zones are present, both in T1-weighted and T2-weighted sequences [46, 66]. Nevertheless, the area of the hyposignal zones is less than that of the hyperdense calcification zones seen on CT. With major disk dehydration, it may be impossible to distinguish an osteophyte from a protrusion or a disk herniation. The presence of hypersignal fat at the level of the adjacent spongy bone is rather in favor of osteophytic lesions.

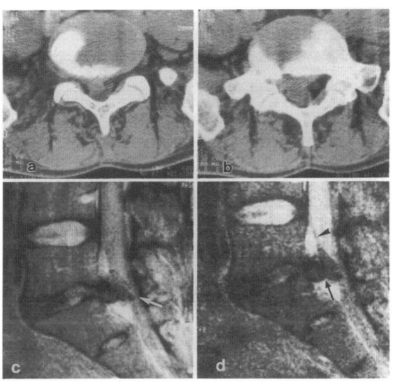

Fig. 229 a–d. Right S1 sciatica of one month's duration. *CT:* **a** *L5-S1 disk:* small, slightly ascending disk herniation. **b** Large free fragment in the right lateral recess; the S1 root is no longer visible and the thecal sac is compressed against the ligamenta flava. Probable ligamentous rupture, especially given the pointed contour of the herniation. *MRI:* Sagittal section; T2 - weighted sequence; TR 1800, TE 80, 120 msec. **c** (80 msec) Anular rupture is evident, with extrusion of nuclear material into the lumbar canal, within the anterior epidural fat. Obvious disk degeneration and collapse, with signal decrease in contrast to the healthy L4–L5 disk. Thecal sac severely compressed, with almost complete stenosis posterior to the herniation (—►). **d** (120 msec) Posterior longitudinal ligament is clearly seen *(arrowhead),* naturally enhanced anteriorly by the epidural fat and posteriorly by the thecal sac CSF. The herniation has two components, one subligamentous and the other transligamentous; the latter is posterior to the epidural fat and squeezed by the posterior longitudinal ligament. There is constriction of the hernia at the site of the ligamentous tear (—►)

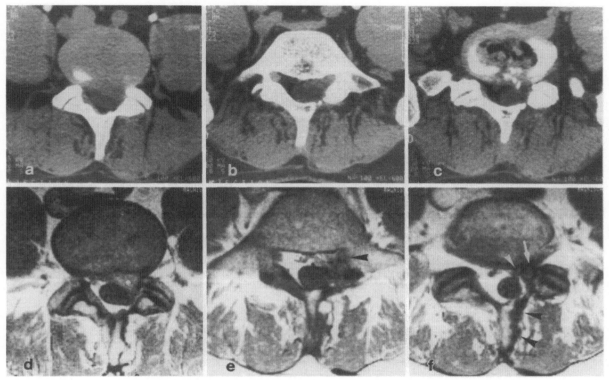

Fig. 230 a–f. 48-year-old man operated for a left L5–S1 disk herniation 2 years previously. Recurrent left L5 sciatica with loss of the Achilles tendon reflex. *CT:* **a** *L4–L5 disk:* left posterolateral herniation migration to the left lateral recess; L5 root is obscured. **b** *Section through midportion of L5:* surgical fenestration, no signs of fibrosis in the soft tissue. Filling-in of L5 axilla (fibrosis or inferior part of herniation?). **c** Intradiskal gas at L5–S1. Small posterior rupture of ring apophysis. Left S1 root is not visible. *MRI:* Transverse oblique section derived from a sagittal scout view, T1 – weighted sequence, TR = 500 msec, TE = 28 msec, 4 excitations. **d** *L4–L5 disk:* evident left posterolateral herniation, with quite a high signal

(✱). **e** *Section through midportion of L5:* left L5 root is clearly visible against the pedicle *(arrowhead).* Its axilla is filled in by soft tissue with a low-intensity signal which differs from that of the herniation. Postoperative fibrosis is present. **f** *L5–S1 disk:* S1 root is easily distinguished, it is large and surrounded by fibrosis with a low-intensity signal (→). *Note* the sequelae tracing the surgical approach along the left aspect of the spinous process, which are undetectable on CT *(black arrowhead).* The tear in the ring apophysis is seen with difficulty *(white arrowhead):* back of signal. This illustrates the difficulties in diagnosing calcifications using MRI

Postoperative MRI

MRI appears to be particularly valuable for the postoperative examination of lumbar spines [7, 14, 15, 31, 49, 51, 61, 72, 84, 86, 87, 98]. As we have seen, these patients often present difficult diagnostic problems and are sources of error in the first 6 months of the posteroperative period. The density of the postoperative fibrosis may be identical to that of the disk, or the fibrosis may not take up the contrast medium, making the diagnosis of recurrent herniation difficult. A combined opacification with intravenous and intrathecal contrast media has been employed to facilitate differentiation. In case of extensive

postoperative fibrosis, the entire spinal canal may have a uniform density blurring the boundaries separating the disk, the fibrosis, the thecal sac and the ligamenta flava.

MRI appears to permit easier differentiation between the fibrosis, the disk and the thecal sac (Fig. 230). The structural criteria applied to CT scans (lack of mass effect and extension distant to the disk, for the fibrosis; mass effect and location adjacent to the intervertebral space, for the herniation) are easier to apply to MRI because of the better contrast resolution (Fig. 231). A recurrent herniation has the same appearance as the initial herniation, whereas the fibrosis has a lower signal intensity than the herniation on

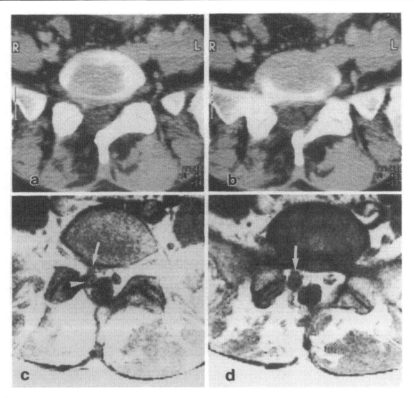

Fig. 231 a-d. 38-year-old woman operated for a right L5-S1 herniation 5 years previously. Now has right L5-S1 recurrence. *CT:* **a-b** *Diskal plane:* small posterolateral asymmetry of L5-S1 disk; displacement of poorly visualized right S1 root. No signs of fibrosis or scar tissue at the fenestration site. In the right lateral recess, the epidural fat is obliterated and the S1 root remains poorly visible. **c-d** MRI: transverse oblique section derived from a sagittal scout view; spin echo; T1 - weighted sequence, TR 600 msec, TE 28 msec, 4 excitations. S1 root is well outlined, increased in size, displaced *(white arrowhead)* and in contact with a small posterolateral disk fragment (→). *Comment:* MRI gives definite proof of a residual fragment

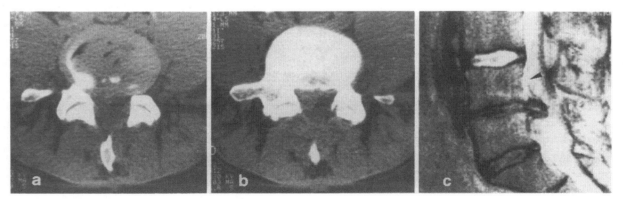

Fig. 232 a-c. 42-year-old man; diskectomy at L4-L5 and L5-S1 16 months previously. Right L5 lumbosciatic pain of 3 months' duration. *CT:* **a,b** Recurrent right L4-L5 herniation. No epidural fibrosis at the neurosurgical approach. *MRI:* **c** Spin echo; T2 - weighted sequence; TR 2000 msec, TE 80, (2nd echo). - Large subligamentous herniation, elevation of posterior longitudinal ligament *(arrowhead).* - *Note* the two components within the herniation. - Loss of signal intensity by the last two disks. *Comment:* MRI completely confirms the recurrent herniation seen on CT

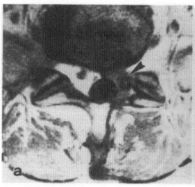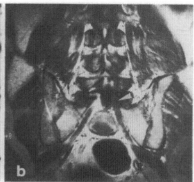

Fig. 233 a, b. 51-year-old man, previously operated for a left L5–S1 disk herniation. Residual sciatica 10 months after surgery. Follow-up CT shows scar tissue (fibrosis) surrounding the left S1 root. **a** Transverse oblique section derived from a sagittal scout view; spin echo; T1 – weighted sequence, TR 600 msec, TE 28 msec. *Diskal plane:* tissue with an isointense signal adjacent to the left lateral portion of the thecal sac and surrounding the S1 root *(black arrowhead).* No partial volume effect; on the contrary, the thecal sac is drawn toward the surgical approach. **b** Frontal section; spin echo; T1 – weighted squence, TR 450 msec, TE 26 msec. There is a large isolated left S1 root *(white arrowhead). Comment:* MRI rules out a possible associated free fragment

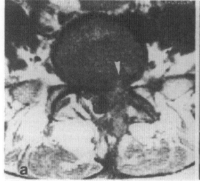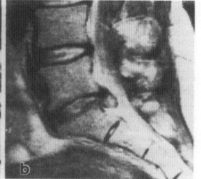

Fig. 234 a, b. 37-year-old man previously operated for a large left L5–S1 herniation. Sudden recurrence of left S1 sciatica 3 weeks after surgery. **a** Transverse oblique section derived from a sagittal scout view; T1 – weighted section; TR 500 msec, TE 28 msec, 4 excitations. Section through the L5–S1 disk. Diskectomy orifice can be seen *(white arrowhead).* Posteriorly, filling-in of epidural fat by considerable material with an isointense signal. In the immediate postoperative period it is difficult to differentiate between a residual or recurrent fragment and scar tissue. Left S1 root is not visible. **b** Sagittal section; spin echo; T2 weighted sequence, TR 2000, TE 80, 120. Recurrent herniation is evident in this sequence; it remains subligamentous

T 2-weighted sequences (Fig. 232). The poor organization of the fibrosis compared with the highly structured aspect of the ligaments may explain the low signal intensity (Fig. 233). It seems necessary to differentiate between scar tissue a few years old, which is slightly active and has a very weak signal similar to that of ligaments, and recent postoperative fibrosis which sometimes has a higher signal intensity than the disk, possibly due to a hemorrhagic component.

The low spatial resolution and poor signal-to-noise ratio of T 2-weighted images have led us to develop rapid T 1-weighted sequences. In such sequences, there is a naturally poor contrast between the fibrosis and the recurrent herniation. In our series of 100 operated patients with both fibrosis and a herniation, the fibrosis was isointense with the herniation in half the cases, hypointense in 40%, and more intense in 10% (Fig. 234). The injection of Gadolinium-DTPA

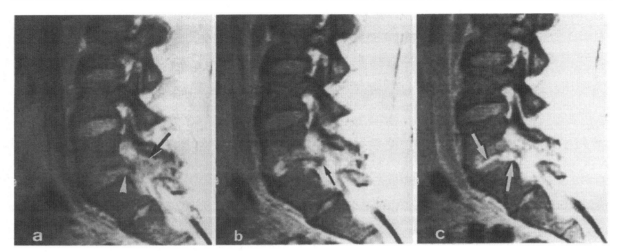

Fig. 235 a–c. 55-year-old man operated 5 years earlier for a left L4–L5 herniation. Now has recurrent left L5 lumbosciatic pain resistant to medical treatment. CT suggests recurrent herniation associated with fibrosis. **a** Left paramedian sagittal section. Gradient echo, T1 – weighted sequence, TE = 450 msec, TE = 17 msec, 4 excitations. Diskectomy sequelae at the level of the anulus fibrosus *(white arrowhead)* and presence of an intermediate-signal soft tissue mass posterior to and below the intervertebral space (→). **b** Identical sequence, *immediately* following the IV injection of DTPA Gadolinium (Schering). Signal enhancement by the fibrosis and epidural veins around and posterior to the recurrent herniation. Herniation appears smaller; its exact size can be determined (→). **c** Identical sequence, *delayed,* following the IV injection of DTPA Gadolinium (Schering). Observe the signal enhancement at the level of the last degenerated and operated disk (→). *Comment:* Value of DTPA Gadolinium in T1 – weighted sequences

(Magnevist) has proved very helpful in increasing the sensitivity of T1-weighted sequences. This paramagnetic contrast medium results in a shortened T1 relaxation time, and has a distribution volume equal to that of iodinated contrast media. It has a mean distribution half-life of 20 minutes. In all instances, we have observed early onset and prolonged enhancement of the fibrosis following injection (Figs. 235, 236). The opacification is usually heterogeneous at first and then tends to become homogeneous. The signal increase is significant in 80% of cases; since the herniation is usually not enhanced, the contrast with it becomes even greater. A slight and belated uptake of contrast medium by a herniated fragment surrounded by scar tissue in only 20% of cases (see Fig. 236). The epidural venous plexuses are also massively enhanced following injection (even more than on CT), which facilitates the interpretation of images (Fig. 237).

In half of the cases, the operated disk exhibits a delayed uptake of contrast medium which may be significant, and seems to be related to post-diskectomy cicatrization (see Fig. 235). This phenomenon is observed more in the posterior third of the disk and at the level of the adjacent cartilaginous end-plates. Analogous to this is the uptake of contrast medium by the periphery of degenerated disks, which is due to fibrovascular remodeling of the endplates. In any event, rapid sequences performed within 20 minutes after injection appear to be the most effective. In our experience, the efficacy of MRI in combination with Gd-DTPA injection (96%) is superior to that of CT coupled with the injection of an iodinated contrast medium (85%).

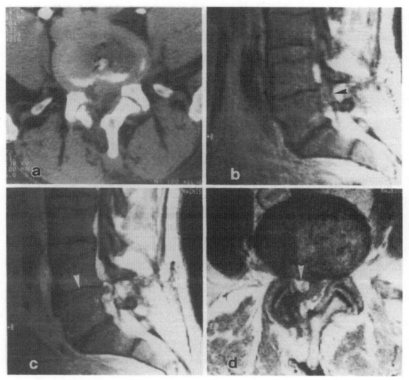

Fig. 236a–d. 50-year-old man operated for a right L4–L5 herniation 16 months earlier. Recurrent sciatica in the same dermatomal distribution. **a** *Follow-up CT:* recurrent herniation with a hypodensity; right L5 root compression. Peripheral enhancement of the fragment (IV injection of Iopamiron 300). *MRI:* **b** Sagittal gradient echo, T1 - weighted sequence, TR = 450 msec, TE = 14 msec, 4 excitations. Right paramedian section: considerable soft tissue next to the intervertebral space *(arrowhead).* **c** Identical sequence, *immediately* following the IV injection of DTPA Gadolinium (Magnevist, Schering). Enhancement of the peripheral scar tissue surrounding the hyposignal of the recurrent herniation. *Note* the peripheral contrast medium uptake by the L4–L5 disk (postoperative appearance *(white arrowhead)* **d** Transverse oblique section derived from a sagittal scout view, *delayed,* after the IV injection of DTPA Gadolinium (spin echo, T1 - weighted sequence, TR = 600 msec, TE = 28 msec). Fibrosis still gives a hypersignal; it surrounds the disk fragment, which shows delayed partial enhancement *(white arrowhead). Comment:* Early sequences following Gadolinium injection are essential for optimal differentiation between fibrosis and herniation

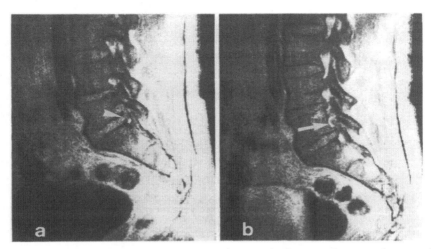

Fig. 237 a, b. 34-year-old man operated for a right L4-L5 herniation 8 months earlier. Now has right L5 sciatica. **CT** scans at L4-L5 are normal, but there is a small ascending, right L5-S1 fragment which compresses the L5 root at the foraminal entrance. **a** Paramedian sagittal section, gradient echo, T1 - weighted section, TR = 450 msec, TE = 14 msec. Filling-in of L5-S1 foramen by disk material in continuity with the intervertebral space: large anular gap *(white arrowhead).* **b** Identical sequence, immediately following the IV injection of DTPA Gadolinium (Schering). Disk fragment can be clearly distinguished among the significantly enhanced venous structures (→). *Comment:* Better evaluation of the true size of the herniation by MRI. L5-S1 chemonucleolysis. Total regression of clinical symptoms

Chemonucleolysis

Since chymopapain acts on the hydrophilic properties of the nucleus, MRI appears to be particularly well-suited for evaluating the effects of chemonucleolysis. Several follow-up studies ranging from 6 weeks to 3 months have attempted to determine correlations between the structural and clinical findings [2, 15, 33, 50, 63, 72].

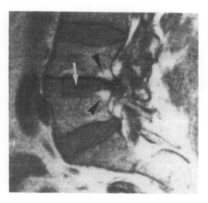

Fig. 238. L4–L5 chemonucleolysis 2 months earlier. Recurrent L5 sciatica. Sagittal oblique sections derived from a transverse scout view. (T1 - weighted images, TR 500 msec, TE 26 msec, 4 excitations). Note degeneration of the L4–L5 and L5–S1 disks, together with a collapsed L4–L5 and a vacuum disk phenomenon (→) at both levels. Considerable increase of peridiskal intensity at the end-plates *(black arrowhead)*. This is due either to inflammation or to localized fibrosis after chemonucleolysis

A decrease in the signal intensity of the disk (especially on T2-weighted sequences) and disk collapse are observed whether the evolution is favorable or not. On the other hand, three anatomic criteria have been shown to have a good clinical correlation:

— A partial reduction in the size of the defect indenting the thecal sac along two dimensions, those of height and width;
— An increase in the intensity of the peridiscal signal at the cartilaginous end-plates. This is due to inflammation or fibrosis. Successful treatment may be due to destruction of the end-plates (Fig. 238);
— A good clinical outcome is accompanied in 88% of cases by 2 or 3 positive criteria, and in 63% by 3 positive criteria. On the other hand, an unfavorable outcome is never accompanied by 3 positive criteria, and only 25% exhibit 2 positive criteria.

Finally, it is important to be aware of the possible signs of discitis, which is just as rare a complication of chemonucleolysis as of surgery. When present, there is an increase in the signal intensity of the adjacent vertebral bodies as well as of the disk, with a disappearance of the intranuclear defect [4, 30] (Fig. 239).

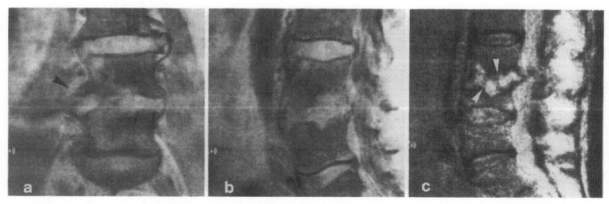

Fig. 239 a–c. Low back pain in a febrile patient L4–L5 diskitis on CT. **a–b** Gradient-echo (T1 - weighted images, TR 450 msec, TE 16 msec) coronal and sagittal sections. Disappearance of bony outlines of L4 and L5 end-plates. Right paravertebral abscess *(arrowhead)*. The signal obtained in this sequence is not very different from that of a normal disk.

c L3–L4 diskitis. Spin echo (T2 - weighted images, TR 2000 msec, TE 120 msec) Intense hypersignal which is characteristic of the disk and adjacent vertebral end-plates, corresponding to diskitis with spread to the adjacent cancellous bone *(white arrowhead)*

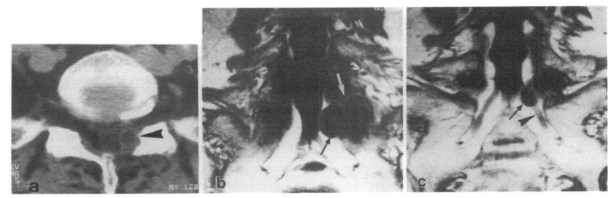

Fig. 240 a–c. 66-year-old patient with left S1 sciatica. *CT:* **a** Cystic structure is seen posterior to the left S1 root and at the level of the facet joint *(black arrowhead).* *MRI:* Spin echo (T1 – weighted images, TR 600 msec, TE 28 msec) **b–c** Coronal sections: cystic formation with a hyposignal (characteristic of fluid (→) attached to the L5-S1 facet joint *(upper part)* *(white arrow).* This structure is in contact with the S1 axilla *(black arrow).* *Comment:* Synovial cyst is a rare differential diagnosis in lumbosciatic pain. Confirmation provided by surgery

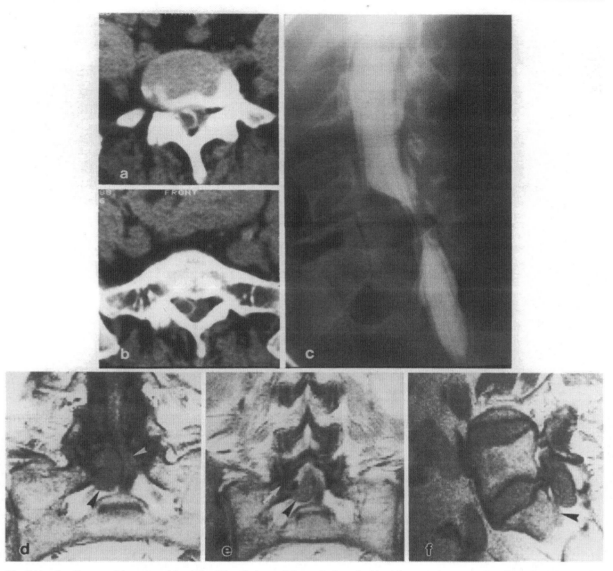

Fig. 241a-f. 61-year-old man with right S1 sciatica. *CT:* **a-b** Hypodense fluid structure with peripheral calcification, found at the facet joint level and descending in the lateral recess. *Lumbar myelogram:* **c** Large impression on the thecal sac. *MRI:* **d-e** Gradient echo (T1 - weighted images, TR 500 msec, TE 16 msec) Hyposignal fluid structure *(black arrowhead)* communicating with the facet joint (→) and displacing the thecal sac *(white arrowhead).* **f** Sagittal oblique section derived from a frontal scout view Spin echo (T1 - weighted images, TR 600 msec, TE 28 msec). Vertical extension of the cystic structure is better evaluated; its lower end is posterior to S1 *(black arrowhead).* *Comment:* Confirmed by surgery

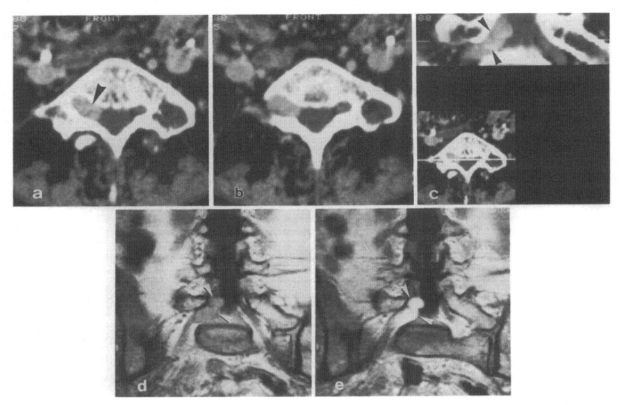

Fig. 242a-e. Right L5 sciatica of several weeks' duration without motor deficit. CT shows an expansive mass located in the right L5-S1 intervertebral foramen, enhanced by the IV injection of contrast (probable right L5 neurinoma). **a** Section through midportion of L5 vertebral body. Filling-in of the right lateral recess and significant erosion of the surrounding bone *(black arrowhead).* **b** Section through upper portion of the right L5-S1 intervertebral foramen. Bone erosion is still visible, even through the section plane is not symmetrical. Right L5 root is not easily distinguished from the hyperdense expansive mass. **c** Frontal reformation: the com-ponents of the expansive mass within and outside the spinal canal are well defined *(black arrowhead).* **d** T1-weighted frontal MRI section (TR = 500 msec; TE = 16 msec; 4 excitations). Hyposignal mass next to and within the axilla of the right L5 root *(white arrowhead).* **e** After the IV injection of Gadolinium-DTPA: tumoral mass has an increased signal intensity on T1 images. *(white arrowhead). Comment:* Neurinoma of the right L5 root was confirmed at operation. The indications for neurosurgery were uncertain since there was no clinical right L5 motor deficit

Evaluation of the role of MRI in disk pathology has only just begun; with increased experience on the part of the radiologist, the interpretations will become more accurate and the indications better defined (especially in the differential diagnosis of synovial cyst [27, 34, 96] (Figs. 240, 241) and neurinoma [92] (Fig. 242). Despite a considerable section thickness and a spatial resolution slightly inferior to that obtained with the latest generation of CT scanners, MRI appears to be particularly well-suited to the diagnosis of disk herniations by using at least two orthogonal planes, and oblique sections if necessary. In addition to being capable of demonstrating disk generation, T2-weighted sequences appear capable of closely examining the posterior longitudinal ligament.

Although CT remains the technique of choice for the initial investigation of the lumbar spine in a patient with sciatic pain, MRI has already made interesting contributions in difficult cases (eg, foramino-lateral herniations, postoperative and postchemonucleolysis examinations).

References

Computed Tomography

1. Abdelwahab I. F., Gould E. S.: The role of diskography after negative post myelography CT scans: retrospective view. AJNR, 1988, Vol. 9, n° 1, 187-190.
2. Abdullah A. F., Ditto E. W., Byrd E. B., Williams R.: Extreme-lateral lumbar disc herniations: Clinical syndrome and special problems of diagnosis. J. Neurosurg., 1974, 41, 229-234.
3. Adamsbaum C., Rolland Y., de Broucker F., Dichy J., Levesque M.: Hypodensité discale et hernie discale. J. Radiol., 1988, 69(11), 671-673.
4. Amundsen P.: Cervical myelography with Amipaque: seven years experience. Radiologe, 1981, 21, 282-287.
5. Anano A. K., Lee B. C. P.: Plain and metrizamide CT of lumbar disc disease: comparison with myelography. AJNR, 1982, 3, 567-571.
6. Angtuaco E. J. C., Holder J. C., Boop W. C., Binet E. F.: Computed tomographic discography in the evaluation of extreme lateral disc herniation. Neurosurgery, 1984, 14, 350-352.
7. Arce C. A., Dohmann G. J.: Thoracic disk herniation: improved diagnosis with computed tomographic scanning and a review of the literature. Surg. Neurol., 1985, 23, 356-361.
8. Aronson N., Merwyn Bagan, Filtzer D. L.: Results of using the Smith-Robinson approach for herniated and extruded cervical discs. Neurosurg., 1970, 32, 721-722.
9. Babin E., Capesius P., Maitrot D.: Signes radiologiques osseux des variétés morphologiques des canaux lombaires étroits. Ann. Radiol., 1977, 20, 491-499.
10. Badami J. P., Norman D., Barbaro N.: Metrizamide CT-myelography in cervical myelopathy and radiculopathy: correlation with conventionnal myelography and surgical findings. AJR April 1985, 144, 675-680.
11. Baleriaux D., Notermann J., Ticket L.: Recognition of cervical soft disk herniation by contrast-enhanced CT AJNR May/June 1983, 607-608.
12. Bard M.: Renseignements fournis pour le diagnostic des névralgies cervico-brachiales par le durolipaque intra-rachidien et la discographie cervicale. Rhumatologie, 1978, 30, 148-151.
13. Barmeir E., Blinder G. E., Sasson A. A., Hirsch M.: Prone computed tomography metrizamide myelography: a technique for improved diagnosis of lumbar disc herniation. Clin. Radiol., 1984, 35 (6), 479-481.
14. Bastin J. M., Claisse R. H., Tellier E.: L'ossification du ligament longitudinal postérieur. Rev. Rhum., 1980, 47, 613-620.
15. Bell G. R., Rothman R. H., Booth R. E., Cuckler J. M., Garfin S., Herkowitz H., Simeone F. A., Dolinskas C., Han S. S.: A study of computer assisted tomography. Comparaison of metrizamide myelography and computed tomography in the diagnosis of herniated lumbar disc and spinal stenosis. Spine, 1984, 9, 552-556.
16. Benoist M.: Principles of chemonucleolysis using chy-
mopapain. Focus on chemonucleolysis. J. F. Bonneville - Springer-Verlag, 1986, 9-16.
17. Benoist M., Deburge A., Busson J.: La chemonucléolyse dans le traitement des sciatiques pour hernie discale. La Presse Méd., 1984, 13 (12), 733-736.
18. Benoist M., Deburge A., Heripret G., Busson J., Rigot J., Cauchoix J.: Treatment of lumbar disk herniation by chymopapain chemonucleolysis. A report of 120 patients. Spine, 1982, 7, 285-290.
19. Benoist M., Deburge A., Rigot J., Busson J., Cauchoix J.: La chimionucléolyse dans le traitement des sciatiques discales: 120 observations. Presse méd., 1982, 11, 2121-2124.
20. Biering-Sorensen F.: Physical measurements as risk indicators for low-back trouble over a one-year period. Spine, 1984, 9, 106-119.
21. Bolender N. F., Schonstrom N. S. R., Spengler D. M.: Role of computed tomography and myelography in the diagnosis of central spinal stenosis. J. Bone Jt Surg., 1985, 67 A, 240-246.
22. Bollini G., Bergoin M., Choux M., Padovani J.: Calcifications discales de l'enfant. Rev. Chir. Orthop., 1984, 70, 377-382.
23. Blomquist H. K., Lindquist M., Mattsson S.: Calcification of intervertebral discs in childhood. Paediatr. Radiol., 1979, 8, 23-26.
24. Bonafe J., Prere J.: Myélographie à l'iopamidol. Ann. Radiol., 1983, 26, 18 bis, 783-788.
25. Bonneville J. F., Runge M.: Le point sur la chimionucléolyse. J. Radiol., 1988, 69 (10), 557-560.
26. Bosacco S. J., Berman A. T., Garbarino J. L., Teplick J. G., Peyster R.: A comparison of CT scanning and myelography in the diagnosis of lumbar disc herniation. Clin. Orthop., 1984, 190, 124 - In J. P., Benjamin M. V., Krcheff I. I. Computed tomography of the asymptomatic post-surgical lumbar spine analysis of the physiologic scar. AJR, 1984, 142, 149-152.
27. Braun I. F., Lin J. P., George A. E., Kricheff I. E., Hoffmann J.: Pitfalls in the computed tomographic evaluation of the lumbar spine in disc disease. Neuroradiology, 1984, 26, 15-20.
28. Bricout J. H., Menegalli D., Guenego O., Ker-Saint-Gilly A. de: Place de la tomodensitométrie dans le diagnostic étiologique d'une sciatique. Sem. Hôp. Paris, 1985, 61, 3209-3217.
29. Brotchi J., Baleriaux D.: Approche diagnostique nouvelle des lombosciatalgies neurochirurgicales. Incidence et thérapeutique. Bulletin et mémoires de l'Académie Royale de Médecine de Belgique, 1983, 138, 467-476.
30. Brown B. M., Bedell J. E., Frank E.: Contrast-enhanced computed tomography scanning of the post operative spine. Surg. Neurol., 1986, 25, 351-356.
31. Brown B. M., Schwartz R. H., Frank E., Blank N. K.: Preoperative evaluation of cervical radiculopathy and myelopathy by surface coil MR Imaging. AJNR, 1988, Vol. 9, n° 5, 859-866.
32. Brown B. M., Stark E. H., Dion G., Ono H.: Computed tomography and chymopapain chemonucleolysis: preliminary findings. AJNR, 1985, 6, 51-54.
33. Brown M. D.: The pathophysiology of disc disease. Orthop. Clin. North. Am., 1971, 2, 359-370.
34. Buchheit F., Maitrot D., Philippides D., Babin E.: Les formes topographiques des hernies discales. Apport de la saccoradiculographie avec zonographie. Neurochirurgie, 1975, 21, 43-54.

35. Buckwalter J. A., Cooper R. R., Maynard J. A.: Elastic fibers in human intervertebral discs. J Bone Joint surg., 1976, *58 A*, 73-76.

36. Bushau C.: Synovial cyst of the lumbar spine simulating extra-dural mass. Neuroradiology, 1979, *18*, 263-268.

37. Byrd S. E., Cohn M. L., Biggers S. L., Hutington C. T., Locke G. E., Charles M. F.: The radiographic evaluation of the symptomatic post-operative lumbar spine patient. Spine, 1985, *10*, 652-661.

38. Capesius P., Bruch J. M., Lemaitre Y., Roilgen A., Sandt G.: Diagnostic scanographique des hernies discales. Radiol. J. Cépur, 1981, *1*, 147-151.

39. Caron J. P., Djindjian R., Julian H., Lebrigand H., Houdart R., Comoy J.: Les hernies discales dorsales. Les modalités de leur retentissement sur la moëlle, leur traitement chirurgical par abord latéral ou postéro-latéral, avec exérèse de la saillie discale. Ann. Méd. Int., 1971, *122*, 675-688.

40. Carrera G. F., Williams A. L., Haughton V. M.: Computed tomography in sciatica. Radiology, 1980, *137*, 433-437.

41. Carruthers C. C., Kousaie K. N.: Surgical treatment after chemonucleolysis failure. Clin. Orthop., 1982, *165*, 172-175.

42. Carson J., Gumpert J., Jefferson A.: Diagnosis and treatment of thoracic intervertebral disk protrusions. J. Neurol. Neurosurg., 1971, *34*, 68-77.

43. Carter H., Pierron D., Georges B.: La sciatique en 1982. Diagnostic et traitement. Conc. Med., 1982, *104*, 329-343.

44. Castan P., Maurel J., Bouzige J. C.: La saccoradiculographie aux hydrosolubles. Maloine S. A. Edit., Paris, 1979.

45. Cauchoix J., Deburge A.: Constatations opératoire et résultats chirurgicaux obtenus après échec de la chimionucléolyse. Acta Orthop. Belg., 1983, *49* (suppl 1), 79-89.

46. Cecile J. P., Descamps C., Vincent G., Debrouker R., Dufour R., Cipel L. Foucart H., Desmarchelier F.: Resultats de la discolyse à la chymopapaïne. 300 observations. Ann. Radiol., 1983, *26* (8), 642-647.

47. Chaquat Y., Ginet C., Zecker B.: Etude de 108 névralgies cervico-brachiales idiopathiques et de névralgies cervico-brachiales cervicarthrosiques. Rev. Rhum., 1978, *45*, n° 2, 111-117.

48. Chaquat Y., Vignaud J., Faures Quenet B., Kanovitch B., Aubin M. L., Breville P.: Notre expérience, sur une courte série de la fiabilité de l'examen tomodensitométrique sans contraste dans le diagnostic des hernies discales lombaires. Rev. Rhum. Mal. Ostéo-Articulaires, 1981, *48* (10), 640.

49. Chevrot A., Bellin M. F., Gires F., Vallee C., Cormier D., Revel M., Menkes C. J., Armor B., Pallardy G.: Discography and nucleolysis with disease. Focus on chemonucleolysis. J. F. Bonneville. Springer-Verlag, 1986, 60-65.

50. Chevrot A., Gires F., Vallee C., Wybier M.: La discographie lombaire. Fiches radiologiques Schering, 1986.

51. Chevrot A., Rousselin B., Gires F., Wybier M., Vallee C., Pallardy G.: Lyse isthmique unilatérale en tomodensitométrie. J. Radiol., 1988, *69* (12), 767-769.

52. Chin L. S., Black K. L., Hoff J. T.: Multiple thoracic disc herniations. J. Neurosurg., 1987, *7* (6), 623-625.

53. Clere P., Runge M., Bonneville J. F.: Results after chemonucleolysis. Focus on chemonucleolysis. J. F. Bonneville. Springer-Verlag, 1986, 79-84.

54. Cloward R. B.: The anterior approach for removal of ruptured cervical disk. J. Neurosurg., 1958, *15*, 6, 602.

55. Cloward R. B.: Cervical discography. Acta Radiol., 1963, *1*, 675-688.

56. Coin Gene C., Jupiter F.: Cervical disk degeneration and herniation: diagnosis by computerised tomography. Southern Med. Journ. August 1984, *77*, n° 8, 980.

57. Cordoliani Y. S., Cosnard G., Ferry M., Bassoulet J., Pharaboz C., Le Gall M.: Dépistage scanographique du neurinome foraminal. J. Radiol., 1985, *66* (11), 673-677.

58. Coventry M. B., Ghormley R. K., Kernohan J. W.: The intervertebral disc: its microscopic anatomy and pathology. J. Bone Joint Surg., 1945, *27*, 105-112.

59. Crouzet G., Vasdev A., Chirossel J. P., Hosatte F., Coulomb M., Geindre M.: Anatomie tomodensitométrique normale du canal rachidien lombaire et méthodologie d'exploration. J. Radiol., 1982, *63*, 249-257.

60. Crouzet G., Vasdev A., Chirossel J. P., Petit C., Geindre M.: Réflexions sur les aspects tomodensitométriques du canal lombaire étroit. J. Radiol., 1983, *64* (6-7), 405-414.

61. Daniels D. L., Grogan J. P., Johansen J. G., Meyer G. A., Williams A. L., Haughthon V. M.: Cervical radiculopathy: computed tomography and myelography compared. Radiology, 1984, *151*, 109-113.

62. Deburge A., Benoist M., Boyer D.: Diagnostic des hernies discales exclues. Rev. Rhum., 1982, *49*, 677-681.

63. Deburge A., Benoist M., Rocolle J.: La chirurgie des échecs de la nucléolyse des hernies discales lombaires. Revue de Chir. Orthop., 1984, *70*, 637-641.

64. Deburge A., Benoist M.: Sciatique et chimionucleolyse. Masson-Paris, 1986.

65. Deeb Z. L., Rosenbaum A. E., Bensy J. J., Scarff T. B.: Calcified intramedullary aneurysm in spinal angioma. Neuroradiology, 1977, *14*, 1-3.

66. Delcoux P., Houcke E., Razemon J. P.: Anatomie pathologique de la hernie discale. Presse médicale, 1958, *40*, 899-905.

67. De Palma A., Rothman R.: The intervertebral disk, in: Computed tomography of the spine, Ed. by Donovan J., Williams and Wilkins, 1984, 390.

68. Deramond H.: Failures of chemonucleolysis. Focus on chemonucleolysis. J. F. Bonneville. Springer-Verlag, 1986, 107-113.

69. De Santis M., Crisi G., Folchi Vici F.: Late contrast enhancement in the CT diagnosis of herniated lumbar disk. Neuroradiology, 1984, *26* (4), 303-307.

70. Dietemann J. L., Dirheimer Y., Wackenheim A.: Lombosciatique. Documentation rhumatologique Rangasil. Département CIBA, 1985.

71. Dillon W. P., Kaseff L. G., Knackstedt V. E., Osborn A. G.: Computed tomography and differential diagnosis of the extruded lumbar disc. J. Comput. Assist. Tomogr., 1983, *7*, 969-975.

72. Dorwart R. H., Genant H. K.: Anatomy of the lumbosacral spine. Radiol. Clin. North Am., 1983, *21*, 201-220.

73. Doyon D., Halimi P., Busy F., Pierron D.: Diagnostic actuel des hernies discales lombo-sacrées (TDM et IRM incluses). Cours de perfectionnement post-universitaire. Société Française de Radiologie, 1985, 1-12.

74. Drape J. L.: Scanographie des hernies discales lombaires Thèse Méd., Strasbourg, 1987, n° 219.

75. Drasin G. F., Daffnet R. H., Sexton R. F., Cheatam W. C.: Epidural venography diagnosis of herniated lumbar intervertebral disc and other disease of the epidural space. AJR, 1976, *126*, 1010-1016.

76. Drouillard J., Duperron P., Philippe J. C., Eresue J., La-

vignolle B., Senegas J., Drouillard N., Leman P., Tavernier J.: La tomodensitométrie des sciatiques. Résultats à propos de 128 cas. Ann. Radiol., 1983, *26* (6), 463.

77. Dublin A. B., McGahan J. P., Reid M. H.: The value of computed tomographic metrizamide myelography in the neuroradiological evaluation of the spine. Radiology, 1983, *146,* 79-86.

78. Dublin A. B., Reid M. H.: Outpatient low-dose computed tomography metrizamide myelography and evaluation of lumbar disk disease. J. Comput. Tomogr., 1984, *8* (2), 113-117.

79. Eckardt J. J., Kaplan D. D., Batzdorf U., Dawson E. G.: Extra-foraminal disc herniation simulating a retroperitoneal neoplasm. Case report. J Bone Joint Surg., 1985, *67* (A), 1275-1277.

80. Edwin C., Mc Cullough P. D., Thomas J. P. D.: Patient dosage in computed tomography. Radiology, 1978, *129,* 457-463.

81. Ellmann M. H., Vazquez T., Ferguson L., Mandel N.: Calcium pyrophosphate deposition in ligamentum flavum. Arthritis rhum., 1978, *21,* 611-613.

82. Elster A., Kenneth M.: Vacuum phenomenon within the cervical spinal canal: CT demonstration of a herniated disk. Journ. Comput. Ass. Tom. 1984, *8,* 533-535.

83. Epstein B. S., Epstein J. A., Jones M. D.: Anatomico-radiological correlations in cervical spine discal disease and stenosis. Clin. Neurosurg., 1978, *25,* 148-173.

84. Epstein J. A., Epstein N. E., Marc J., Rosenthal A. D., Lavine L. S.: Lumbar intervertebral disk herniation in teen-age children: recognition and management of associated anomalies. Spine, 1984, *9* (4), 427-432.

85. Fanell J. B., Twomey L. T.: Acute low-back pain. Comparison of two conservative treatment approaches. Med. J. Assist. 1, 1982, 160-164.

86. Farfan H. F., Huberdeau R. M., Dubow H. I.: Lumbar intervertebral disc degeneration. J Bone Joint Surg., 1972, *54 A,* 492-510.

87. Farnarier P., Grisoli F., Vincentelli F., Tonon C., Couailler J. F.: Exploration par le métrizamide des névralgies cervico-brachiales. J. Neuroradiology, 1980, *7,* 133-143.

88. Firooznia H., Benjamin V., Kricheff I. I., Rafii M., Golimbu C.: CT of lumbar spine disk herniation: correlation with surgical findings. AJR, 1984, *142,* 587-592.

89. Firooznia H., Kricheff I. I., Rafii M., Golimbu C.: Lumbar spine after surgery: examination with intravenous contrast-enhanced CT. Radiology, 1987, *163,* 221-226.

90. Fitzer P. M.: Anterior herniation of the nucleus pulposus: radiologic and clinical features. South Med J., 1985, *78* (11), 1296-1300.

91. Fon G., Sage M.: Computed tomoraphy in cervical disc disease when myelography is unsatisfactory. Clinical Radiology 1984, *35,* 347-350.

92. Fox A., Lin J., Richard S., Kricheff I.: Myelographic cervical nerve root deformities. Radiology August 1975, *116,* 355-361.

93. Fries J. W., Abodecly D. A., Vijungo J. G., Yearger V. L., Gaffey R.: Computed tomography of herniated and extruded nucleus pulposus. J. Comput. Assist. Tomogr., 1982, *6,* 874-887.

94. Fries J. W., Abodegly D. A., Vijungo J. G., Gaffey R.: Lateral L3/L4 herniated nucleus pulposus: clinical and imaging considerations. Comput. Radiol., 1984, *8* (6), 341-354.

95. Frocrain L., Duvauferrier R., Chales G., Ramee A., Paw-

lotsky Y.: Intérêt de l'imagerie par résonance magnétique dans le diagnostic des lombosciatiques récidivantes post opératoires. J. Radiol., 1987, *68* (5), 381-385.

96. Fuentes J. M., Maupoux R., Bourdotte G., Gras M., Castan P., Vlahovitch B., Choucair Y.: L'épidurographie. Place dans l'exploration de la lombo-sciatique et en traumatologie rachidienne. J. Neuroradiologie, 1981, *8,* 21-33.

97. Gado M., Patel J., Hodges F. J.: Lateral disk herniation into the lumbar intervertebral foramen: differential diagnosis. AJNR, 1983, *4,* 598-600.

98. Garrera G. F., Williams A. L., Haughton W. M.: Computed tomography in sciatica. Radiology, 1980, *137,* 433-437.

99. Gasquet C., Drouineau J., Goubault F., Hurmic A., Lavigne B., Vander Marcq P.: Etude de l'irradiation du patient et du coût dans les procédures diagnostiques usuelles de hernies discales. Radiculographie. Phlébographie rachidienne et tomodensitométrie. J. Radiol., 1983, *64,* 459-464.

100. Gentry L. R., Turski P. A., Strother C. M., Javid M. J., Sackett J. F.: Chymopapaïn chemonucleolysis: CT changes after treatment. AJR, 1985, *145* (2), 361-369.

101. Gentry L. R., Turski P. A., Strother C. M., Javid M. J., Sackett J. F.: Chymopapaïn chemonucleolysis: CT changes after treatment. AJNR, 1985, *6,* 321-329.

102. Gerhater R., Holgate R.: Lumbar epidural venography in the diagnosis of disc herniations. AJR, 1976, *126,* 992-1002.

103. Gertzbein S. D.: Degenerative disk disease of the lumbar spine. Immunological implications. Clin. Orthop., 1977, *12,* 68-71.

104. Gertzbein S. D., Tile M., Gross A., Falk R.: Autoimmunity in degenerative disc disease of the lumbar spine. Orthop. Clin. (Am.), 1975, *6* (1), 67-73.

105. Ghosh P., Bushell G. R., Taylor T. F. K., Akeson W. H.: Collagens, elastin and non collagenous protein of the intervertebral disk. Clin. Orthop., 1977, *12,* 124-132.

106. Gibson M. D., Buckley J., Maukinney R., Mulholland R. G., Worthington B. S.: Magnetic resonance imaging and discography in the diagnosis of disc degeneration. Comparative study of 50 discs. J. Bone Joint Surg., 1986, *68,* 369-373.

107. Glenn W. V. Jr, Rhodes M. L., Altschuler E. R., Wiltse L. L., Kostanek C., Kuo Y. M.: Multiplanar display computerized body tomography applications in the lumbar spine. Spine, 1979, *4,* 282-319.

108. Godersky J. C., Erickson D. L., Seljeskog E. L.: Extreme lateral disc herniation: diagnosis by computed tomographic scanning. Neurosurgery, 1984, *14* (5), 549-542.

109. Goubault F., Drouineau J., Hurmic A., Vandermarcq P., Gasquet C.: Valeur de l'examen tomodensitométriques dans le diagnostic des hernies discales lombaires. A propos de 155 disques opérés. J. Radiol., 1984, *65,* 71-77.

110. Graves V. B., Finney H. L., Mailander J.: Intradural lumbar disk herniation. AJNR, 1986, *7,* 495-497.

111. Guilbeau J. C., Morvan G., Nahum H.: Les calcifications intra-rachidiennes. Sémiologie, valeur pathologique. J. Radiol., 1982, *83,* 453-463.

112. Guinto F. C. Jr, Hashim H., Stumer M.: CT demonstration of disk regression after conservative therapy. AJNR, 1984, *5* (5), 632-633.

113. Gulati A. N., Weinstein R., Studdard E.: CT scan of the spine for herniated disc. Neuroradiology, 1981, *2,* 57-60.

114. Hall S., Bartleson J. D., Onofrio B. M., Baker H. L., Oka-

saki H., O'Duffy J. D.: Lumbar spinal stenosis. Ann. Int. Med., 1985, *103*, 271–275.

115. Hamilton E., Rothman R.: Lumbar disc disease: clinical and CT evolution in CT of the Spine ed. by Donovan J., Williams and Wilkins, 1984, 334.

116. Hammerschlag S. B., Wolpert S. M., Carter B.: Computed tomography of the spinal canal. Radiology, 1976, *121*, 361–367.

117. Hankinson H. L., Wilson C. B.: Use of the operating microscope in anterior cervical discectomy without fusion. J. Neurosurg., 1975, *43*, 452–456.

118. Harris R. I., Macnab I.: Structural changes in the lumbar intervertebral discs. Their relationship to low back pain and sciatica. J Bone Joint Surg., 1954, *36 B*, 304–322.

119. Hartjes H., Roosen U., Grote W., Buch A., Brenner A., Ruhman U., Hitche H.: Cervical disk syndrome. Value of metrizamide myelography and discography. AJNR, 1983, *4*, 644–645.

120. Haughton V. M., Eldevik O. P., Ho Khang-Cheng, Larson S. J., Unger G. F.: Arachnoiditis from experimental myelography with aqueous contrast media. Spine, 1978, *3*, 65–69.

121. Haughton V. M., Eldevik O. P., Magnares B., Amundsen P.: A prospective comparison of computed tomography and myelography in the diagnosis of herniated lumbar disks. Radiology, 1982, *192*, 103–110.

122. Haughton V. M., Ho Khang-Cheng, Unger C. F.: Arachnoiditis following myelography with water-soluble agents. The role of contrast medium osmolality. Radiology, 1977, *125*, 731–733.

123. Haughton V. M., Syversten A., Williams A. L.: Soft tissue anatomy within the spinal canal as seen on computed tomography. Radiology, 1980, *134*, 649–655.

124. Hayashi K., Yabuti T., Durokawa T., Seiki H., Hogaki M., Noura S.: The anterior and the posterior longitudinal ligaments of the lower cervical spine. J. Anat., 1977, *124*, 633–636.

125. Heintz E., Yeates A., Burger P., Drayer B. P., Osborne D., Hill R.: Opacification of epidural venous plexus and dura in evaluation of cervical nerve root: CT technique. AJNR, Sept/Oct 1984, *5*, 621–624.

126. Helms C. A., Dowartz M. R., Gray M.: The C. T. appearance of conjoined nerve roots and differentiation from a herniated nucleus pulposus. Radiology, 1982, *144*, 803–807.

127. Hemminghytt S., Daniels D. L., Williams A. L., Haughton V. M.: Intraspinal synovial cysts: natural history and diagnosis by CT. Radiology, 1982, *145*, 375–376.

128. Herman G. T., Coin C. G.: The use of three-dimensional computer display in the study of disk disease. J. Comput. Assist. Tomogr., 1980, *4*, 564–567.

129. Higuchi M., Abe K.: Ultrastructure of the nucleus pulposus in the intervertebral disc after systemic administration of hydrocortisone in mice. Spine, 1985, *10* (7), 638–643.

130. Hiramatsu Y., Nobechi T.: Calcification of the posterior longitudinal ligament of the spine among Japanese. Radiology, 1971, *100*, 307–312.

131. Hirschy J. C., Leve W. M., Berninger W. H., Hamilton R. H., Abbott G. F.: CT of the lumbosacral spine: importance of tomographic planes parallel to vertebral endplate. AJR, 1981, *126*, 47–52.

132. Ho P. S. P., Ho K. C., Yu S. et al.: Calcification of the nucleus pulposus with pathologic confirmation in a premature infant. AJNR, 1989, Vol. 10, n° 1, 201.

133. Hoddich W. K., Helms C. A.: Bony spinal changes that differentiate conjoined nerve roots from herniated nucleus pulposus. Radiology, 1985, *154*, 119–120.

134. Holt E. P. J.: Fallacy of cervical discography. Report of 50 cases in normal subjects. Jama, 1964, *188* (9), 799–801.

135. Houser O. W., Onofrio B. M., Forbes G. S., Baker H. L.: Correlation of radiological features to failure of lumbar intervertebral disc chemonucleolysis. J. Neurosurg., 1986, *64*, 736–742.

136. Houtteville J. P., Toumi K.: Surgical findings and results after chemonucleolysis failure in sciatica. Focus on chemonucleolysis. J. F. Bonneville. Springer-Verlag, 1986, 115–121.

137. Hubault A.: Névralgies cervico-brachiales. EMC Paris App. locomoteur, 1983, 14370-C 10.

138. Husag L., Probst C.: Microsurgical anterior approach to cervical disk. Review of 60 consecutive cases of discectomy without fusion. Acta Neurochirgica, 1984, *73*, 229–242.

139. Hyman R. A., Merten C. W., Liebeskind A. L., Naidich J. B., Stein H. L.: Computed tomography in ossification of the posterior longitudinal spinal ligament. Neuroradiology, 1977, *13*, 227–228.

140. Jesel M.: Lombocruralites et lombosciatiques. Conf. de neurol., 1974, *12*, 67–77.

141. Jesel M.: Syndromes de la queue de cheval. Conf. de neurol., 1973, *6*, 23–38.

142. Jiddane M., Bartoli J. M., Diaz P., Nicoli F., Grisoli F., Salamon G.: Les hernies discales lombaires latérales. J. Radiol., 1985, *66* (11), 679–682.

143. Johansen J. G.: Demonstration of anterior intervertebral disc herniation by CT. Neuroradiology, 1987, *29*, 214.

144. Johnson E. F., Mitchell R., Berryman H., Cardoso S., Veal O., Patterson D.: Secretory cells in the nucleus pulposus of the adult human intervertebral disc. A preliminary report. Acta Anatomica, 1986, *125*, 161–164.

145. Jomin M., Lesoin F., Losez G., Clarisse J.: Les hernies cervicales. Deux cent trente observations. Sém. Hôp. Paris, 1985, *61*, n° 21, 1479–1485.

146. Kadoya S., Nakamura T., Tada A.: Neuroradiology of ossification of the posterior longitudinal spinal ligament. Comparative studies with computed tomography. Neuroradiology, 1978, *16*, 357–358.

147. Kaiser M. C., Capesius P., Veiga-Pires J. A., Sandt G.: A sign of lumbar disk herniation recognizable on lateral CT-generated digital radiograms. J. Comput. Assist. Tomogr., 1984, *8* (6), 1066–1071.

148. Kaiser M. C., Sandt G., Roilgen A., Capesius P., Poos D., Ohanna F.: Intradural disk herniation with CT appearance of gas collection. AJNR, 1985, *6*, 117–118.

149. Karnaze M. G., Gado M. H., Sartor K. J., Hodges F. J.: Comparison of MR and CT myelography in imaging the cervical and thoracic spine. AJNR, 1987, Vol. 8, n° 6, 983–991.

150. Kawano N., Yoshida S., Ohwada T., Yada K., Sasaki K., Matsuno T.: Cervical radiculomyelopathy caused by deposition of calcium pyrophosphate dihydrate crystals in the ligamenta flava. J. Neurosurg., 1980, *52*, 279–283.

151. Keeneesi C., Lesur E.: Orientation of the articular processes at L4, L5, and S1. Possible role in pathology of the intervertebral disc. Anat. Clin., 1985, *7* (1), 43–47.

152. Kempe L. G.: Operative Neurosurgery, vol. 2. Posterior fossa, spinal cord, and peripheral nerve disease. Springer-Verlag, Berlin – Heidelberg – New-York, 1970.

153. Kieffer S. A., Cacayorin E. D., Sherry R. G.: The radiological diagnosis of herniated lumbar intervertebral disk. A current controversy. Jama, 1984, *251* (9), 1192–1195.

154. Kikuchi S., Mac Nab I., Moreau P.: Localisation of the level of symptomatic cervical disc degeneration. J Bone Joint Surg., 1981, *63 B*, 272.

155. Klafa L. A., Collis J. S.: An analysis of cervical discography with surgical verification. J. Neurosurg., 1969, *30*, 38–41.

156. Konings J. G., Williams F. J. B., Deutman R.: The effects of chemonucleolysis as demonstrated by computerized tomography. J Bone Surg., 1984, *66* (B), 417–421.

157. Konings J. G., Williams F. J. B., Deutman R.: Computed tomography (CT) analysis of the effects of chemonucleolysis. Clin. Orthop. Rel. Research, 1986, *206*, 32–36.

158. Kornberg M., Rechtine G. R.: Quantitative assessment of the fifth lumbar spinal canal by computed tomography in symptomatic L4/L5 disc disease. Spine, 1985, *10* (4), 328–330.

159. Kornberg M., Rechtine G. R., Dupuy T. E.: Computed tomography in the diagnosis of the herniated disk at the L5–S1 level. Spine, 1984, *9* (4), 433–436.

160. Krause D., Maitrot D., Buchheit F., Tongio J.: Hernies cervicales molles. Scanner et chirurgie. J. Neuroradiol., 1985, *12*, 271–280.

161. Krause D., Maitrot D., Veillon F., Genin P., Drape J. L., Benhaim M., Buchheit F., Tongio J.: Hernies lombaires migratrices. Scanner et chirurgie. J. Neuroradiol., 1986, *13*, 39–52.

162. Krause D., Woerly B., Drape J. L., Benhaim M., Boyer P., Maitrot D., Rabischong P., Buchheit F., Tongio J.: Soft cervical disc herniations. Acta Radiologica, supp. 369, XIII Symposium Neuroradiologicum Stockholm, 1986, 236–238.

163. Krause D., Woerly B., Drape J. L., Boyer P. et Coll.: Evolution des hernies cervicales molles non-opérées. Communication à la Société Française de Neuroradiologie, Paris, Décembre 86.

164. Krayenbuhl H.: Zur diagnose und differential diagnose der intervertebral disk hernie. Practis, 1942, *31*, 19.

165. Landmann J. A., Hoffmann J. C., Braun I., Barrow D. L.: Value of computed myelography in the recognition of cervical herniated disk. AJNR July/August 1984, *5*, 391–394.

166. Laredo J. D., Bard M., Morvan G.: Bases anatomiques de l'interprétation du scanner lombaire, images pièges. Cours de perfectionnement post-universitaire, 1986, Société Française de Radiologie.

167. Lassale B., Benoist M., Morvan G., Massare C., Deburge A., Cauchoix J.: Sténose du canal lombaire. Etude nosologique et sémiologique. A propos de 163 cas opérés. Rev. Rhum. Mal Ostéo-artic., 1983, *50* (1), 39.

168. Lassale B., Morvan G., Gottin M.: Anatomy and radiological anatomy of the lumbar radicular canals. Anat. Clin., 1984, *6*, 195–201.

169. Lazorthes G.: Le système nerveux périphérique. Masson 3e édit., 1981, 175–182.

170. Lazorthes Y., Verdie J. C., Richard J., Theron J., Houtteville J. P., Courtheaux P.: Chemonucleolysis of cervical disk. Preliminary results in 15 cases of root compression. "Current concepts in chemonucleolysis". Published by the Royal Society of Medicine, International Congress and Symposium, London 1985.

171. Lazorthes Y., Zadeh J. O., Larrigue J.: Les hernies discales cervicales. Rev. Méd. Toulouse, 1970, *VI*, 647.

172. Le Gall R., Jestin Y., Pabot du Chatelard P., Ferry M., Cosnard G.: Etude comparative du scanner et de la saccoradiculographie dans le diagnostic des hernies discales lombaires inaugurales. A propos de 50 cas vérifiés chirurgicalement. J. Radiol., 1984, *65* (3), 165–172.

173. Lesoin F., Viaud C., Di Paola S., Vilette L., Autricque A., Clarisse J., Janin M.: Traitement des hernies cervicales molles par injection intradiscale percutanée d'aprotinine. Neurochi., 1986, *32* (3), 272–275.

174. Lesoin F., Rousseaux M., Autricque A. et al.: Thoracic disc herniations: evolution in the approach and indications. Acta Neurochir., 1986, *80*, 30–34.

175. L'Hermine C., Duquesnoy B., Flament J. F., Chastanet P., Delcambre B.: Intérêt de la radiculographie de profil en station verticale pour le diagnostic de canal lombaire étroit. J. Radiol., 1985, *66* (5), 355–360.

176. L'Huillier F., Chevrot A., Vallee C., Gires F., Wybier M., Pallardy G.: Lomboradiculalgie et hernie discale calcifiée. J. Radiol., 1988, *69* (12), 763–766.

177. Lindblom K., Haltquist J.: Absorption of protruded disk tissue. J. Bone Jt. Surg., 1950, *32 A*, 557–561.

178. Lucantoni D., Galzio R., Zenobii M., Cristuib L., Magliani V., Caffagni E.: Involvement of lumbosacral roots caused by lateral recess stenosis. J. Neurosurg. Sci., 1984, *28* (2), 93–96.

179. Lunsford L. D., Bissonette D. J., Jannetta J. P., Sheptak P. E., Zorub D. S.: Anterior surgery for cervical disc disease: treatment of lateral cervical disc herniation in 253 cases. J. Neurosurg., 1980, *53*, 1–11.

180. Mac Cullough J. A.: Chemonucleolysis. Experience with 2000 cases. Clin. Orthop., 1980, *146*, 128–135.

181. Mac Gregor J. C., Butler P.: Disc calcifications in childhood: computed tomographic and magnetic resonance imaging appearances. B. J. Radiol., 1986, *59*, 180–182.

182. Mac Ray D. L.: Asymptomatic intervertebral disc protusions. Acta Radiol., 1956, *46*, 9–27.

183. Mainzer F.: Herniation of the nucleus pulposus: a rare complication of intervertebral disk calcification in children. Radiology, 1973, *107*, 167–170.

184. Maitrot D.: Hernies discales lombosacrées (analyse clinique, radiologique et chirurgicale à propos de 700 cas). Thèse Méd., Strasbourg, 1973, n° 5.

185. Malghem J., Nagant de deux Chaisnes C., Romboutslin-Demans C., Dory M. Maldague B.: Ossification of the posterior longitudinal ligament of the cervical spine: report of a case with computed tomography study and associated with Forestier's disease. J. Belge Radiol., 1979, *62*, 69–77.

186. Mall J. C., Kaiser J. C.: Post-chymopapaïn (chemonucleolysis): clinical and computed tomography correlation: preliminary results. Skeletal Radiol., 1984, *12* (4), 270–275.

187. Mani R. J.: The computed tomographic differential diagnosis of disc disease. Chapter 20 in: Computed tomography of the spine. Edited by M. J. Donovan, 1984, Williams and Wilkins. Baltimore, U. S. A., 1984, 340–386.

188. Marsault C., Larde D., Utzamann O., Menu Y., Avonac B., Williaumey J.: Intérêt de la tomodensitométrie dans le diagnostic des hernies discales lombaires. Rev. Rhum., 1981, *48*, 457–462.

189. Martin N., Guilbeau J. C., Murat M., Debroucker T., Bouali I., Nahum H.: Hernie discale intradurale lombaire. Diagnostic scanographique. J. Radiol., 1988, *69* (11), 681–684.

190. Massare C.: Discographie. In: Traité de Radiodiagnostic. H. Fischgold. Ed. Masson Paris, 15, 39-49, 1971.

191. Massare C.: Scanner et hernie discale lombaire in: La tomodensitométrie ostéo-articulaire. Morvan G., Massare C. Lequesne M. Documenta Geigy, Paris, 1985, 39-61.

192. Massare C., Bard M.: La discographie cervicale. Journ. Radiol., 1974, 55, 395.

193. Massare C., Benoist M., Cauchoix J.: Le diagnostic des hernies discales lombaires et lombo-sacrées. Intérêt de la discographie. Revue de Chir. Ortho., 1973, 59, 61-67.

194. Massare C.: CT examination of a subject presenting with common sciatica. J. Belge Radiol., 1982, 65, 403-413.

195. Massare C.: Les échecs du traitement chirurgical des sciatiques discales communes paralysantes. Place du scanner. Revue Chir. Ortho., 1982, 68, 233-240.

196. Meijenhorst G. C. H.: Computed tomography of the lumbar epidural veins. Radiology, 1982, 145, 687-691.

197. Menkes C. J.: Indications and contraindications of nucleolysis. Focus on chemonucleolysis. J. F. Bonneville. Springer-Verlag, 1986, 24-26.

198. Metzger J., Hirsch J. F., Duttine G., Poirier M., Feldmann L., Haddad K., Allal M.: Radiculographie au métrizamide avec épreuve dynamique simplifiée. Nouv. Presse Méd., 1980, 9, 1219-1222.

199. Meyer G. A., Haughton V. A., Williams A. L.: Diagnosis of herniated lumbar disc with computed tomography. N. Engl. J. Med., 1979, 301, 1166-1167.

200. Miyasaka K., Isu T., Abe S., Takei H., Tsuru M.: High resolution computed tomography in the diagnosis of cervical disc disease. Neuroradiology, 1983, 24, 253-257.

201. Moneret-Vautrin D. A., Martar C., Laxenaire M. D., Roland J., Aussedat P., Oulli G., Gerard H.: Détection d'une sensibilisation à la chymopapaïne. Bilan chez 111 candidats à la chimonucléolyse. Sém. Hôp. FRA, 1986, 62 (44), 3499-3504.

202. Moore W. W., Walker E.: Intraspinal epidermoid tumor. Case report and discussion. J. Neurosurg., 1951, 8, 343-347.

203. Morvan G.: Les examens complémentaires dans la sciatique. La Vie Médicale, 1985, 30/31, 2/3.

204. Morvan G., Busson J., Massare C., Bard M., Seguy E.: Exploration tomodensitométrique des névralgies cervico-brachiales avec injection intra-veineuse de produit de contraste. Journal de Radiologie, 1984, n° 3, 65, 159-164.

205. Morvan G., Massare C.: Tomodensitometric measurements of the lumbar spinal canal. J. Belge Radiol., 1982, 65, 397-402.

206. Morvan G., Massare C., Frija G.: Le scanner ostéo-articulaire. Techniques d'utilisation, indications, résultats. Editions Vigot, Paris, 1986.

207. Moufarrif N. A., Hardy R. W., Weinstein M. A.: Computed tomographic, myelographic, and operative findings in patients with suspected herniated lumbar discs. Neurosurgery, 1983, 12 (2), 184-188.

208. Nagakawa H., Okumara T., Sugiyama T.: Discrepancy between metrizamide CT and myelography in diagnosis of cervical disk protusions. AJNR 1983, 4, 604-606.

209. Naidich T. P., King D. G., Moran C. J., Sagel S. S.: Computed tomography of the lumbar thecal sac. J. Comput. Assist. Tomogr., 1980, 4, 37-41.

210. Nainkin L.: Arachnoidis ossificans. Report of a case. Spine, 1978, 3, 83-86.

211. Naylor A., Happey F., Turner R. L., Shentall R. D., Richardson C.: Enzymatic and immunological activity in the intervertebral disc. Orthop. Clin. North Am., 1975, 6, 51-58.

212. Neave V. C. D., Wycoff R. R.: Case report: computed tomography of cystic nerve root sleeve dilatation. J. Comput. Assist. Tomogr., 1983, 7, 881-885.

213. Nicolau A., Diard F., Darrigade J. M., Dorcier F., Vital J. M.: Hernie postérieure d'un disque calcifié chez l'enfant. A propos de 2 observations. J. Radiol. 66 (11), 683-688.

214. Nixon J.: La mécanique des disques intervertébraux. J. R. Soc. Med., 1986, 79, 100-104.

215. Nordby E. J.: Current concepts review. Chymopapain in intradiscal therapy. J. Bone Joint Surg. (Am), 1983, 65 (A), 1350-1353.

216. Novetsky G. J., Berlin L., Lobo N., Miller H. S.: The extraforaminal herniated disk: Detection by Computed tomography. AJNR, 1982, 3, 653-655.

217. Orrisson W., Hohansen J., Eldevik O., Haughton V.: Optimal computed tomographic techniques for cervical spine imaging. Radiology, 1982, 144, 180.

218. Osborn A. G., Hood R. S., Sherry R. G., Smoker W. R. K., Harnsberger H. R.: CT/MR Spectrum of far lateral and anterior lumbosacral disk herniations. AJNR, 1988, Vol. 9, n° 4, 775-778.

219. Palacios E., Brackett C. E., Leary D. J.: Ossification of the posterior longitudinal ligament associated with a herniated intervertebral disk. Radiology, 1971, 100, 313-314.

220. Pallardy G., Chevrot A. et Coll.: Discographie cervicale in: Arthrographies opaques. Masson Ed., 1988, 215-219.

221. Payne E. E., Spillane J. D.: The cervical spine. An anatomico-pathological study of 70 specimens with particular reference to the problem of cervical spondylosis. Brain, 1957, 80, 571-596.

222. Pech P., Daniels D., Williams A., Haughton V.: The cervical neural foramina: correlation of microtomy and CT anatomy. Radiology, 1985, 155, 143-146.

223. Pennings L., Wilmink J. T.: Biomechanics of lumbosacral dural sac. A study of flexion-extension myelography. Spine, 1981, 6, 398-408.

224. Penning L., Wilminck J. T., Woerden H. H., Knol E.: CT myelographic findings in degenerative disorders of the cervical spine: clinical significance. AJR April 1986, 146, 793-801.

225. Pere P., Delgoffe C., Vinet E.: L'apport du scanner en rhumatologie. La Pratique Médicale, 1984, 14, 39-43.

226. Perves A., Massare C.: Confrontation radioclinique et tomodensitométrique de 50 sténoses lombaires dégénératives opérées. Rev. Chir. Orthop., 1983, 69 (2), 129.

227. Pierron D., Fahim R., Halimi P., Doyon D.: La place de l'examen tomodensitométrique dans le diagnostic des complications de la chirurgie discale lombaire. J. Radiol., 1985, 66 (8-9), 497-501.

228. Pillard D., Masse P., Taussig G.: Discopathie calcifiante de l'enfant. Rev. Chir. Orthop., 1980, 66, 515-521.

229. Post M. J. D.: The impact of time, metrizamide and high resolution on the diagnosis of spinal pathology. Radiographic evaluation of the spine. Current Advances with Emphasis on Computed Tomography. Edited by MJD Post New York Masson. 259-294, 1980.

230. Postacchini F.: Chemonucleolysis in the treatment of prolapsed intervertebral disc. Early results. Ital. J. Orthop. Traumatol., 1984, 10 (1), 5-19.

231. Postachinni F., Bellocci M., Massobrio M.: Morphologic changes in annulus fibrosus during aging. An ultrastructural study in rats. Spine, 1984, 9 (6), 596-603.

232. Postachinni F., Facchini M., Palieri P.: Efficacy of various forms of conservative treatment in low back pain. A comparative Study. Neuro-Orthopedics, 1988, Vol. 6, n° 1, 28-35.

233. Rabischong P., Louis R., Vignaud J., Massare C.: Le disque intervertébral. Anat. Clin., 1978, 1, 55-64.

234. Raininko R., Torma T.: Contrast enhancement around a prolapsed disk. Neuroradiology, 1982, 24, 49-51.

235. Raskin S. P.: Demonstration of nerve roots on unenhanced computed tomographic scans. J. Comput. Assist. Tomogr., 1981, 5, 281-284.

236. Raskin S. P., Keating J. W.: Recognition of lumbar disk disease: comparison of myelography and computed tomography. AJR, 1982, 139, 349-355.

237. Rauschning W.: Computed tomography and cryomicrotomy of lumbar spine specimens. A new technique for multiplanar anatomic correlation. Spine, 1983, 8 (2) 170-180.

238. Raynor R. B.: Symptomatic disc herniation into vertebral body. Surg. Neurol., 1985, 23 (6), 621-625.

239. Reid J. D.: Effects of flexion-extension movements of the head and spine upon the spinal cord and nerve roots. Neurol. Neurosurg. Psychiat., 1960, 23, 216-221.

240. Renier J. C.: Physio-pathologie et anatomopathologie de la radiculalgie cervico-brachiale commune. Rhumathologie, 1978, 30, 9-14.

241. Renier J. C., Bontoux L.: Le disque intervertébral lombaire. Encycl. Méd. Chir., Paris, Appareil locomoteur, 15840 A¹⁰, 3 - 1984.

242. Resnick D., Niwayama G.: Radiographic and pathologic features of spinal involvement in diffuse idiopathic skeletal hyperostosis (DISH). Radiology, 1976, 119, 559-568.

243. Resnick D., Guerra J., Robinson C. A., Vint V. C.: Association of diffuse idiopathic skeletal hyperostosis (DISH) and calcification and ossification of the posterior longitudinal ligament. Am. J. Roentgenol., 1978, 131, 1049-1053.

244. Ritchie W. G. M., Davison A. M.: Dural calcification: a complication of prolonged periodic haemodialysis. Clin. Radiol., 1974, 25, 349-353.

245. Roberson G. H., Hatten H. P. Jr, Hesseling J. H.: Epidurography: selective catheter technique and review of 53 cases. AJR, 1979, 132, 787-794.

246. Roland J., Bracard S., Forlodou D., Moret C., Picard L.: Anatomical aspects of the intervertebral disc. Focus on chemonucleolysis. J. F. Bonneville, Springer-Verlag, 1986, 1-6.

247. Roland J., Larde D., Masson J. P., Picard L.: Les veines lombaires épidurales. Radio-anatomie normale. J. Radiol., 1977, 58, 35-38.

248. Rouviere H., Delmas A.: Anatomie humaine. Masson, 11th edn., 1974, Vols. 1 and 2.

249. Rosenthal D. I., Stauffer A. E., Davis K. R., Ganott M., Taveras J. M.: Evaluation of multiplanar reconstruction in CT recognition of lumbar disk disease. AJR, 1984, 143, 160-176.

250. Runge M., Clere P., Bonneville J. F.: Computed tomography and chemonucleolysis. Focus on chemonucleolysis. J. F. Bonneville. Springer-Verlag, 1986, 29-35.

251. Russel E., D'Angelo C., Zimmermann R., Czervionke L., Huckmann M.: Cervical disk herniation: CT demonstration after contrast enhancement. Radiology 1984, 152, 703-712.

252. Ryan R. W., Lally J. F., Kozic Z.: Asymptomatic calcified herniated thoracic disks: CT recognition. AJNR, 1988, Vol. 9, n° 2, 363-366.

253. Ryckewaert A.: Détérioration structurale des disques intervertébraux. Traité de Médecine, Godeau P., 2 vol. 2873 p., Paris, 1981, Flammarion édit. p. 2092-2102.

254. Sachsenheimer W., Hamer J., Muller M. A.: The value of spinal computed tomography in diagnosis of herniated lumbar discs. Acta Neurochir., 1982, 60, 107-114.

255. Sackett J., Strother C.: New techniques in myelography. New York, Harper and Row, 1979, 109-123.

256. Saillant G., Berteaux D., Roy-Camille R.: Le traitement chirurgical des névralgies cervico-brachiales. Rhumatologie 1978, 30, 31-32.

257. Salvi V.: Computerized axial tomography in the diagnosis of lumbar disc hernia. Ital. J. Orthop. Traumatol., 1985, 11 (1), 43-50.

258. Sartoris D. J., Resnick D., Guerra J.: Vertebral venous channels: CT appearance and differential considerations. Radiology, 1985, 155, 745-749.

259. Schaik Van J. P. P., Verbiest H., Schaik Van F. D. J.: Morphometry of lower lumbar vertebrae as seen on CT scans: newly recognised characteristics. AJR, 1985, 145, 327-335.

260. Schimer M.: Thoracic intervertebral disk prolapse. Orthopade, 1985, 14, 112-117.

261. Schmit P., Favre C., Denarnaud L.: Les calcifications discales de l'enfant. J. Radiol., 1985, 66 (5) 339-343.

262. Schneidermann G., Flanningan B., Kingston S., Thomas J., Dillin W. H., Watkins R. G.: Magnetic resonance imaging in the diagnosis of disk degenerative correlation with discography. Spine, 1987, 12, 276-291.

263. Schubiger O., Valavanis A.: CT differentiation between recurrent disk herniation and post-operative scar formation: the value of contrast enhancement. Neuroradiology, 1982, 22, 251-254.

264. Schubiger O., Valavanis A.: Post-operative lumbar CT. Technic, results, and indications. AJNR, 1983, 4, 595-597.

265. Schubiger O., Valavanis A., Hollmann J.: Computed tomography of the intervertebral foramen. Neuroradiology, 1984, 26 (6), 439-444.

266. Schwartz H. G.: Anastomoses between cervical nerve roots. Neurosurg., 1956, 13, 190-194.

267. Scotti G., Scialfa G., Pieralli S., Boccardi E., Valsecchi F., Torron C.: Myelography and radiculopathy due to cervical spondylosis: myelographic-CT correlations. AJNR, 1983, 4, 601-603.

268. Scoville W. B., Dohmann G. J., Corkill G.: Late results of cervical disk surgery. J. Neurosurg., 1976, 45 (2), 203-210.

269. Shapiro R.: Myelography. Year Book Médical Publishing, Chicago: 1975, 348-462.

270. Siala M., Bellamine B., Abdelkafi A., Hamza R., Slimane N., Chevrota A.: La hernie pré-marginale postérieure isolée. A propos de 6 cas. J. Radiol., 1988, 69 (10), 581-586.

271. Sigal R., Bittoun J., Halimi P., Blas C., Doyon D.: Comment lire une image IRM? Feuillets de radiol., 1986, 5, 299-306.

272. Simon L., Barjon M. C.: La sciatique commune: vérités d'hier et d'aujourd'hui. Tempo Médical, 1985, 186, 9-22.

273. Smith L.: Enzyme dissolution of nucleus pulposus in humans. Jama, 1964, *187*, 137–140.

274. Sobel D., Barkovich A., Munderloh S.: Metrizamide myelography and post-myelographic computed tomography: comparative adequacy in the cervical spine. AJNR 1984, *5*, 385–390.

275. Sonnabend D. H., Taylor T. K. F., Chapman G. K.: Intervertebral disc calcification syndromes in children. J. Bone Joint Surg. (Br. Vol.), 1982, *64*, 25–31.

276. Statemeier P. H.: Evaluation of the lumbar spine. A comparison between computed tomography and myelography. Radiol. Clin. North Am., 1983, *21*, 221–257.

277. Sunderland S.: Meningeal-neural relations in the intervertebral foramen. J. Neurosurg., 1974, *40*, 756–763.

278. Taylor T. K. F., Akeson W. H.: Intervertebral disk prolapse: a review of morphologic and biochemic knowledge concerning the nature of prolapse. Clin. Orthop. Rel. Research, 1971, *76*, 54–79.

279. Teal J. S., Ahmadi J., Zee C. S., Tsai F. Y., Segall H. D., Becker T. S.: Inconsistent venous opacification: a pitfall of épidural venography. AJR, 1982, *138*, 1149–1154.

280. Teplick J. G., Haskin M. E.: CT and lumbar disc herniation. Radiol. Clin. North. Am., 1983, *21*, 259–288.

281. Teplick J. G., Haskin M. E.: Computed tomography of the post-operative lumbar spine. AJNR, 1983, *4*, 1053–1072. AJR, 1983, *141*, 865–884.

282. Teplick J. G., Haskin M. E.: Intravenous contrast-enhanced CT of the post-operative lumbar spine: improved identification of recurrent disk herniation, scar, arachnoïditis and diskitis. AJR, 1984, *143*, 845–855.

283. Teplick J. G., Haskin M. E.: Spontaneous regression of herniated nucleus pulposus. AJNR, 1985, *6*, 331–335.

284. Teplick J. G., Teplik S. K., Goodman L., Haskill M. E.: Pitfalls and unusual findings in computed tomography of the lumbar spine. J. Comput. Assist. Tomogr., 1982, *6*, 888–893.

285. Theron J.: Cervico-vertebral phlebography: pathological results. Radiology, 1976, *118*, 73–81.

286. Theron J., Blais M., Casasco A., Courtheoux P., Adam Y., Derlon J. M., Houtteville J. P.: Therapeutic radiology of the lumbar spine. Chemonucleolysis, infiltration and coagulation of posterior spinal articulations. J. Neuroradiology, 1983, *10*, 209–230.

287. Theron J., Djindjan R.: Cervicovertebral phlebography using catheterization: a preliminary report. Radiology, 1973, *108*, 325–331.

288. Theron J., Moret J.: Correlations between phlebography and surgery. In: Theron J., Moret J. Spinal Phlebography. Berlin: Springer, 67–70, 1978.

289. Tondury: Zur anatomie des Halswirbelsäule. Z. Anat. Entwe. GSH, 1943, *112*, 448.

290. Tournade A., Braun J. P.: Morphological study of the action of chymopapain on the intervertebral disc. Focus on chemonucleolysis. J. F. Bonneville. Springer-Verlag, 1986, 17–22.

291. Troisier D., Goslane E., Durey A., Rodineau B.: Traitement des lombosciatiques par injection intradiscale d'enzymes protéolytiques. 80 Observations. La Nouv. Presse Ed., 1980, *9*(4), 227–229.

292. Troisier O.: Technique de la discographie extra-durale. J. Radiol., 1982, *63*, 571–578.

293. Troisier O., Cypel D.: Discography: an element of decision. Surgery versus chemonucleolysis. Clin. Orthop. Rel. Research, 1986, *206*, 70–78.

294. Troup J. D. G., Martin J. W., Lloyd D. C. E. F.: Back pain in industry. A prospective survey. Spine, 1981, *6*, 61–69.

295. Urban J. P. G., Holm S., Maroudas A., Nachemson A.: Nutrition of the intervertebral disk. Clin. Orthop., 1977, *27*, 101–114.

296. Vadala G., Dore R., Garbagna P.: Unusual osseous changes in lumbar herniated disks: CT features. J. Comput. Assist. Tomogr., 1985, *9*(6), 1045–1049.

297. Varughese G.: Lumbosacral intradural periradicular ossification: case report. J. Neurosurg., 1978, *49*, 132–137.

298. Verbiest H.: The significance and principles of computerized axial tomography in idiopathic developmental stenosis of the bony lumbar vertebral canal. Spine, 1979, *4*, 369–378.

299. Wackenheim A., Dietemann J. L.: Radiodiagnostic du rachis lombaire. Collection d'Imagerie Radiologique, Masson, Paris, 1987. Hernies discales, 25–52, Canal lombaire étroit, 61–72, Chimionucléolyse, 73–75, Spondylolyse et spondylolisthésis, 85–96.

300. Wang A., Zanani A. A.: Intradural herniation of thoracic disc: CT metrizamide myelography. Comput. Radiol., 1986, *2*, 115–118.

301. Weiss T., Treisch J., Kazner E., Kohler D., Collmann H., Claussen C.: CT of the post-operative lumbar spine: the value of intravenous contrast. Neuroradiology, 1986, *28*, 241–245.

302. Weisz G. M.: The value of CT in diagnosing post-operative lumbar conditions. Spine, 1986, *11*(2), 164–166.

303. Wilkinson H. A., Schuman N.: Intradiscal corticosteroids in the treatment of lumbar and cervical disk problems. Spine, 1980, *5*(4), 385–389.

304. Williams A. L.: CT diagnosis of degenerative disc disease. The bulging annulus. Radiol. Clin. North. Am., 1983, *21*, 289–300.

305. Williams A. L., Haughton V. M.: CT recognition of lateral lumbar disk herniation. AJR, 1982, *139*, 345–347.

306. Williams A. L., Haughton V. M., Daniels D. L., Grogan J. P.: Differential CT diagnosis of extruded nucleus pulposus. Radiology, 1983, *148*, 141–148.

307. Williams A. L., Haughton V. M., Daniels D. L., Thornton R. S.: CT recognition of lateral lumbar disc herniation. AJNR, 1982, *3*, 211–213.

308. Williams A. L., Haughton V. M., Meyer G. A., Ho C. C.: Computed tomographic appearance of the bulging annulus. Radiology, 1982, *142*, 403–408.

309. Williams A. L., Haughton V. M., Syvertsen A.: Computed tomography in the diagnosis of herniated nucleus pulposus. Radiology, 1980, *135*, 95–99.

310. Woerly B.: Scanographie des hernies cervicales molles – corrélations radio-chirurgicales à propos de 45 cas. Thèse Méd., Strasbourg, 1987, n° 149.

311. Yamamoto I., Kageyama N., Nakamura K., Takahashi T.: Computed tomography in ossification of the posterior longitudinal ligament in the cervical spine. Surg. Neurol., 1979, *12*, 414–418.

312. Yang P. J., Seeger J. F., Dzioba R. B., Carmody R. F., Burt T. B., Komar N. N., Smith J. R.: High dose IV contrast in CT scanning of the post operative lumbar spine. AJNR, 1986, *7*, 703–707.

313. Yu Y. L., Du Boulay G. H., Stevens J. M., Kendall B. E.: A reappraisal of the diagnostics in cervical disc disease: the posterior longitudinal ligament perforated or not. Neuroradiology, 1983, n° 3, *28*, 215.

314. Zufferey J. de Preux J.: Tomodensitométrie lombaire, saccoradiculographie et réalités neurochirurgicales dans les lombo sciatalgies d'origine discale et osseuse. Médecine et Hygiène, 1984, *42*, 1000–1008.

Magnetic Resonance Imaging

1. Abdelwahab I. F., Gould E. S.: The role of diskography after negative post-myelography CT scans: retrospective review. AJNR, 1988, Vol. 9, n° 1, 187-190.
2. Aguila L. A., Piraino D. W., Modic M. T., Dudley A. W., Duchesneau P. M., Weinstein M. A.: The intranuclear cleft of the intervertebral disk: Magnetic resonance imaging. Radiology, 1985, 155, 155-158.
3. Almefty O., Harkey L. H., Middleton T. H., Smith R. R., Fox J. L.: Myelopathy in cervical spondylotic lesions demonstrated by MRI. J. Neurosurg., 1988, 68, 217-222.
4. Arrington J. A., Martagh F. R., Silbiger M. L., Techtine G. R., Nokes S. R.: Magnetic resonance imaging of postdiscogram discitis and osteomyelitis in the lumbar spine: case report. J. Fla. Med. Assoc., 1986, 73, 192-194.
5. Axel L.: Surface coil magnetic resonance imaging. J. Comput. Assist. Tomogr., 1984, 8, 381-384.
6. Baleriaux D., Deroover N., Hernanus N., Segebarth C.: MRI of the spine. Diag. Imag. Clin. Med., 1986, 55, 66-71.
7. Babyn P. S., Chuang S. H., Daneman A., Davidson G. S.: Recurrent post-diskectomy low back pain: MR-surgical correlation. AJNR, 1988, Vol. 9, n° 4, 769-774.
8. Beyer H. K., Uhlenbrock D., Steiner G.: Disk hernia of the lumbar spine. Radiologic study with special reference to the technic and value of nuclear magnetic resonance tomography. Rontgen-Blatter, 1986, 39 (2), 47-52.
9. Beyer H. K., Uhlenbrock D., Steiner G.: Diagnosis of lumbar disk hernia. Possibilities and limitations of nuclear magnetic resonance tomography. Rontgenpraxis, 1986, 39, 122-126.
10. Breger R. K., Czerviouke L. F., Kass E. G. et al.: Truncation artifact in MR images of the intervertebral disk. AJNR, 1988, Vol. 9, n° 5? 825-828.
11. Bronskill M. J., Mc Veigh E. R., Kucharczyk W., Henkelman R. C.: Syrinx-like artifacts on MR images of the spinal cord. Radiology, 1988, 166, 485-488.
12. Brown B. M., Schwartz R. H., Frank E., Blank N.: Preoperative evaluation of cervical radiculopathy and myelopathy by surface-coil MR imaging. AJNR, 1988, 9 (5), 859-866.
13. Brown B. M., Schwartz R. H., Frank E., Blank N.: Preoperative evaluation of cervical radiculopathy and myelopathy by surface-coil MR imaging. AJR, 1988, 151, 1205-1212.
14. Bundschuh C. V., Modic M. T., Ross J. S., Masaryk T. J., Bohlmann H.: Epidural fibrosis and recurrent disk herniation in the lumbar spine: MR imaging assessment. AJNR, 1988, vol. 9, n° 1, 169-178.
15. Chafetz N. I., Genant H. K., Moon K. L., Helms C. A., Morris J. M.: Recognition of lumbar disk herniation with NMR. AJNR, 1984, 141, 1153-1156.
16. Chevalier J.: La résonance magnétique nucléaire permet de distinguer une hernie discale franche d'une protrusion. Journées technologiques du Cesta, Paris. Panorama du médecin, 1985, 10, 2021.
17. Chevrot A., Gires F., Leroy-Willig A., Barbery P., Wybier M., Vallee C., Roucayrol J. C., Pallardy G.: IRM du rachis lombaire. Feuillets de Radiologie, 1988, 28 (6), 461-477.
18. Clarke L. P., Schwintzlein H. N., Murtagh F. R., Silbiger M. L.: High resolution MRI: imaging anatomy of the lumbosacral spine. Magn. Res. Imag., 1986, 4, 515-523.
19. Czervionke L. F., Daniels D. L., Ho P. S. P., Yu S., Pech P., Strandt J., Williams A. L., Haughton V. M.: Cervical neural foramina: correlative anatomic and MR imaging study. Radiology, 1988, 169, 753-759.
20. Daniels D. L., Hyde J. S., Kneeland J. B.: The cervical nerves and foramina: local coil MR imaging. AJNR, 1986, 7, 129-133.
21. Doyon D., Aubert B., Merlino-Aubert N.: Pratique de l'IRM. Journées d'IRM de Bicetre, 1987, 32-40.
22. Doyon D., Halimi P., Busy F., Pierron D.: Diagnostic actuel des hernies discales lombo-sacrées (TDM et IRM incluses). Cours de perfectionnement post-universitaire. Société Française de Radiologie, 1985, 1-12.
23. Edelman R. R., Shoukimas G. M., Stark D. D., Davis K. R., New P. F. J., Saini S., Rosenthal D. I., Wismer G. L., Brady T. J.: High - resolution surface - coil imaging of lumbar disk disease. AJNR, 1985, 6, 479-485.
24. Edelman R. R., Stark D. D., Saini S.: Oblique planes of section in MR imaging. Radiology, 1986, 159, 807-810.
25. Enzmann D. R., Rubin J. B., Wright A.: Use of cerebrospinal fluid gating to improve T2 - weighted images. Part I. The spinal cord. Radiology, 1987, 162, 763-767.
26. Enzmann D. R., Rubin J. B., Wright A.: Cervical spine MR imaging: generating high signal CSF in sagittal and axial images. Radiology, 1987, 163, 233-238.
27. Feldman R., Mc Culloch J.: Juxta-facet cysts of the lumbar spine. Neuro-orthopedics, 1987, 4, 31-35.
28. Feuzi G., Heywang S. H., Vogl T., Obermuller J., Einhaupl K., Clados D., Steinhoff H.: Nuclear magnetic resonance tomography of the spine and spinal cord compared with computed tomography and myelography. R. O. F. O., 1986, 144, 636-643.
29. Flannigan B. D., Lufkin R. B., McGlade C., Winter J. et al.: MR imaging of the cervical spine: neurovascular anatomy. AJR, 1987, 148, 785-790.
30. Frocrain L., Duvauferrier R., Charles G., Martin A., Moisan A., Romee A., Pawlotsky Y.: Une nouvelle méthode diagnostique de la spondylodiscite. L'imagerie par résonance magnétique. J. Radiol., 1987, 68, 373-380.
31. Frocrain L., Duvauferrier R., Charles G., Ramee A., Pawolotsky Y.: Intérêt de l'imagerie par résonance magnétique dans le diagnostic des lombosciatiques récidivantes post-opératoires. J. Radiol., 1987, 68, 371-385.
32. Gibson M. J., Buckley J., Maukinney R., Mulholland R. G., Worthington B. S.: Magnetic resonance imaging and discography in the diagnosis of disc degeneration. Comparative study of 50 discs. J. Bone Joint Surg., 1986, 68, 369-373.
33. Gibson M. J., Buckley J., Mulholland R. G., Worthington B. S.: The changes in the intervertebral disc after chemonucleolysis demonstrated by magnetic resonance imaging. J. B. J. S., 1986, 5, 719-723.
34. Granat O., Jeanbouquin D., Perfettini C., Pernot P., Ducolombier A., Cosnard G.: Kyste synovial articulaire inter-apophysaire du rachis lombaire. Confrontations tomodensitométriques et imagerie par résonance magnétique. J. Radiol., 1987, 68, 387-390.
35. Grenier N., Grossman R. I., Schiebler M. L., Yeager B. A., Goldberg H. I., Kressel H. Y.: Degenerative lumbar disk disease: pitfalls and usefulness of MR imaging in detection of vacuum phenomenon. Radiology, 1987, 164, 861-865.

36. Grenier N., Kressel H. Y., Schiebler M. L., Grossman R. I., Dalinka M. K.: Normal and degenerative posterior spinal structures: MR imaging. Radiology, 1987, *165*, 517-525.

37. Hajek P. C., Baker L. L., Goobar J. E., Sartoris D. J., Hesselink J. R., Haghighi P., Resnick D.: Focal fat deposition in axial bone marrow: MR characteristics. Radiology 1987, 162: 245-249.

38. Halimi P., Marcus C., Doyon D., Sigal R., Blas C.: Imagerie par résonance magnétique de la moelle. Journées d'IRM de Bicetre, 1987, 41-51.

39. Han J. S., Kaufman B., El Yousef S. J., Benson J. E., Bonstelle C. T., Alfidi R. J., Haaga J. R., Yeung H., Huss R. G.: MR imaging of the spine. AJNR, 1983, *4*, 1151-1159. AJR, 1983, *141*, 1137-1145.

40. Haughton V. M., Daniels D. L., Czervionke L. F., Williams A. L.: Cervical spine in magnetic resonance imaging. Mosby Company, 1988, 614-633.

41. Haughton V. M., Feuerich D. O.: Oblique plane MR imaging of the cervical spine. J. Comput. Assist. Tomogr., 1987, *10*(5), 823-826.

42. Hedberg M. C., Drayer B. P., Flom R. A., Hodak J. A., Bird C. R.: Gradient echo (Grass) MR imaging in cervical radiculopathy. AJNR, 1988, *9*, 145-151.

43. Hedberg M. C., Drayer B. P., Flom R. A., Hodak J. A., Bird C. R.: Gradient echo (Grass) MR imaging in cervical radiculopathy. AJR, 1988, *150*, 683-689.

44. Heller H., Braitinger S., Petsch R., Dornemann H.: Disk processes in MR. European J. Radiol., 1986, *6* (1), 59-64.

45. Hickey D. S., Aspden R. M., Hukins D. W. L., Jenkins J. P. R., Isherwood I.: Analysis of magnetic resonance images from normal and degenerated lumbar intervertebral discs. Spine, 1986, *11*, 702-708.

46. Ho P. S. P., Ho K. C., Yu S. et al.: Calcification of the nucleus pulposus with pathologic confirmation in a premature infant. AJNR, 1989, Vol. 10, n° 1, 201.

47. Ho P. S. P., Yu S., Sether L. A., Wagner M., Ho K. C., Haughton V. M.: Ligamentum flavum: Appearance on sagittal and coronal MR images. Radiology, 1988, 168: 469-472.

48. Ho P. S. P., Yu S., Sether L. A., Wagner M., Ho K. C., Haughton V. M.: Progressive and regressive changes in the nucleus pulposus. Part I. The neonate. Radiology, 1988, *169*, 87-91.

49. Hochhauser L., Kieffer S. A., Cacayorin E. D., Petro G. R., Teller W. F.: Recurrent postdiskectomy low back pain: MR-Surgical correlation. AJNR, 1988, 9: 769-774.

50. Huckman M. S., Clark J. W., Mc Neil T. W., Whisler W. W., Hejna W. F., Russell E. J., Ramsey R. G., Turner D.: Chemonucleation and changes observed on lumbar MR scan: preliminary report. AJNR, 1987, *8*(1), 1-4.

51. Hueftle M. G., Modic M. T., Ross J. S. et al.: Lumbar spine: postoperative MR imaging with Gd-DTPA. Radiology, 1988, 167: 817-824.

52. Hyman R. A., Edwards J. H., Vacirca S. J., Stein H. L.: 0.6 T MR imaging of the cervical spine: multislice and multiecho techniques. AJNR, 1985, *6*, 229-236.

53. Idy I., Bittoun J., Desgrez A.: L'IRM et la Spectroscopie par RMN: principes physiques et mesures des paramètres. Journées d'IRM de Bicetre, 1987, 7-31.

54. Jenkins J. R. P., Hickey D. S., Zhu X. P., Machin M., Isherwood I.: MR imaging of the intervertebral disk: a quantitative study. Br. J. Radiol., 1985, *58*, 705-709.

55. Karnaze M. G., Gado M. H., Sartor K. J., Hodges III F. J.: Comparison of MR and CT myelography in imaging the cervical and thoracic spine. AJR, 1988, *150*, 397-403.

56. Kelly W. M.: Image artefacts and technical limitations. In: Magnetic Resonance Imaging in the Central Nervous System. Brant-Zawadzki M., Norman D. - Raven Press - New-York, 1987, 43-82.

57. Kjos B. O., Norman D.: Strategies for efficient imaging of the lumbar spine. In: Magnetic Resonance Imaging of the Central Nervous System, Brant-Zawadzki M., Norman D. - Raven Press - New-York, 1987, 279-287.

58. Krause D., Drape J. L., Woerly B., Kardous N., Tongio J.: Hernies discales lombaires. Intérêt des coupes obliques en résonance magnétique nucléaire. J. Neuroradiol., 1988, 15: 305-324.

59. Le Bihan D.: Imagerie par Résonance Magnétique - Bases physiques. Collection d'Imagerie Médicale. Masson Paris, 1985.

60. Levy L. M., Di Chiro G., Brooks R. A., Dwyer A. J., Wener L., Frank J.: Spinal cord artifacts from truncation errors during MR imaging. Radiology, 1988, *166*, 479-483.

61. Maravilla K. R., Lesh P., Weinreb J. C., Selby D. K., Mooney V.: Magnetic resonance imaging of the lumbar spine with CT correlation. AJNR, 1985, *6*, 237-245.

62. Margulis A. R., Higgins C. B., Kaufman L., Crooks L. E.: Clinical Magnetic Resonance Imaging. Radiology Research and Education Foundation, San-Francisco, 1983.

63. Masaryk T. J., Boumphrey F., Modic M. T., Tamborello C., Ross J. S., Brown M. D.: Effects of chemonucleolysis demonstrated by MR imaging. J. Comput. Assist. Tomogr., 1986, *10*(6), 917-923.

64. Masaryk T. J., Modic M. T., Geisinger M. A. et al.: Cervical myelopathy: a comparison of magnetic resonance and conventional myelography. J. Comput. Assist. Tomogr., 1986, *10*, 184-194.

65. Masaryk T. J., Ross J. S., Modic M. T., Boumphrey F., Bohlman H., Wilber G.: High resolution MR imaging of sequestrated lumbar intervertebral disks. AJNR, 1988, Vol. 9, n° 2, 351-358.

66. McGregor J. C., Butler P.: Disc calcifications in childhood: Computed tomographic and magnetic resonance imaging appearances. Br. J. Radiol., 1986, *59*, 180-182.

67. Mikhael M. A., Ciric I. S., Kudrna J. C., Hindo W. A.: Recognition of lumbar disc disease with magnetic resonance imaging. Computerized Radiol., 1985, *9*, 213-222.

68. Modic M. T., Masaryk T. J., Boumphrey F., Goormastic M., Bell G.: Lumbar herniated disk disease and canal stenosis: prospective evaluation by surface coil MR, CT and myelography. AJNR, 1986, *7*, 709-717.

69. Modic M. T., Masaryk T. J., Mulopulos G. P., Bundschuh C. et al.: Cervical radiculopathy: prospective evaluation with surface coil MR imaging, CT with metrizamide and metrizamide myelography. Radiology, 1986, *161*, 753-759.

70. Modic M. T., Masaryk T. J., Ross J. S., Carter J. R.: Imaging of degenerative disk disease. Radiology, 1988, 168: 177-186.

71. Modic M. T., Masaryk T. J., Ross J. S., Mulopulos G. P., Bundschuh C. V., Bohlman H.: Cervical radiculopathy: value of oblique MR imaging. Radiology, 1987, *163*, 227-231.

72. Modic M. T., Pavlicek W., Weinstein M. A., Boumphrey F., Ngo F., Hardy R., Duscheneau P. M.: Magnetic

resonance imaging of intervertebral disk disease. Clinical and pulse sequence considerations. Radiology, 1984, *152* (1), 103–111.

73. Modic M. T., Steinberg P. M., Ross J. S., Masaryk T. J., Carter J. R.: Degenerative disk disease: Assessment of changes in vertebral body marrow with MR imaging. Radiology, 1988, 166: 193–199.

74. Modic M. T., Weinstein M. A., Pavlicek W., Boumphrey F., Starnes D., Duchesneau P. M.: Magnetic resonance imaging of the cervical spine: technical and clinical observations. AJR, 1983, *141,* 1129–1136.

75. Norman D.: The Spine. In: Magnetic Resonance Imaging of the Central Nervous System. Brant-Zawadzki M., Norman D. - Raven Press. New-York, 1987, 289–328.

76. Norman D., Mills C. M., Brant-Zawadzki M., Yeates A., Crooks L. E., Kaufman L.: Magnetic resonance imaging of the spinal cord and canal: potentials and limitations. AJR, 1983, *141,* 1147–1152.

77. Osborn A. G., Hoods R. S., Sherry R. G., Smoker W. R. K., Harnsberger H. R.: CT/MR spectrum of far lateral and anterior lumbosacral disk herniations. AJNR, 1988, Vol. 9, n° 4, 775–778.

78. Partain C. L., James A. E., Rollo F. D., Price R. R.: Nuclear Magnetic Resonance Imaging. W. B. Saunders Company, Philadelphia, 1983.

79. Paushter D. M., Modic M. T., Masaryk T. J.: Magnetic resonance imaging of the spine: applications and limitations. Radiol. Clin. North Am., 1985, *23,* 551–562.

80. Pech P., Haughton V. M.: Lumbar intervertebral disk: correlative MR and anatomic study. Radiology, 1985, *156,* 699–701.

81. Petsch R., Heller H., Braintinger S., Dornemann H.: MR imaging of the cervical spine using special coils. Digital bilddiagn. 1985, *5,* 173–180.

82. Raynor R. B.: Symptomatic disc herniation into vertebral body. Surg. Neurol., 1985, *23* (6), 621–625.

83. Roos A., Kressel H., Spritzer C., Dalinka M.: MR imaging of marrow changes adjacent to end-plates in degenerative lumbar disk disease. AJR, 1987, *149,* 531–534.

84. Ross J. S., Delamarter R. R., Hueftle M. G. et al.: Gadolinium-DTPA enhanced MR imaging of the post-operative lumbar spine: Time course and mechanism of enhancement. AJNR, 1989, Vol. 10, n° 1, 37–47.

85. Ross J. S., Hueftle M. G., Masaryk T. J., Modic M. T.: Imaging decisions in low back pain. MRI Decisions, 1987, *1* (1), 16–30.

86. Ross J. S., Masaryk T. J., Modic M. T., Bohlman H., Delamater R., Wilber G.: Lumbar spine: post-operative assessment with surface-coil MR imaging. Radiology, 1987, *164,* 851–860.

87. Ross J. S., Masaryk T. J., Modic M. T., Delamater R., Bohlman H., Wilber G., Kaufman B.: MR imaging of lumbar arachnoiditis. AJR, 1987, *149,* 1025–1032.

88. Rubin J. B., Enzmann D. R.: Optimizing conventional MR imaging of the spine. Radiology, 1987, *163,* 777–783.

89. Rubin J. B., Enzmann D. R., Wright A.: CSF-gated MR imaging of the spine: theory and clinical implementation. Radiology, 1987, *163,* 784–792.

90. Rubin J. B., Wright A., Enzmann D. R.: Lumbar spine: motion compensation for cerebrospinal fluid on MR imaging. Radiology, 1988, *166,* 225–231.

91. Schneidermann G., Flannigan B., Kuigston S., Thomas J., Dillin W. H., Watkins R. G.: Magnetic resonance imaging in the diagnosis of disk degeneration. Correlation with discography. Spine, 1987, *12,* 276–291.

92. Scotti G., Scialfa G., Colombo N., Landoni L.: MR imaging of intradural extramedullary tumors of the cervical spine. J. Comput. Assist. Tomogr., 1985, *9* (6), 1037–1041.

93. Sigal R., Bittoun J., Halimi P., Blas C., Doyon D.: Comment lire une image IRM? Feuillets de radiol., 1986, *5,* 299–306.

94. Slone R. M., Buck L. L., Fitzsimmons J. R.: Varying gradient angles and offsets to optimize imaging planes in MR. Radiology, 1986, *158,* 531–536.

95. Teresi L. T., Lufkin R. B., Reicher M. A. et al.: Asymptomatic degenerative disc disease and spondylosis of the cervical spine MR imaging. Radiology, 1987, *164,* 83–88.

96. Vallee G., Chevrot A., Benhamard A., Gires F., Wyber M., Cellier B., Pallardy G.: Aspects tomodensitométriques des kystes synoviaux articulaires lombaires à developpement intra-rachidien. J. Radiol., 1987, *68,* 519–526.

97. Wehrli F. W., MacFall J. R., Shutts D., Breger R., Herfkens R. J.: Mechanisms of contrast in NMR Imaging. J. Comp. Assist. Tomogr., 1984, *8,* 369–380.

98. Weisz G. M., Kitchener P. N.: The use of magnetic resonance imaging in the diagnosis of postoperative lumbar conditions. Med. J. Australia, 1987, *146* (2), 99–101.

99. Wimmer B., Friedburg H., Henning J., Kaufmann G. W.: Diagnostic imaging potentialities of nuclear resonance tomography. Changes in vertebrae, ligaments and intervertebral disks in comparison with computed tomography. Radiology 1986, *26,* 137–143.

100. Wood M. L., Henkelman R. M.: Truncation artifacts in magnetic resonance imaging. Magn. Reson. Med., 1985, *2,* 517–526.

101. Yu S., Haughton V. M., Ho P. S. P., Sether L. A., Wagner M., Ho K. C.: Progressive and regressive changes in the nucleus pulposus. Part. II. The adult. Radiology, 1988, *169,* 93–97.

102. Yu S., Haughton V. M., Sether L. A., Wagner M.: Anulus fibrosus in bulging intervertebral disks. Radiology, 1988, *169,* 761–763.

103. Yu S., Sether L. A., Ho P. S. P., Wagner M., Haughton V. M.: Tears of the anulus fibrosus: Correlation between MR and pathologic findings in cadaver. AJNR, 1988, Vol. 9, n° 2, 367–370.

Subject Index

Printed in Great Britain
by Amazon.co.uk, Ltd.,
Marston Gate.